Health and Gender

Ilaria Tarricone • Anita Riecher-Rössler
Editors

Health and Gender

Resilience and Vulnerability Factors For Women's Health in the Contemporary Society

Springer

Editors
Ilaria Tarricone
Bologna Transcultural Psychosomatic Team (BoTPT), Department of Medical and Surgical Sciences
Alma Mater Studiorum, University of Bologna
Bologna
Italy

Anita Riecher-Rössler
Center for Gender Research and Early Detection
University of Basel Psychiatric Hospital
Basel
Switzerland

ISBN 978-3-030-15037-2 ISBN 978-3-030-15038-9 (eBook)
https://doi.org/10.1007/978-3-030-15038-9

This Springer imprint is published by the registered company Springer Nature Switzerland AG
The registered company address is: Gewerbestrasse 11, 6330 Cham, Switzerland

Foreword

We accepted with enthusiasm the possibility to present this book, which was written by a multidisciplinary team and is intended not only for colleagues but also for students of medicine and other healthcare professions, with the aim of providing an updated overview of health issues dealing with sex and gender issues at all stages of life.

There is scientific evidence that gender and sex, having different and complementary meanings, are substantial variables, which strongly affect clinical presentation of disease and response to treatment.

This book starts with a few chapters aimed at making the point on these issues and their practical implications and also contains a section dedicated to the organization of social and health services, taking into account specifics related to sex and gender differences and questions dealing with achievement of gender equality in science. Equality, not a "neutral" model, is based on a full appreciation of the differences, given that it is a strong approximation to consider the world populated by a single subject, namely, male. The cultural changes and genuine perception of the importance of this effort can hopefully be achieved through sharing real experiences. For this reason, we considered it a good opportunity to also include some personal paradigmatic histories in the book, providing insights into the many possible ways to practically deal with gender and sex issues.

As members of a university having a long tradition and history, it is important for us to remember that academic institutions are, and should always remain, on the front line to promote cultural changes, acting particularly on the new generation who needs to face the global challenges of future society together with policymakers and other stakeholders in many and sometimes conflicting fields. In our view, promotion of careful consideration of sex and gender variables in research and training and consideration of the gender equality as a founding issue are ways to provide our society with a good catalyst for a more adherent and in-depth promotion of well-being.

Progress along the path of gender equality can be achieved in a number of ways in academic institutions: first, by introducing gender and sex variables in teaching, which can be easier through case studies in the biomedical field, but is now increasingly important in all disciplines. However, other drivers are strongly related with the promotion of a new attitude towards gender equality aspects in existing and newly recruited staff through the role of the Guarantee Committees; the prevention of violence and daily activities of emergency services; the need to give social weight at the care work, which should be not relegated to a question of mothers; and, eventually, the active participation in international research projects such as the EU-funded PLOTINA[1] project, coordinated by the University of Bologna. We take this opportunity to mention PLOTINA as a paradigm, intended to enable the development, implementation and assessment of self-tailored Gender Equality Plans with innovative and sustainable strategies for participating research performing organizations (RPOs). This can be achieved in several ways: (1) stimulating gender-aware cultural change; (2) promoting career development of both female and male researchers to prevent waste of talent, particularly for women; and (3) ensuring that different views and methods are taken into account in research and teaching, actively considering the gender/sex dimension and analysis.

In conclusion, gender issues have now come of age in medicine, and this book is a timely initiative not only to promote knowledge of what has already been achieved but also to stimulate new awareness that progress, along this path, can certainly bring new ways of caring for the health and well-being of all individuals. Hopefully, this book can contribute to increasing the number of female researchers; promote and empower their careers; stimulate the integration of the gender/sex dimension into the design, evaluation and implementation of research; enrich its quality and relevance; and enhance the social value of any medical and, in general, scientific innovation.

School of Medicine
Alma Mater Studiorum, University of Bologna,
Bologna, Italy

Fabrizio De Ponti

Guarantee Committee for Equal Opportunities,
Employee Well-Being and Non-Discrimination
at Work (CUG)
Alma Mater Studiorum, University of Bologna
Bologna, Italy

Welfare at Work, Department of Agricultural
and Food Sciences
Alma Mater Studiorum, University of Bologna
Bologna, Italy

Tullia Gallina Toschi

Department of Medical and Surgical Sciences
University of Bologna
Bologna, Italy

Marco Zoli

[1] PLOTINA—Promoting gender balance and inclusion in research, innovation and training—GA n° 666008 (www.plotina.eu)

Preface

This handbook, Women's Health in Contemporary Society: Risk and Resilience Factors, adopts the WHO definition of gender as a condition which interacts with, but is distinct from, the binary of biological sex. For the purposes of this book, "gender refers to socially constructed roles that shape behaviours, activities, expectations, and opportunities considered appropriate in a particular socio-cultural context for all people" [1]. Gender is an important determinant of not only illness and symptom presentation but also of access to healthcare, response to treatment and careers in health systems.

"Gender also refers to the relationships between people, and the distribution of power in those relationships. Gender is not static but changes across time and place. When individuals or groups do not conform to established gender norms (including concepts of being masculine or feminine), roles, responsibilities or relations, they often face stigma, discriminatory practices, or social exclusion—all of which can adversely affect health" in several ways [1]. There is a disparity between genders for life expectancy, healthy life years and health behaviours as well as mortality and morbidity risk [2]. On average, women live longer but spend fewer years in good health due to specific underlying causes which arise, at least partially, from gender inequality [3].

"Gender equality is a fundamental human right, grounded in the Universal Declaration of Human Rights, and is core to achieving all Sustainable Development Goals" [1]. Specifically, gender equality refers to equal rights, responsibilities and opportunities for all people [4]. "It is a necessary foundation for a world that is sustainable, peaceful, prosperous, healthy, and where no- one is left behind" [1].

In the absence of gender equality, several factors arise which have adverse effects on women's well-being and long-term health as well as their career development. These factors include gender role conflicts, heavy total workload and additional unpaid work [4]. Unemployment and lower occupational and social status of women, which stems from female labour market exclusion, result in a wide range of negative outcomes in the realm of developmental and child health [5]. The unemployment rate of women is 30%, almost double that of men which is 17%; a fifth of women living in poverty are not active in the labour market due to domestic and caretaking responsibilities [4].

Women who do participate in the labour market face a pay gap. This gender-based disparity in pay for the same work also affects pensions, meaning that the inequality persists throughout working years and into retirement [3]. The gender gap in pensions is estimated at 38% for the EU27 [3]. The accumulation of gender-based discrimination over their lifetimes renders older women particularly vulnerable to poverty and social exclusion, creating a risk for income barriers to healthcare [3].

Unsurprisingly, gender also determines career pathways within health systems [1]. "Women make up over 70% of the paid health workforce in many countries, and are often the main providers of home and community-based care as well as unpaid care. However, women are under-represented in management and decision-making positions within health systems. As a result, the gender pay gap in the health and social sectors is even bigger than the overall gap of 20%. For these fields, the average pay difference between genders is 26% in high-income countries and 29% in upper-middle income countries" [1]. Moreover, gender biases, physical and sexual violence and harassment remain important challenges for workers in the health and social sectors.

Therefore, we believe that future generations of medical doctors and healthcare workers should be trained to develop an awareness of gender differences in health promotion and disease prevention as well as in organizations of health systems. This text is intended to be a handbook for medical students and health graduates who offer a rereading of the major health problems, the protective and risk factors for health and the organization of care in a gender-oriented perspective, by adopting the point of view of women.

The handbook is composed of six sections: Part I is an introduction, Part II covers the biological and psychosocial determinants of health for women, Part III focuses on women's health at all stages of life, Part IV examines gendered aspects in medical disorders and care, Part V considers cures and organization of services from a gendered perspective, and Part VI presents a historical point of view and epilogues. Every chapter explores some aspects of the domains covered and offers a list of references for further insights.

"As the non-governmental organization CHANGE says, "the world has already developed a consensus on women's importance to development". National and international policies moved away from demographic-centred population and development programmes towards putting human rights and women's equality at the centre" [5]. We are very grateful to all the authors who give their important contributions to this book. We hope that our work contributes to increasing students' awareness of gender disparities and interest in making gender-oriented health promotion and care a priority in our contemporary society.

Bologna, Italy — Ilaria Tarricone
Basel, Switzerland — Anita Riecher-Rössler

References

1. WHO gender and health. 2018. http://www.who.int/news-room/fact-sheets/detail/gender.
2. Payne S. How can gender equity be addressed through health systems? WHO Regional Office for Europe and European Observatory on Health Systems and Policies. 2009. ISSN 1997-8065.
3. EuroHealthNet. Gender equality and health POLICY PRÉCIS. Data from the European Institute for Gender Equality's Gender Equality Index 20. https://eurohealthnet.eu/media/news-releases/impact-gender-inequality-health.
4. UN Women. Gender equality glossary. https://trainingcentre.unwomen.org/mod/glossary/view.php?id=36.
5. http://www.genderhealth.org/about_us/.

More References

https://www.rush.edu/health-wellness/discover-health/how-gender-affects-health.

https://www.childfund.org/The-Health-Impact-of-Gender-Inequality/?no_redirect=true.

https://www.usaid.gov/what-we-do/global-health/cross-cutting-areas/gender-equality.

https://www.ncbi.nlm.nih.gov/pubmed/7801161.

Acknowledgements

I would like to fully thank all the authors of this book who contributed with competence and sensitivity to carry out the effort of describing several of the main issues related to women health in contemporary society. I am particularly grateful to my co-Editor Prof Anita Riecher for her huge contribution. I would like to thank Dr Francesca Tronconi for her patient and outstanding assistance in chapters' revision and Dr Ralph Nisbet for his precious linguistic revision of my last chapter. Finally, I thank the readers and the students who wish to read this handbook to reinforce their attitudes and skills for growing a gender-sensitive health care.

Ilaria Tarricone

Contents

Part I

Introduction

Fairness, Equality and Health: Towards a Gender-Oriented Perspective

1

Elena Luppi

Key Points
- The gender perspective includes not only sex differences among human beings but rather social, cultural and economic attributes related with femininity and masculinity in a certain culture.
- Gender inequalities mean disadvantages and marginalisation caused by social norms and stereotypes. Most of gender inequalities impact on women; but this can happen also towards men and LGBT people.
- Gender equity is the process of being fair to women and men, while gender equality is the equal enjoyment by women and men of socially valued goods, opportunities, resources and rewards.
- Gender equity and gender equality are part of the international policy agendas since long time, but in the last decades, the emphasis on this issue has increased: UN, OECD, the European Commission and other international or national governmental organisms put in their agendas important issues concerning gender equity and equality.
- Gender equality is related with the protection of human rights, the functioning of democracy, the respect for the rule of law and the economic growth and competitiveness. Gender equality is a condition for human health, well-being and fulfilment.

The notion of gender refers to the social, cultural and economic attributes, implications and opportunities associated with being male or female [1, 2]. When talking about gender instead of simply mentioning sex differences, we recognise that biological and physical characteristics are not the only determinant of female and male life paths. Whether in private life, in the workplace or in the public sphere, men and

E. Luppi (✉)
Department of Education Studies, University of Bologna, Bologna, Italy
e-mail: elena.luppi@unibo.it

I. Tarricone, A. Riecher-Rössler (eds.), *Health and Gender*,
https://doi.org/10.1007/978-3-030-15038-9_1

women encounter different expectations that are determined more from social issues rather than from personal characteristics or talents. We refer to gender identities as an outcome of biological and cultural dimensions affecting the ways individuals perform their sex and gender. We can consider in fact gender as the first dimensions characterising human identities, the first form of diversity in human beings, strongly interrelated with ethnicity, age, health and social and cultural diversities, as well as many other variables that design the kaleidoscope of human race [3].

The assumption of a gender-oriented perspective in investigating human phenomena takes into account the impact of gender-based differences in social rules and conventions; in status and power; in politics and policies; in prejudices, stereotypes and segregation mechanisms; and in any other aspect of human life determining equality or inequality. Equalities and inequalities represent the core of the gender issue discourse and policies and therefore the notion of gender equality and gender equity: two concepts that are often used interchangeably but rather imply two different perspectives to the problem. According to the definition provided by the United Nations Population Fund, we consider that "*Gender Equity is the process of being fair to women and men and Gender Equality is the equal enjoyment by women and men of socially-valued goods, opportunities, resources and rewards (UNPF).*[1]"

Gender inequality mainly means disadvantage and marginalisation for women; but this can impact on men as well and also on LGBT people. For instance, social norms and stereotypes tend to segregate men that are employed in traditionally feminine work fields, such as child education. Therefore gender equality, as defined by the UNPF, does not often lead to equal outcomes for men and women. Being given the same chances in life is not sufficient to come to equal results. This is true simply because women and men are different, biologically and socially: they have different needs and encounter different experiences. Compared to *gender equality*, the notion of *gender equity* is more comprehensive and complete because it implies fairness in the way women and men are treated. The different life paths of men and women are taken into account, and working for gender equity means providing compensations for the ones that are afflicted by disadvantages (mostly women, historically and socially). Giving women and men the same opportunities is the first step; but for true gender equality to be achieved, there is a need for gender equity.

To ensure fairness to women and men, *gender equity* policies plan strategies and measures for compensating inequalities, different opportunities, starting points, access to goods and possibilities. Women empowerment is an example of such compensating measures that can identify and redress power imbalances to give women more consciousness and means to manage their own lives. In fact, the social inequalities that afflict women in society often constitute a hindrance to their full access to the possibilities related with their talents, and equality cannot be guaranteed if such obstacles are not removed first. A process starting from gender equity to reach gender equality implies that men and women will not become the same neither will be treated as the same, but their opportunities to access to resources and experiences will to their choices and talents, not by their gender. In our societies, where male

[1] https://www.unfpa.org/resources/frequently-asked-questions-about-gender-equality.

norms are considered as a measure for women's positions, gender equality requires women's empowerment. This measure of gender equity can help in ensuring that decision-making at private and public levels and access to resources are no longer weighted in men's favour, so that both women and men can fully participate as equal individuals in society.

Gender equity and gender equality are part of the international policy agendas since long time, but in the last decades, the emphasis on this issue has increased. In 2010 the European Commission approved the "Strategy for equality between women and men 2010–2015". Such an important statement comes from the recognition of gender equality as a core value for Union, a principle affirmed in the EU Charter of Fundamental Rights. In March 2010 the Commission adopted the Women's Charter, in order to renew its commitment to gender equality and to strengthen the gender perspective in all its policies. The actions are focused on the assumption of a gender mainstreaming approach, in order to integrate the gender dimension in any area of EU policy but also foresee specific measures and interventions. According to gender mainstreaming policies and the related legislations, programmes or actions must be assessed considering their implications and impacts on both women and men. Gender mainstreaming represents a perspective that is necessary to achieve the goal of gender equity and equality [4, 5].

After the "Council of Europe Convention on Action against Trafficking in Human Beings" [6] and the "Council of Europe Convention on Preventing and Combating Violence against Women and Domestic Violence (Istanbul Convention)" [7], the Council of Europe formulated a Gender Equality Strategy 2014–2017 [8], with the intention to achieve the advancement and empowerment of women and the effective realisation of gender equality in the Council of Europe member states, through different actions: combating gender stereotypes and sexism; preventing and combating violence against women; guaranteeing equal access of women to justice; achieving balanced participation of women and men in political and public decision-making; and achieving gender mainstreaming in all policies and measures.

Even in this case, the notion of gender equity and equality is recognised as the baseline for human growth. The document states: "*Gender equality means equal visibility, empowerment, responsibility and participation for both women and men in all spheres of public and private life. It also means an equal access to and distribution of resources between women and men. Although the legal status of women in Europe has undoubtedly improved during recent decades, effective equality is far from being a reality*" ([8], p. 4).

This programme recognises the multidimensional origins and impacts of discriminations and insists on the importance of addressing to it in a systematic and comprehensive way.

In 2013 the OECD Council on Gender Equality in Education, Employment and Entrepreneurship launched a recommendation document, known as the "OECD 2013 Gender Recommendation", setting out a number of measures that OECD members and non-members who adhered to it should consider implementing in order to tackle gender inequalities in education, employment and entrepreneurship [9]. In particular it is recommended that adherents should, through appropriate legislation,

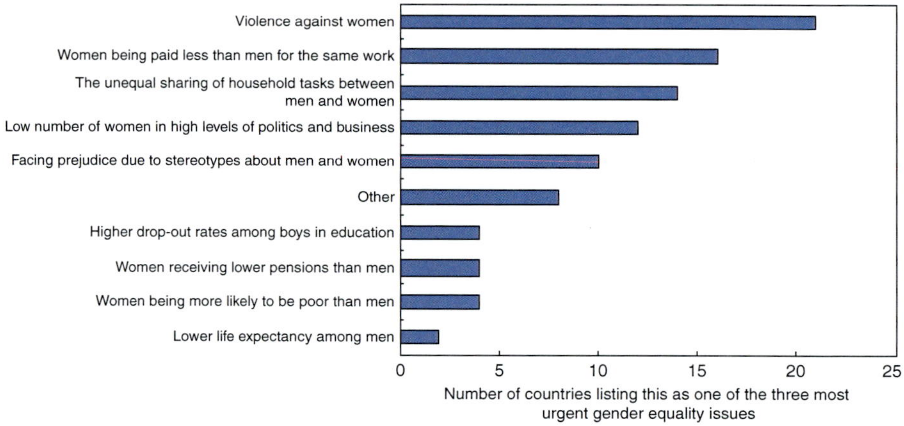

Fig. 1.1 OECD countries priority ranking on gender equality: number of adherent countries to the 2013 Gender Recommendation listing the following as one of the three most urgent gender equality issues needing to be addressed in their country. *Note*: 35 countries responded. Each country could select up to three priority issues. *Source*: OECD Employment, Labour and Social Affairs Committee (ELSAC), Questionnaire on Progress in Implementing the 2013 Gender Recommendation. StatLink https://doi.org/10.1787/888933573886

policies, monitoring and campaigning, provide equal access to education, better enable female labour force participation, promote family-friendly policies, foster greater male uptake of unpaid work, work to a better gender balance in public and private leadership positions and promote entrepreneurship among women. The two following figures synthetize the most urgent gender equality issues selected as a priority by the participant and the adherent countries (Figs. 1.1 and 1.2).

One of the most recent OECD's reports on gender equality states "*Gender equality is not only a fundamental human right. It is also a keystone of a prosperous, modern economy that provides sustainable inclusive growth. Gender equality is essential for ensuring that men and women can contribute fully at home, at work and in public life, for the betterment of societies and economies at large*" ([9], p. 3).

In January 2016, the United Nations adopted the 17 Sustainable Development Goals of the 2030 Agenda for Sustainable Development[2] whose purpose is to mobilise efforts to end all forms of poverty, fight inequalities and tackle climate change while ensuring that no one is left behind. The Goal no. 5 is dedicated to gender equity and equality: "*Achieve gender equality and empower all women and girls*". This goal follows the Millennium Development "*Promote gender equality and empower women*" and is based upon the conviction that gender equality is not only a fundamental human right but also a necessary foundation for a peaceful, prosperous and sustainable world. UN considers that equal access to education, healthcare and decent work and representation in political and economic decision-making processes for women and girls are conditions for sustainable economies and a benefit

[2] http://www.un.org/sustainabledevelopment/sustainable-development-goals/.

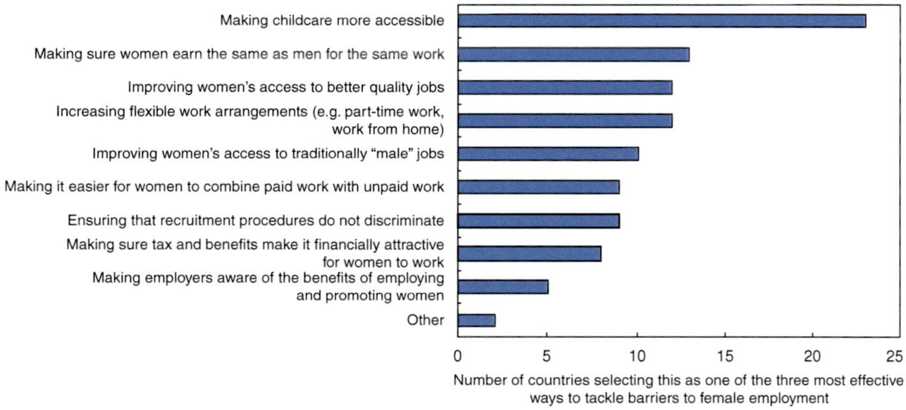

Fig. 1.2 OECD countries priority ranking on gender equality: number of adherent countries to the 2013 Gender Recommendation listing the three most effective ways to tackle barriers to female empowerment. *Note*: 35 countries responded. Each country could select up to three priority issues. *Source*: OECD Employment, Labour and Social Affairs Committee (ELSAC), Questionnaire on Progress in Implementing the 2013 Gender Recommendation. StatLink https://doi.org/10.1787/888933573905

for societies and humanity at large. Even in the UN policies, equity is a requisite for reaching the final goal of equality. Moreover, the forms and impacts of gender segregations and inequalities are recognised as multifaceted and transversal to different countries, human conditions and access to instruction and wealth. Due to this complexity and intersectionality, the policies dedicated to tackle the obstacles to gender equality should be integrated, coherent and comprehensive.

According to the analysis of the most recent and relevant reports and documents provided by international organisms and policy makers, Sörlin et al. synthesise the most urgent issues concerning gender equity and equality as follows: *1. Equal distribution of power and influence between women and men [...]; 2. Economic equality between women and men [...] regarding education and paid work providing lifelong economic independence; 3. Equal distribution of unpaid care and household work [...] equal responsibility for household work and [...] equality in giving and receiving care; 4. Men's violence against women should cease. Women and men, girls and boys, should have equal rights and opportunities to physical integrity* ([10], p. 2).

The issue of gender equality is related, as we have seen, with the protection of human rights, the functioning of democracy and the respect for the rule of law and economic growth and competitiveness, but it is also a condition for human health, well-being and fulfilment. A culture of gender segregation is not simply a win-lose game between men and women but a lose-lose game for humanity. We need to switch the cultures and policies of inequality into paradigms that affirm a win-win culture, both in private and public life, for our organisations and institutions. If we decide to neglect gender issues and the urgency for gender equality, we need to be aware of what we risk and of the price we will pay and will let future generations pay.

References

1. Butler J. Gender trouble. Feminism and the subversion of identity. New York, NY: Routledge; 1990.
2. Connell RW. Gender and power. Stanford, CA: Stanford University Press; 1987.
3. Hankivsky O, Reid C, Cormier R, Varcoe C, Clark N, Benoit C, Brotman S. Exploring the promises of intersectionality for advancing women's health. Int J Equity Health. 2010;9:5.
4. True J, Shepherd LJ, editors. Gender mainstreaming in international institutions. New York, NY: Routledge; 2010.
5. Palmary I, Nunez L. The orthodoxy of gender mainstreaming: reflecting on gender mainstreaming as strategy for accomplishing the millennium development goals. J Health Manag. 2009;11(65):65–78.
6. Council of Europe Treaty Series. Council of Europe Convention on Action against trafficking in human beings No. 197, Warsaw, 16.V.2005.
7. Council of Europe. Council of Europe Convention on preventing and combating violence against women and domestic violence. 2011.
8. Council of Europe. Council of Europe Gender equality strategy 2014-2017. Strasbourg: Council of Europe; 2014.
9. OECD. The pursuit of gender equality: an uphill battle. Paris: OECD Publishing; 2017.
10. Sörlin A, et al. Can the impact of gender equality on health be measured? a cross-sectional study comparing measures based on register data with individual survey-based data. BMC Public Health. 2012;12:795.

Suggested Reading

Carbado DW, Crenshaw KW, Mays VM, Tomlinson B. Intersectionality: mapping the movements of a theory. Du Bois Rev. 2013;10(2):303–12.

Esping-Andersen G. Incomplete revolution: adapting welfare states to women's new roles. Princeton, NJ: Princeton University Press; 2017.

Flood M, Howson R, editors. Engaging men in building gender equality. London: Cambridge Scholars Publishing; 2017.

Harvey VL, Bell GC. Health care disparities and the LGBT population. Lanham: Lexington Books; 2014.

Lewis J, Ostner I. Gender and the evolution of European social policies, ZE-S, Arbeitspapier nr. 4/94. Bremen: University of Bremen; 1994.

Nussbaum M. Sex and social justice. Oxford: Oxford University Press; 2000.

Sen A. The many faces of gender inequality. Frontline. 2001;18:22.

UN. Review and appraisal of the implementation of the Beijing Declaration and Platform for Action and the outcomes of the twenty-third special session of the General Assembly. 2014. http://www.un.org/ga/search/view_doc.asp?symbol=E/CN.6/2015/3.

The Woman in the History of Health 2

Annagiulia Gramenzi

After centuries of dormancy, young women
can now look toward a future moulded by their own hands
Rita Levi Montalcini, Nobel Prize for Physiology and Medicine

Key Points

- The role of women has been largely neglected by historians of medicine, who have primarily focused on the great male university-trained physicians. This attitude has changed in the past few decades.
- Women have always engaged in healing from the beginning of history. With the founding of medieval universities, medicine became a profession, and women were formally excluded from medicine, but they did not stop healing.
- Even midwifery would become masculinized during the later years of the early modern era with the rise of the "man-midwife."
- Over the last few decades, the medical profession in the West has moved toward a situation where females comprise the majority of new medical graduates, even though career paths are still gender biased to the disadvantage of female physicians.
- It is not completely clear if "women's health was women's business," but the care of women during pregnancy was prominently controlled by other women.

A. Gramenzi (✉)
Dipartimento di Scienze Mediche e Chirurgiche, Alma Mater Studiorum - Università di Bologna, Bologna, Italy
e-mail: annagiulia.gramenzi@unibo.it

I. Tarricone, A. Riecher-Rössler (eds.), *Health and Gender*,
https://doi.org/10.1007/978-3-030-15038-9_2

The entrance of women in history and in history of science and medicine, both as objects and subjects, has been extremely slow. By the origins of women's studies in the early twentieth century, the heritage of women in healthcare only began to receive significant historical attention from the 1970s [1], when both the second wave feminist movement and the new study of social history contributed to the development of both women's history and history of medicine. Prior to this period, medicine and its history were mostly written solely by and about men emphasizing the scientific developments and the men who had made them possible. The ordinary everyday practice of medicine, let alone the kinds of domestic or marginal healing often performed by women, was simply not part of the discipline.

Discrimination toward women in medicine can be traced back to the legend of Agnodice told by the Roman author Hyginus (c. 64 BC–17 AD) [2]. Agnodice entered medicine some 2000 years ago by dressing as a man to circumvent the restrictions of her gender. However, in order to gain the trust of her female patients, she would undress enough to prove to her patients that she was indeed a woman. Following the gender ambiguity highlighted by Agnodice, this chapter will briefly focus on two "hot" topics that are central to studies of women in the history of medicine:

1. Women as healthcare workers
2. Women as patients

2.1 Women as Healthcare Workers

Since the beginning of human history, women have been crucial to medical service provision and have been responsible for the care of children as well as of the sick and the dying. Increasingly historians acknowledge the presence of women in the broader medical spectrum, although there are very few studies which document who such women were, what their specific practices and theories were, and how their medical work was perceived.

"Official" Western medicine has been widely dominated by men. Across antiquity, admission to medical school was denied to females, and the medical profession was considered exclusively male-centered. Women were barred from cathedral schools first and then from universities and thereby they could not participate in the professionalization of medicine [3]. Valuable historical studies have shown that between 1500 and 1800, female medical practitioners were increasingly marginalized and relegated to the "*sphere of compassionate and charitable activity*" [4]. Crucial to the marginalization of women as healers was the denigration of their empirical knowledge and activities by university-trained physicians and powerful surgeon guildsmen. However, during this time women did continue to practice even without formal training or recognition especially in domestic and household medicine but also in the setting of emerging structures of public health such as hospitals and charitable institutions [3, 4]. But still during the nineteenth century, women were generally considered too frivolous, delicate, and unable to act as rational beings to deal with medical education, with special emphasis on human anatomy and diseases. In his 1873 book *Sex in education*, Dr. E. H. Clarke warned that "*higher education in women produces monstrous brains and puny bodies, abnormally active cerebration and abnormally weak digestion, flowing thought and constipated bowels*" [5]. In one field alone throughout history women were always accepted and even preferred: midwifery, even though starting with the introduction of obstetrical and surgical instruments such as forceps in the 1600s the proportion of female midwives gradually reduced over time. During this time it became fashionable for women to have "man-midwives" as there was a presumption that male practitioners possessed more technical skills and superiority in matters of medicine [6]. Consequently, until the early twentieth century, women's role as healers and obstetricians had been relegated to that of the passive assistant or hand maiden to the male doctor.

By the mid-1800s, increasing numbers of women were admitted to several all-male medical schools, and, finally, in the past four decades, the proportion of women entering medical school around the world has progressively increased to outnumber males in most Western countries. This changing gender composition of the medical workforce is known as the feminization of medicine, but that doesn't mean equal treatment [7]. Compared to men, women doctors are underrepresented in leadership positions in medicine, despite similar levels of skills or experience (Fig. 2.1). In addition, women are more likely to choose specialties that are still conventionally seen as "feminine," such as family medicine, pediatrics, psychiatry, dermatology, and obstetrics/gynecology. These long-standing gender differences have important practical and social implications and represent a priority to ensure that women should be equally represented across all spheres and hierarchies of medicine.

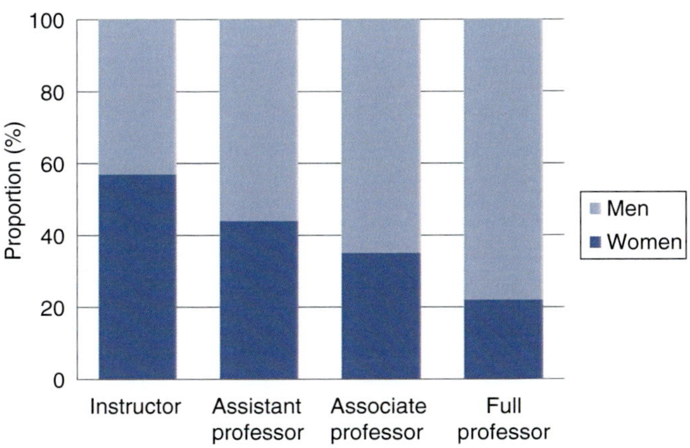

Fig. 2.1 Medical school full-time faculty distribution by rank and gender–United States, 2015. From: Association of American Medical Colleges www.aamc.org/members/gwims/statistics/

2.2 Women as Patients

Despite the growing interest in female health and medicine over the past decades, up to now there has been no comprehensive study on the history of women as patients.

For centuries, women have been perceived as weak, sickly creatures on the basis of both the church doctrines about the inferiority of women due to Eve and many ancient texts about women and their bodies full of distortions and misinformation. According to the humoral theory, men were hot and dry, indicating the perfection and nobility of their bodies, while women were cold and moist, indicating their imperfection [8]. In most schools of thought, women were held to be inferior copies of the male organism. The same female reproductive system heavily influenced these ideas. The second century Roman physician Galen—probably the most influential physician of all time—described the female genitalia as being an inverse of the male: male, having the hotter body, necessarily carried his organs on the outside, whereas the woman, being cooler, carried hers on the inside [9]. How the female reproductive system functioned was also a mystery and a matter of debate. The most famous example was the idea of the "wandering uterus" causing various female medical problems, which has its origins in ancient Greece. The belief that the uterus was responsible for a variety of illnesses—known collectively as "hysteria"—persisted until the early twentieth century [10].

It should be pointed out that throughout the history women have been subject to the same general diseases and injuries that afflict men and children. Therefore, women's need for healthcare was more or less constant, and at least some of this need was addressed by specialized caretakers. Some historians claim that "*women's health was women's business*". Others provide plenty of evidence that women medical practitioners treated men and men treated women even in gynecology and obstetrics (though a female intermediary would be employed for manual examinations) [11]. The care of women during pregnancy does not appear to be exclusively controlled by other women; however women figured prominently there.

By the early 1800 with the advent of modern medical degrees and physical examinations, the pelvic exam began to be performed by male physicians, as women were not allowed to enroll in medical school, as we have already seen. It seems that this examination consisted of a "compromise" since the physician kneeled before the woman but did not directly inspect her genitals, only palpated them [12]. In this period, a chaperone began to be used to attend gynecological visits.

As the role of women in healthcare grew, so did the profession's understanding of the particular health needs of women. Nevertheless, until 1950 the risk of dying in childbirth (mainly for puerperal sepsis and hemorrhage) was still as high as it had been just in the 1850s [13, 14]. The wider use of antisepsis; asepsis and the introduction of antibiotics; better health and nutrition and the better education of women; the effects of body awareness; the wider use of contraception, including the pill; the improvement in obstetric anesthesia and midwifery practices; and the spread of antenatal care have undoubtedly reduced the dramatic number of women dying in childbirth to almost zero [15]. Although the safety of childbirth and of women is now generally taken for granted in developed wealthy world, in developing poor countries, the maternal mortality remains unacceptably high, and women's health needs are still denied. So far, the health institutions have failed to confront these inequalities. It's time they did so.

References

1. Lerner G. Placing women in history: definitions and challenges. Femin Stud. 1975;3:5–14.
2. Hyginus GJ. Fabula CCLXXIV. In: Marshall P, editor. Fabulae. 2nd revised ed. Munich: K.G. Saur; 2002. (Bibliotheca scriptorum Graecorum et Romanorum Teubneriana).
3. Green MH. Gendering the history of women's healthcare. Gend Hist. 2008;20:487–518.
4. Strocchia ST. Women and healthcare in early modern Europe. Renaissance Stud. 2014;28:496–514.
5. Clarke EH. Sex in education, or, a fair chance for the girls. Boston, MA: James R. Osgood and Company; 1873.
6. McTavish L. Blame and vindication in the early modern birthing chamber. Med Hist. 2006;50:447–64.
7. Riska E. Gender and medical careers. Maturitas. 2011;68:264–7.
8. Laqueur TW. Making sex: body and gender from the Greeks to Freud. Cambridge, MA: Harvard University Press; 1990.
9. Gourevitch D. Quelques fantasmes érotiques et perversions d'objet dans la littérature gréco-romaine. MEFR Antiquité. 1982;94:823–42.
10. Gilman SL, King H, Porter R, Rousseau GS, Showalter E. Hysteria beyond Freud. Los Angeles, CA: University of California Press; 1993.
11. Green M. Women's medical practice and health care in medieval Europe. Signs. 1989;14:434–73.
12. Balayla J. Male physicians treating female patients: issues, controversies and gynecology. Mcgill J Med. 2011;13:72–6.
13. Loudon I. The transformation of maternal mortality. BMJ. 1992;305:1557–60.
14. Ruiz JI, Nuhu K, McDaniel JT, Popoff F, Izcovich A, Criniti JM. Inequality as a powerful predictor of infant and maternal mortality around the world. PLoS One. 2015;10:e0140796.
15. WHO. World health statistics 2017: monitoring health for the SDGs, sustainable development goals. Geneva: World Health Organization; 2017.

Suggested Reading

Bergström S. Global maternal health and newborn health: looking backwards to learn from history. Best Pract Res Clin Obstet Gynaecol. 2016;36:3–13.

King H. Hippocrates' woman: reading the female body in ancient Greece. London; New York, NY: Routledge; 1998.

Libbon SE. Pathologizing the female body: phallocentrism in western science. J Int Women's Stud. 2007;8:79–92.

Pomata G. Practicing between heaven and earth: women healers in seventeenth-century Bologna. Dynamis. 1999;19:119–43.

The Trotula: an English translation of the medieval compendium of women's medicine. Edited and translated by Monica H. Green. University of Pennsylvania Press. 2002.

Whaley L. Women and the practice of medical care in early modern Europe, 1400–1800. Basingstoke: Palgrave Macmillan; 2011.

Gender Violence: Risk Factors and Social Vulnerability

3

Barbara Ferrari

Key Points

- **Gender violence**: Vienna Declaration and Programme of Action Adopted by the World Conference on Human Rights, in Vienna on 25 June 1993.
- **Social vulnerability**: The term "social vulnerability" refers to a situation in which one lives a daily life that becomes insecure.
- **Women**: The etymology of the word woman is undoubtedly linked to the syncopated form dŏmna of the Latin domĭna (female of dominus) meaning lady or mistress.

Violence is a very difficult concept to define. It is changeable and elusive; the word violence is commonly used in everyday language to describe a series of very different social facts, so that there are differences in the use of this term and in the meanings that are attributed to it.

Violence can therefore be defined as a form of constriction and as an imposition of force that is affirmed through concrete and physical acts but also psychological, for example, through threats, plagiarism, and fear.

> [...] Violence against women is perhaps the most shameful human rights violation. It does not know either geography, culture, or wealth. As long as it continues, we cannot claim to have made real progress towards equality, development and peace [...] [1].

Domestic violence means when in a marital or similar family relationship, there are people who use physical, sexual, or psychological violence. Violent are all behaviors or acts that put the woman in power and control by the partner.

B. Ferrari (✉)
Department of Biomedical and Neuromotor Sciences-Psychiatry,
University of Bologna, Bologna, Italy
e-mail: barbara.ferrari4@unibo.it

I. Tarricone, A. Riecher-Rössler (eds.), *Health and Gender*,
https://doi.org/10.1007/978-3-030-15038-9_3

The dynamics of domestic violence, violence driven by the partner within the family, presents the characteristics of a set of behaviors that tend to establish and to keep control of the woman and sometimes on the daughters.

These are real strategies for exercising power over the other person, using different modes of behavior such as the destruction of objects or the killing of animals belonging to the woman; the exploitation or denigration of his/her behaviors and ways of being; the threat of violence; the imposition of controls or restrictions on seeing friends, relatives, or leaving home alone; unleashing jealousy totally unmotivated; dealing with partners as a housekeeper; etc.

Violence against women is a widespread phenomenon and independent of culture, social development, and religion.

Gender differences, therefore, often socially attributed to the sexes on the basis of natural biological diversity, have the task of directing the choice and the assumption of "male" or "female" behaviors. Masculinity is often linked to the concepts of domination and aggression, understood as a free path to the use of violence and the way to resolve conflicts.

The female role, however, is usually oriented toward understanding and tolerating, disposing of their own needs with respect to others, and therefore remains linked to the stereotype of the person who has to take care of others.

From this it follows that the reference to gender roles could explain the reason for "acceptance of violence" by some women it is probably due to "[…] the fact that since girls have internalized as feminine qualities to endure … There is thus an acceptance of the violence arising from the idea that the *command* should be the *male*, interiorized conception during a gendered socialization that has placed man, whether father or partner, in a position of superiority […]" [2].

It happens that women who are unable to escape the violent partner have lived in the shadow of violence as little girls, obeying a master father who taught them the rule of total submission to the man of the home "[…] The context of life and relationship in which these women grow up is thus of particular importance in the structure of women's role … which causes them to mortify, if necessary, their own identity in favor of that of a wife (even if the wife of a violent husband), capable of canceling herself in order to safeguard what remains of family […]" in relation to the deep-rooted social expectations of having to satisfy the will of one's partner [2].

The various disagreeable situations experienced by women who have suffered violence may therefore lose the benchmarks and the secrecy they trusted in the couple relationship.

They are in a condition of *social vulnerability*, that is, "[…] as a possible transition place for individual careers, crippled by precariousness and fragility both at work and in the social relationships in which the individual is placed […]" [3].

In addition, *vulnerability* involves a number of processes of social dissociation that jeopardize the stability of patterns of organization of daily life even in its relational dimension.

We can therefore argue that *social vulnerability* is due to a combination of factors such as the shortage of available resources, the weakness of the social networks that it has entered, and the difficulty of developing appropriate strategies to cope with the difficulties [4].

References

1. United Nations General Assembly. Declaration on the elimination of violence against women. Proceedings of the 85th Plenary Meeting, Geneva, 20 December 1993.
2. Cersosimo G, Marra P, Rauty R. L'amore negato. Con-vivere con la violenza? In: Corradi C, editor. I modelli sociali della violenza contro le donne. Rileggere la violenza nella modernità. 3rd ed. Milano: Franco Angeli; 2016.
3. Castel R. De l'indigence à l'exclusion, la désaffiliation. Précarité du travail et vulnérabilité relationelle. In: Donzelot J, editor. Face à l' exclusion, le modèle française. Paris: Esprit; 1991.
4. Ferrari B. Periurbano e vulnerabilità sociale. In: Sociologia urbana e rurale n, vol. 62. Milano: Franco Angeli; 2000.

Suggested Reading

Alisic E, Groot A, Snetselaar H, Stroeken T, van de Putte E. Parental intimate partner homicide and its consequences for children: protocol for a population-based study. BMC Psychiatry. 2015;15:177. https://doi.org/10.1186/s12888-015-0565-z.

Berzenski SR, Yates TM. Research on intimate partner violence: a developmental process analysis of the contribution of childhood emotional abuse to relationship violence. J Aggress Maltreat Trauma. 2010;19:180–203. https://doi.org/10.1080/10926770903539474.

Campbell JC, Webster D, Koziol-McLain J, Block C, Campbell D, Curry MA, Gary F, Glass N, McFarlane J, Sachs C, Sharps P. Risk factors for femicide in abusive relationships: results from a multisite case control study. Am J Public Health. 2003;93(7):1089–97.

Devries KM, Mak JY, Garcia-Moreno C, et al. Global health. The global prevalence of intimate partner violence against women. Science. 2013;340(6140):1527–8. https://doi.org/10.1126/science.1240937.

Eisman AB, Ngo QM, Kusunoki YY, Bonar EE, Zimmerman MA, Cunningham RM, Walton MA. Sexual violence victimization among youth presenting to an urban emergency department: the role of violence exposure in predicting risk. Health Educ Behav. 2017;1:1090198117741941. PMID:29199476.

Foshee VA, Bauman KE, Linder GF. Family violence and the perpetration of adolescent dating violence: examining social learning and social control processes. J Marriage Fam. 1999;61:331–42. https://doi.org/10.2307/353752.

Stöckl H, Devries K, Rotstein A, et al. The global prevalence of intimate partner homicide: a systematic review. Lancet. 2013;382(9895):859–65. https://doi.org/10.1016/S0140-6736(13)61030-2.

Storey JE, Strand S. The influence of victim vulnerability and gender on police officers' assessment of intimate partner violence risk. J Fam Viol. 2017;32(1):125–34. https://doi.org/10.1007/s10896-016-9905-0.

Gender Violence: Protective Factors and Resilience

4

Santa D'Innocenzo

Key Points

- **RESILIENCE** reflects the ability to maintain a stable equilibrium and relatively stable healthy level of psychological and physical functioning, even in the face of highly disruptive stressful and traumatic events.
- Adequate **PUBLIC POLICY** programs can contribute to strengthen resilience in childhood creating supportive environments that help to build skills tackling future disparities.
- Resilience arises from everyday life as a process that regulates stressor events, in this sense its strengthening can also have positive effects on mental **HEALTH**.
- Research on adolescent risk factors for delinquency suggested that, due to **SEX** and genetic differences, some youth displaying resilience and others a heightened vulnerability.
- Building resilience needs to be achieved with specific **GENDER**-sensitive programs.

Sex and gender shape health [1] by way of both biological and sociocultural factors, but difficulties still persist in understanding the origins of the differing factors and the connections between them. Despite growing recognition of the importance of these issues, progress needs to be made to further implement sex and gender integration as standard practice, because the assumptions and the models that are built on them can have specific consequences that are relevant not only to research and healthcare but also to public policy.

In effect, the complexity of gender differences in health extends beyond notions of either social or biological disadvantage. These issues become critical when they

S. D'Innocenzo (✉)
Forensic Foundation Study Research Office, Bologna, Italy
e-mail: santa@santadinno.com

I. Tarricone, A. Riecher-Rössler (eds.), *Health and Gender*,
https://doi.org/10.1007/978-3-030-15038-9_4

expose vulnerable individuals to a greater danger in facing the sudden changes that are typical of our times. Only individuals considered more resilient are able to satisfactorily face the daily challenges of life today.

In this context, the concept of resilience [2] is usually intended as the capacity to buffer change and to learn and develop tenacity. It is a framework for understanding how to sustain and enhance adaptive capabilities in a complex world of rapid change. Its broad use in different disciplines has motivated social scientists and policy researchers to adopt its patterns and concepts in specific analyses [3].

Some authors [4] described how resilience arises from everyday life as a process that regulates stressor events. In this model, the ability to react successfully when coped with the greatest stresses is acquired day by day when faced with life's smaller daily problems. In recent years more concrete theories of the concept of resilience have been developed based on this understanding, from a theoretical perspective of both the treatment and above all the prevention of underdeveloped resilience.

Literature teaches us that individuals can learn skills to improve their resilience and that this can, in part, be achieved by using public policy tools. However, the most fruitful investment for any public policy program is to promote social and emotional abilities and prevent vulnerability by contributing to structure a capacity for resilience in the early stages of development, preferably in childhood.

In fact, resilience is not a stable human attribute. It is strongly influenced by external social factors, and therefore it can be adjusted, and above all it can be easily learned. The most appropriate public policies work at various levels to change the environment by implementing protective factors that enable children to navigate adverse events constructively through articulated prevention strategies that include school, after-school programs, and, where necessary, social services and mental health practitioners.

Children exposed to maltreatment or other forms of abuse should benefit from early prevention interventions directed at the treatment of the mother-child relationship, through which a more adaptable personality can be developed. Children with lower ego control and ego resilience levels [5] need interventions focused on the development of flexible adaptive skills in different situations and contexts. Preadolescence prevention efforts should focus on strengthening social skills and emotional and behavioral regulation skills in order to reduce both socially and individually destructive behavior.

Effective parenting and good teaching practice can increase resilience in children, but adults can learn to become more resilient as well. While the importance of establishing resilience in childhood cannot be emphasized enough, there are programs for promoting resilience in adults that offer promising results, such as the Promoting Adult Resilience (PAR) program [6] and REsilience and Activity for each DaY (READY) program [7]: the research on psychological resilience suggests that it is largely a malleable phenomenon, and as such it is suitable for intervention even in the workplace [8].

In general, working on protective factors in childhood seems to be a useful strategy for children at risk of domestic violence as well, since there are individual and familial characteristics that predict resilience levels among children exposed to domestic violence [9].

Public policy social programs such as Positive Youth Development [10] help to strengthen resilience and self-control and have demonstrated that they can generate a relevant improvement to the attitudes of individuals, also with respect to gender differences, and with a relevant impact on the health sector [11].

In conclusion, the cognitive skills that underpin resilience seem like they can indeed be learned over time, creating resilience where there was none, but unfortunately, the opposite may also be true. This is why the fact that protective factors operate across different levels interacting with different environments gives a relevant responsibility to public policy programs in order for researching models to be realistic and interventions to be effective, especially considering how individual capacity interplays with external protective factors. In many cases levels of mental distress among communities need to be understood less in terms of individual pathology and more as a physiological response to relative deprivation, poor environments, and social injustice, which erode the developing of emotional, spiritual, and intellectual resources essential to psychological well-being and good outcomes as adults.

There is a need for more research on the interactions between adversities, internal and external protective factors, and public policy interventions to foster individuals to tolerate stressor events in order to build resilience, as well as to tackle gender inequalities in health.

Program	Ref.	Aim
Promoting Adult Resilience (PAR) program	Liossis et al. [6]	The cost of lost working time from mental health problems extends from costs on family, to employers, through lost productivity, and to the community. A mentally healthy workforce has benefits for individuals, employers, and the community alike [12]
REsilience and Activity for each DaY (READY) program	Burton et al. [7]	Potentially, it is aimed to promote well-being targeting five protective factors identified from empirical evidence: positive emotions, cognitive flexibility, social support, life meaning, and active coping
Public policy social programs such as Positive Youth Development	Sanders et al. [10]	It is directed to tackle the increasingly diverse society and underlying disparities that impair the health and well-being of a number of populations and youth development and create the conditions by which young people from all populations have opportunities to develop skills and habits that lead to long-term good health

Mentioned programs/Table drafted by Santa D'Innocenzo

References

1. Birda CE, Riekerb PP. Gender matters: an integrated model for understanding men's and women's health. Soc Sci Med. 1999;48(6):745–55.
2. Southwick SM, Bonanno GA, Masten AS, Panter-Brick C, Yehuda R. Resilience definitions, theory, and challenges: interdisciplinary perspectives. Eur J Psychotraumatol. 2014;5:25338. https://doi.org/10.3402/ejpt.v5.25338.
3. Capano G, Jie Woo J. Resilience and robustness in policy design: a critical appraisal. New York, NY: Springer; 2017. http://ash.harvard.edu/files/ash/files/resilience_and_robustness.pdf.
4. Masten AS. Ordinary magic: resilience processes in development. Am Psychol. 2001; 56(3):227.
5. Huey SJ Jr, Weisz JR. Ego control, ego resiliency, and the five-factor model as predictors of behavioral and emotional problems in clinic-referred children and adolescents. J Abnorm Psychol. 1997;106(3):404–15.
6. Liossis PL, Shochet IM, Millear PM, Biggs H. The promoting adult resilience (PAR) program: the effectiveness of the second, shorter pilot of a workplace prevention program. Behav Chang. 2009;26(02):97–112.
7. Burton NW, Pakenham KI, Brown WJ. Feasibility and effectiveness of psychosocial resilience training: a pilot study of the READY program. Psychol Health Med. 2010;15(3):266–77.
8. Sarkar M, Fletcher D. How resilience training can enhance wellbeing and performance. In: Crane MF, editor. Managing for resilience: a practical guide for employee wellbeing and organizational performance. London: Routledge; 2017. p. 227–37.
9. Martinez-Torteya C, Bogat GA, Von Eye A, Levendosky AA. Resilience among children exposed to domestic violence: the role of risk and protective factors. Child Dev. 2009;80(2):562–77. Michigan State University.
10. Sanders J, Munford R, Thimasarn-Anwar T, Liebenberg L, Ungar M. The role of positive youth development practices in building resilience and enhancing wellbeing for at-risk youth. Child Abuse Negl. 2015;42:40–53. https://doi.org/10.1016/j.chiabu.2015.02.006.
11. Catalano RF, Hawkins JD, Toumbourou JW. Positive youth development in the United States: history, efficacy, and links to moral and character education. Handbook of moral and character education. London: Routledge; 2008. p. 459–83.
12. WHO (2000) Mental health and work. Impact, issues and good practices, Geneva. https://www.who.int/mental_health/media/en/712.pdf

Suggested Reading

Chandler D. Resilience: the governance of complexity. Abingdon: Routledge; 2014.

Joseph J. Resilience as embedded neoliberalism: a governmentality approach. Resilience. 2013;1(1):38–52.

Lombardo E, Meier P, Verloo M. Stretching and bending gender equality: a discursive politics approach. In: Lombardo E, Meier P, Verloo M, editors. The discursive politics of gender equality: stretching, bending and policymaking. Oxon: Routledge; 2009. p. 1–18.

Masten AS. Global perspectives on resilience in children and youth. Child Dev. 2014;85(1):6–20.

Public Health England. Local action on health inequalities: building children and young people's resilience in schools. London: TSO; 2014.

Shonkoff JP, Boyce WT, McEwen BS. Neuroscience, molecular biology, and the childhood roots of health disparities: building a new framework for health promotion and disease prevention. JAMA. 2009;301:2252–9.

Part II

The Bio-psicho-social Determinants of Health for the Women

5 Vulnerability and Protective Factors for Mental Health: A Rereading in Gender Perspective

Anita Riecher-Rössler

Key Points

- Sex and gender are increasingly recognized as important factors influencing mental health, since both are associated with specific vulnerabilities, risk, and protective factors.
- As regards "sex" on the biological side, it is mainly the female sex hormone estradiol which seems to have various protective effects.
- Regarding "gender" on the psychosocial side, men and women seem to have different vulnerabilities and a different distribution of risk factors mainly due to "gender-typical" socialization and behavior, differing social roles and gender role stereotypes, but also due to factors like gender-based violence, abuse or discrimination.
- Taking these influences into account could, on the one hand, help to better understand the pathogenetic processes leading to mental disorders with marked gender differences in incidence and prevalence, such as depression or anxiety disorders.
- On the other hand, it could improve our diagnostic processes and therapies, making them more gender-sensitive in the sense of a more personalized medicine.

Sex and gender differences in mental disorders are among the most intriguing and stable findings in psychiatry. Differences have been shown regarding incidence and prevalence, symptomatology, or course in many disorders. But we still do not really understand the causes of these differences. Most likely, they are mainly

A. Riecher-Rössler (✉)
Center for Gender Research and Early Detection, University of Basel Psychiatric Hospital, Basel, Switzerland
e-mail: Anita.Riecher@upkbs.ch

I. Tarricone, A. Riecher-Rössler (eds.), *Health and Gender*,
https://doi.org/10.1007/978-3-030-15038-9_5

due to different vulnerabilities and a different distribution of risk and protective factors in women and men [1–6]. Evidence for this will be discussed in the following chapter.

5.1 Gender Differences in Incidence, Prevalence, and Age of Onset of Mental Disorders

All major epidemiological studies show gender differences in the incidence and prevalence of mental disorders [2, 3, 5, 6]. Women suffer much more frequently from eating disorders, depression, anxiety disorders, somatoform disorders, and also from borderline personality disorders. After a trauma women develop more often a posttraumatic stress disorder. Also, suicide *attempts* occur more often in women. Men, on the other hand, show more *completed* suicides, have higher rates of substance abuse, and most of the other personality disorders, especially antisocial ones. A large worldwide study, conducted on 72,933 participants in 15 countries of all continents, has shown this quite impressively (see Table 5.1) [5].

Table 5.1 Lifetime risk of mental disorders, odds ratios women/men (OR)

Mental disorder	Number of countries	All-country OR
Mood disorders	15	1.9
Major depressive disorder	10	1.9
Dysthymic disorder	6	0.9
Bipolar disorder	15	1.8
Any mood disorder		
Anxiety disorders	12	1.9
Panic disorder	15	1.7
Generalized anxiety disorder	8	2.0
Agoraphobia	13	1.3
Social phobia	12	2.0
Specific phobia	4	1.6
Separation anxiety disorder	14	2.6
Posttraumatic stress disorder	15	1.7
Any anxiety disorder		
Externalizing disorders	5	0.6
Attention-deficit/hyperactivity	3	0.5
disorder	6	0.7
Conduct disorder	3	0.8
Intermittent explosive disorder	12	0.7
Oppositional defiant disorder		
Any externalizing disorder		
Substance disorders	15	0.2
Alcohol abuse	11	0.3
Alcohol dependence	5	0.4
Drug abuse or dependence	14	0.3
Any substance disorder		
Any disorder	15	1.1

Adapted according to [5]

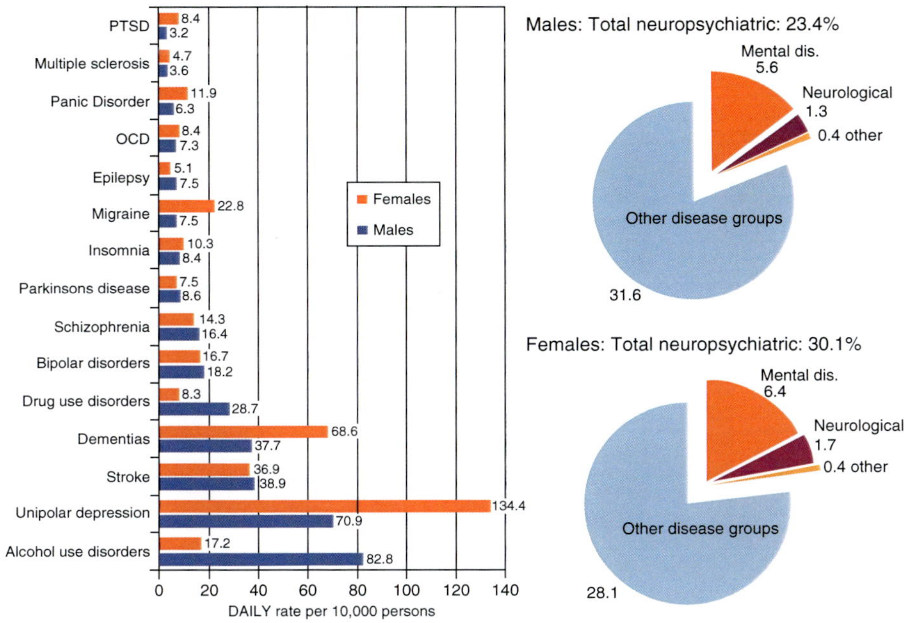

Fig. 5.1 Summary of DALY∗ estimates
∗Disability adjusted life years: number of years lost due to ill-health, disability, or early death. Reprinted from Wittchen HU et al. The size and burden of mental disorders and other disorders of the brain in Europe 2010. Eur Neuropsychopharmacol. 2011;21(9):655–79 [89]; Copyright (2011), with permission from Elsevier

And a meta-analysis including 174 surveys across 63 countries has recently confirmed this [6]. The consequences regarding ill-health, disability, and early death are shown in Fig. 5.1.

As regards schizophrenic psychoses, the cumulative lifetime risk seems to be roughly the same in both sexes if the upper age limit of the studies is 60 [7] or possibly slightly higher in men [8]. Most strikingly, they begin on average 4–5 years later in women than in men [9, 10], and women have a second peak of onset after age 40 with about 20% of all women having their first inpatient episode after age 40, but only 10% of all men [7, 11] (see Fig. 5.2).

5.2 Vulnerability, Risk, and Protective Factors Associated with Sex and Gender

Men and women on average have different vulnerabilities, risk, and stress factors that can influence not only the outbreak, but also the course of mental disorders and the treatment options. This involves biological as well as psychosocial factors.

Two caveats have to be made: First, there is a big overlap between women and men regarding these factors. Not all men are a "prototype man" and not all women

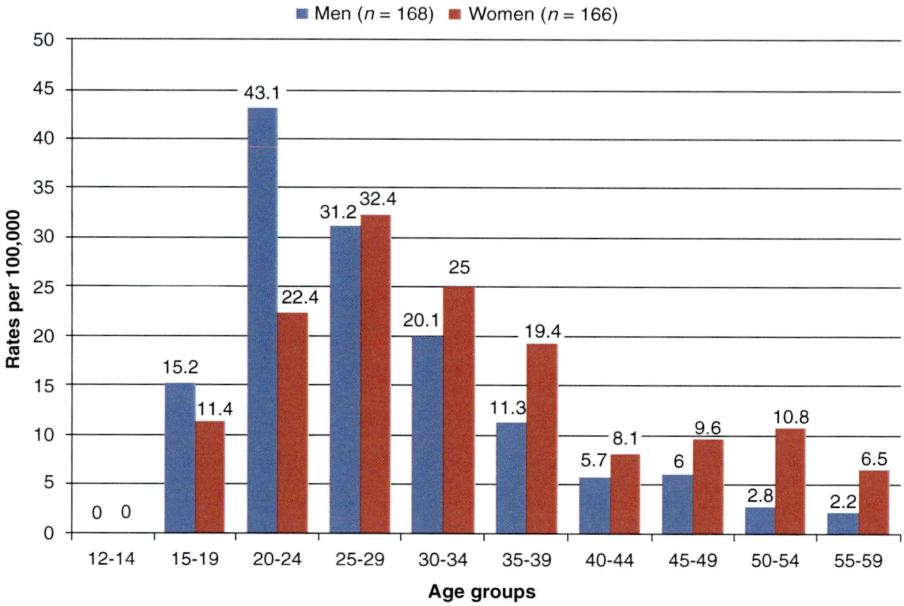

Fig. 5.2 Sex-specific age distribution at first admission for schizophrenia (ICD-9: 295). Source [9]

a "prototype woman." Second, it is difficult to disentangle biological from psychosocial or sociocultural influencing factors. Thus, e.g., human behavior which influences our mental well-being is influenced by biologically determined sex-specific traits, but also by sex-specific cultural stereotypes [12]. Furthermore, gender differences in life experiences might vice versa influence biological differences via epigenetics [13, 14].

5.2.1 Biological Factors

On the biological side, we do not only deal with genetic influences, which can arise from effects of sex chromosome genes [15] (not further discussed in this chapter), but also from hormonal influences on brain development, brain morphology, and brain functioning, showing neuro- and psychoprotective properties.

5.2.1.1 Sex Hormones

Estrogens and testosterone strongly affect brain development during gestation, in the early postnatal period, and around puberty [15–18]. The most active in the brain, 17-β-estradiol, promotes neuronal sprouting and myelination, enhances synaptic density and plasticity, facilitates neuronal connectivity, acts anti-inflammatory and as an antioxidant, inhibits neuronal cell death, and improves cerebral blood flow and glucose metabolism [16, 17, 19–22]; for review, see [10, 18].

Circulating estrogens modulate many neurotransmitter systems relevant to mental disorders, such as the dopaminergic, serotonergic, glutamatergic, noradrenergic, and cholinergic systems [18, 23–28]. Estrogen receptors are expressed in several areas of the human brain that are associated with emotion, memory, and cognition [18, 21, 29, 30].

Clinically, estrogens, especially 17-β-estradiol, seem to have antipsychotic properties [10, 31, 32], to improve affective symptoms [22, 32, 33], aggressive and suicidal behavior [22, 29, 34], and cognitive functioning [20, 30, 35–37], and have stress protective properties [38].

Several intervention studies with estrogens, especially with 17-β-estradiol, have shown positive results in women with schizophrenic psychoses [32, 39–42] or in women with peri-/postmenopausal depressive symptoms [43] or major depression [44–47]. It is therefore astonishing that depression is more frequent in women, because they should actually be protected by estrogens. The higher frequency might, however, be due to the fluctuation of estradiol levels during the female menstrual cycle as well as in the postpartum and perimenopause [18, 48–50]. Thus, estrogen withdrawal has been shown to have a destabilizing effect regarding depression on at least a subgroup of estrogen-sensitive vulnerable women [51, 52]. Perimenopause has been shown to be associated with an increase of depressive symptoms and disorders (overview [15, 44, 53]), although not without contradiction [53]. Women might also be more prone to anxiety, trauma, and stress-related disorders because of their greater monthly and lifespan fluctuations of sex hormones [54].

Also, schizophrenic psychoses more often occur or exacerbate in the premenstrual low estrogen phase of the cycle, with postpartum loss of high estradiol levels of pregnancy and with the perimenopausal loss of estrogens [10, 32, 42]. It has been suggested that estrogens via their antidopaminergic properties might protect women from the outbreak of psychosis during their fertile years, and they only fall ill when they lose this protective factor during menopause [10, 42]. This would not only explain women's later age of onset in schizophrenic psychoses, but also their second peak of incidence after menopause [10, 42].

5.2.2 Psychosocial Factors

Psychosocial risk factors seem to be even more important in explaining the gender gap in the incidence of mental disorders, especially regarding depression, since many well-known risk factors of depression are highly associated with the female gender (for review, see, e.g., [4, 55]).

5.2.2.1 Early Socialization and Coping Style

Gender-specific early socialization and upbringing are supposed to have a distinct impact on the later risk for a mental disorder, on coping strategies, help-seeking behavior, and the course of diseases. For example, it seems that girls tend to be educated more toward passivity, helplessness, and low self-esteem, whereas boys are more encouraged to active coping. Possibly resulting from this, women tend to cope differently with conflicts and problems with more internalizing, ruminating, brooding, feelings of guilt, and depression. Men, on the other hand, are more likely to externalize and blame others for their problems, choose active and sometimes aggressive coping strategies, use addictive drugs or even commit suicide (overview in [4, 15, 55, 56]). Correspondingly, internalizing disorders are more common in women, externalizing more in men, as not only the worldwide WHO Survey [5], but also a recent large European population-based study has shown [2].

5.2.2.2 Social Status and Social Roles

The often different roles men and women still have in our societies, their different social status, and the differences in social stress and social support also seem to distinctly influence their mental health [57, 58].

Women often get less social recognition than men, partly because of their on average lower professional status. For the same work they earn on average less than their male counterparts. As a result, they are more likely to live below the poverty line, especially when they are single-parent mothers [59]. Both factors can impair their mental well-being.

Thus, women are often exposed to numerous stressors and a general overload due to multiple roles—for example, as a mother, wife, housekeeper, professional, carer for parents/in-laws, etc. Even more importantly, they often suffer considerable role conflicts as a result of all these partially competing roles. The social development in the last 50–100 years has given women an enormous increase in opportunities and additional social roles. They now can and should become professionals. At the same time, many women and men were still educated with and exposed to very traditional gender role stereotypes, in which mainly the woman is held responsible for home, hearth, children, well-being of the husband, family, etc. Especially young mothers, when they do not critically reflect these traditional gender roles, may take on a role that does not correspond to their actual desires and needs—such as abandoning their career aspirations or even their entire professional activity—which ultimately may lead to internal conflicts and mental ill-health. Thus, the fact that women suffer from depressive disorders more than men may well be due to the different social roles of the sexes. This conclusion can, e.g., be drawn from a study within the WHO Mental Health Survey with 72,933 respondents in 15 countries of all continents. It revealed gender differences in the depression rate in all countries. In countries, however, where traditional gender roles were dissolving, these differences decreased in the younger age-cohorts [5].

5.2.2.3 Dependency, Harassment, and Violence

Women's lives are often marked by strong dependencies, be it in their partnerships or in the workplace. Furthermore, women, more often than men, experience different forms of gender-based, esp. domestic and partner violence [60–62], which may be another reason for an increased prevalence of depression, posttraumatic stress and anxiety disorders, and suicidality [62–65].

In Europe 20% of all women aged over 15 years have been physically or sexually abused by their (ex)partners [60]. The devastating psychological consequences of sexual abuse and sexual violence are well known [66–68]. A topic still more taboo is women's abuse in the therapeutic relationship [69–71].

Other forms of violence against women influencing their health are human trafficking, female genital mutilation, forced and early marriage, and "honor" crimes [62, 72].

In migrant families, young girls and women are often subjected to a "clash of cultures" between the traditional upbringing and gender role on the one hand and modern western role ideals on the other, which can drive them to attempt suicide [73, 74].

Another important area is gender-based harassment in the workplace [75, 76], which implies not only sexual harassment, but also disadvantages due to rejection of sexual advances or simply gender-based discrimination. For women, this can lead to heavy inner conflicts, fears, and depression.

In the context of mental illness, also the occupation with the body and with beauty is gaining in importance, particularly in women. Modern media suggest ideals that in vulnerable girls and women can lead to bizarre eating habits and eating disorders or to cosmetic surgery, which sometimes is followed by complications and has psychological consequences [55, 77–80].

5.3 Gender Roles and Illness Behavior

On average, women tend to show a better emotional expressiveness than men, report symptoms more willingly, seek help earlier, and demonstrate better compliance (overview in [4, 28, 59]). In contrast, men are often reluctant to seek help due to a traditional "hegemonic" self-concept of masculinity (reviews [81–83]). This does not only apply to mental, but also to physical problems or, e.g., early detection and prevention programs for cancer [84].

The higher rate of completed suicides in men in contrast to the higher rate of suicide attempts in women not only seems to be due to men's worse help-seeking behavior and their negative attitude toward antidepressive therapy, but also to the fact that men choose more aggressive, lethal methods for suicide (reviews [85, 86]).

5.4 Conclusions

Although there is a big overlap between men and women, their mental health is influenced by different vulnerabilities, risk and protective factors. Unfortunately, research so far has often ignored these differences [87]. This is all the more regrettable because it might hamper the detection of potentially differing causal pathways and treatment responses in both women and men and result in a failure to deliver optimal personalized, gender-sensitive treatment. Further research, education, and practice should much more integrate sex and gender aspects. At the same time prevention in the field of mental health should be taken more seriously.

This should include more gender-sensitive prevention programs allowing, e.g., men with traditional ideals of masculinity nevertheless to seek help. And it should also include medical professionals to engage for more gender equality in order to reduce risk factors for mental disorders, as recently proposed by a European Parliament Report [88].

References

1. Riecher-Rössler A. Sex and gender differences in mental disorders. Lancet Psychiatry. 2017;4(1):8–9.
2. Boyd A, Van de Velde S, Vilagut G, de Graaf R, O'Neill S, Florescu S, et al. Gender differences in mental disorders and suicidality in Europe: results from a large cross-sectional population-based study. J Affect Disord. 2015;173:245–54.
3. Jacobi F, Hofler M, Strehle J, Mack S, Gerschler A, Scholl L, et al. Twelve-months prevalence of mental disorders in the German Health Interview and Examination Survey for Adults - Mental Health Module (DEGS1-MH): a methodological addendum and correction. Int J Methods Psychiatr Res. 2015;24(4):305–13.
4. Riecher-Rössler A. Prospects for the classification of mental disorders in women. Eur Psychiatry. 2010;25(4):189–96.
5. Seedat S, Scott KM, Angermeyer MC, Berglund P, Bromet EJ, Brugha TS, et al. Cross-national associations between gender and mental disorders in the World Health Organization World Mental Health Surveys. Arch Gen Psychiatry. 2009;66(7):785–95.
6. Steel Z, Marnane C, Iranpour C, Chey T, Jackson JW, Patel V, et al. The global prevalence of common mental disorders: a systematic review and meta-analysis 1980-2013. Int J Epidemiol. 2014;43(2):476–93.
7. Häfner H, Riecher A, Maurer K, Fatkenheuer B, Löffler W, an der Heiden W, et al. Sex differences in schizophrenic diseases. Fortschr Neurol Psychiatr. 1991;59(9):343–60.
8. van der Werf M, Hanssen M, Kohler S, Verkaaik M, Verhey FR, Investigators R, et al. Systematic review and collaborative recalculation of 133,693 incident cases of schizophrenia. Psychol Med. 2014;44(1):9–16.
9. Häfner H, Riecher A, Maurer K, Fatkenheuer B, Löffler W, an der Heiden W, et al. Geschlechtsunterschiede bei schizophrenen Erkrankungen. Fortschr Neurol Psychiatr. 1991;59(9):343–60.
10. Riecher-Rössler A. Oestrogens, prolactin, hypothalamic-pituitary-gonadal axis, and schizophrenic psychoses. Lancet Psychiatry. 2017;4(1):63–72.
11. Riecher-Rössler A. Die Spätschizophrenie - eine valide Entität? Eine empirische Studie zu Risikofaktoren, Krankheitsbild und Verlauf. Habilitationsschrift. Fakultät für klinische Medizin Mannheim, Universität Heidelberg. 1994.
12. Carter R, Silverman WK, Jaccard J. Sex variations in youth anxiety symptoms: effects of pubertal development and gender role orientation. J Clin Child Adolesc Psychol. 2011;40(5):730–41.
13. Curley JP, Jensen CL, Mashoodh R, Champagne FA. Social influences on neurobiology and behavior: epigenetic effects during development. Psychoneuroendocrinology. 2011;36(3):352–71.
14. Springer KW, Mager Stellman J, Jordan-Young RM. Beyond a catalogue of differences: a theoretical frame and good practice guidelines for researching sex/gender in human health. Soc Sci Med. 2012;74(11):1817–24.
15. Altemus M, Sarvaiya N, Neill Epperson C. Sex differences in anxiety and depression clinical perspectives. Front Neuroendocrinol. 2014;35(3):320–30.
16. Melcangi RC, Panzica G, Garcia-Segura LM. Neuroactive steroids: focus on human brain. Neuroscience. 2011;191:1–5.
17. McCarthy MM. Estradiol and the developing brain. Physiol Rev. 2008;88(1):91–124.

18. Barth C, Villringer A, Sacher J. Sex hormones affect neurotransmitters and shape the adult female brain during hormonal transition periods. Front Neurosci. 2015;9:37.
19. Weickert TW, Weinberg D, Lenroot R, Catts SV, Wells R, Vercammen A, et al. Adjunctive raloxifene treatment improves attention and memory in men and women with schizophrenia. Mol Psychiatry. 2015;20(6):685–94.
20. Pompili A, Arnone B, Gasbarri A. Estrogens and memory in physiological and neuropathological conditions. Psychoneuroendocrinology. 2012;37(9):1379–96.
21. DonCarlos LL, Azcoitia I, Garcia-Segura LM. Neuroprotective actions of selective estrogen receptor modulators. Psychoneuroendocrinology. 2009;34(Suppl 1):S113–22.
22. Riecher-Rössler A. Oestrogens and schizophrenia. Curr Opin Psychiatry. 2003;16:187–92.
23. Gogos A, Sbisa AM, Sun J, Gibbons A, Udawela M, Dean B. A role for estrogen in schizophrenia: clinical and preclinical findings. Int J Endocrinol. 2015;2015:16.
24. Riecher-Rössler A. Estrogens and schizophrenia. In: Bergemann N, Riecher-Rössler A, editors. Estrogen effects in psychiatric disorders. Wien: Springer; 2005. p. 31–52.
25. Garcia-Segura L, Azcoitia I, Doncarlos L. Neuroprotection by estradiol. Prog Neurobiol. 2001;63:29–60.
26. Fink G, Sumner BE, Rosie R, Grace O, Quinn JP. Estrogen control of central neurotransmission: effect on mood, mental state, and memory. Cell Mol Neurobiol. 1996;16(3):325–44.
27. Maki PM, Freeman EW, Greendale GA, Henderson VW, Newhouse PA, Schmidt PJ, et al. Summary of the National Institute on Aging-sponsored conference on depressive symptoms and cognitive complaints in the menopausal transition. Menopause. 2010;17(4):815–22.
28. Riecher-Rössler A, Bitzer J, editors. Frauengesundheit. Ein Leitfaden für die ärztliche und psychotherapeutische Praxis. Elsevier; Urban & Fischer: München; Jena; 2005.
29. Carlson LE, Sherwin BB, Chertkow HM. Relationships between mood and estradiol (E2) levels in Alzheimer's disease (AD) patients. J Gerontol B Psychol Sci Soc Sci. 2000;55(1):P47–53.
30. Oesterlund M. The role of estrogens in neuropsychiatric disorders. Curr Opin Psychiatry. 2002;15:307–12.
31. Seeman MV. Menstrual exacerbation of schizophrenia symptoms. Acta Psychiatr Scand. 2012;125(5):363–71.
32. Riecher-Rössler A, Kulkarni J. Estrogens and gonadal function in schizophrenia and related psychoses. Curr Top Behav Neurosci. 2011;8:155–71.
33. Kahn L, Halbreich U. Estrogen's effect on depression. In: Bergemann N, Riecher-Rössler A, editors. Estrogen effects in psychiatric disorders. New York, NY: Springer; 2005. p. 145–73.
34. Kyomen HH, Hennen J, Gottlieb GL, Wei JY. Estrogen therapy and noncognitive psychiatric signs and symptoms in elderly patients with dementia. Am J Psychiatry. 2002;159(7):1225–7.
35. Boss L, Kang DH, Marcus M, Bergstrom N. Endogenous sex hormones and cognitive function in older adults: a systematic review. West J Nurs Res. 2014;36(3):388–426.
36. Azcoitia I, Arevalo M-A, De Nicola AF, Garcia-Segura LM. Neuroprotective actions of estradiol revisited. Trends Endocrinol Metab. 2011;22(12):467–73.
37. Sherwin BB. Estrogen and memory in women: how can we reconcile the findings? Horm Behav. 2005;47(3):371–5.
38. Goldstein JM, Jerram M, Abbs B, Whitfield-Gabrieli S, Makris N. Sex differences in stress response circuitry activation dependent on female hormonal cycle. J Neurosci. 2010;30(2):431–8.
39. Heringa SM, Begemann MJ, Goverde AJ, Sommer IE. Sex hormones and oxytocin augmentation strategies in schizophrenia: a quantitative review. Schizophr Res. 2015;168(3):603–13.
40. Sommer IE, van Westrhenen R, Begemann MJ, de Witte LD, Leucht S, Kahn RS. Efficacy of anti-inflammatory agents to improve symptoms in patients with schizophrenia: an update. Schizophr Bull. 2014;40(1):181–91.
41. Begemann MJ, Dekker CF, van Lunenburg M, Sommer IE. Estrogen augmentation in schizophrenia: a quantitative review of current evidence. Schizophr Res. 2012;141(2-3):179–84.
42. Riecher-Rössler A, Häfner H. Schizophrenia and oestrogens - is there an association? Eur Arch Psychiatry Clin Neurosci. 1993;242(6):323–8.

43. Zweifel JE, O'Brien WH. A meta-analysis of the effect of hormone replacement therapy upon depressed mood. Psychoneuroendocrinology. 1997;22(3):189–212.
44. Riecher-Rössler A, de Geyter C. The forthcoming role of treatment with oestrogens in mental health. Swiss Med Wkly. 2007;137(41-42):565–72.
45. Gordon JL, Girdler SS. Hormone replacement therapy in the treatment of perimenopausal depression. Curr Psychiatry Rep. 2014;16(12):517.
46. Rubinow DR, Johnson SL, Schmidt PJ, Girdler S, Gaynes B. Efficacy of estradiol in perimenopausal depression: so much promise and so few answers. Depress Anxiety. 2015;32(8):539–49.
47. Toffol E, Heikinheimo O, Partonen T. Hormone therapy and mood in perimenopausal and postmenopausal women: a narrative review. Menopause. 2015;22(5):564–78.
48. Newhouse P, Albert K. Estrogen, stress, and depression: a neurocognitive model. JAMA Psychiat. 2015;72(7):727–9.
49. Calvete E, Camara M, Estevez A, Villardon L. The role of coping with social stressors in the development of depressive symptoms: gender differences. Anxiety Stress Coping. 2011;24(4):387–406.
50. Naninck EF, Lucassen PJ, Bakker J. Sex differences in adolescent depression: do sex hormones determine vulnerability? J Neuroendocrinol. 2011;23(5):383–92.
51. Bloch M, Schmidt PJ, Danaceau M, Murphy J, Nieman L, Rubinow DR. Effects of gonadal steroids in women with a history of postpartum depression. Am J Psychiatry. 2000;157(6):924–30.
52. Schmidt PJ, Ben Dor R, Martinez PE, Guerrieri GM, Harsh VL, Thompson K, et al. Effects of estradiol withdrawal on mood in women with past perimenopausal depression: a randomized clinical trial. JAMA Psychiat. 2015;72(7):714–26.
53. Rössler W, Ajdacic-Gross V, Riecher-Rössler A, Angst J, Hengartner MP. Does menopausal transition really influence mental health? Findings from the prospective long-term Zurich study. World Psychiatry. 2016;15(2):146–54.
54. Li SH, Graham BM. Why are women so vulnerable to anxiety, trauma-related and stress-related disorders? The potential role of sex hormones. Lancet Psychiatry. 2017;4(1):73–82.
55. Kuehner C. Why is depression more common among women than among men? Lancet Psychiatry. 2017;4(2):146–58.
56. Nolen-Hoeksema S. Emotion regulation and psychopathology: the role of gender. Annu Rev Clin Psychol. 2012;8:161–87.
57. Glynn K, Maclean H, Forte T, Cohen M. The association between role overload and women's mental health. J Womens Health (Larchmt). 2009;18(2):217–23.
58. Riecher-Rössler A. Gender-Aspekte. In: Rössler W, Kawohl W, editors. Soziale Psychiatrie: das Handbuch für die psychosoziale praxis. Stuttgart: Kohlhammer; 2013. p. 127–41.
59. Belz M, Riecher-Rössler A. Geschlechtsspezifische Aspekte in der Psychotherapie. In: Herpertz S, Caspar F, Lieb K, editors. Psychotherapie. München: Elsevier GmbH/Urban & Fischer; 2017. p. 553–65.
60. Violence against women: an EU-wide survey. Results at a glance 2014. Available from: http://fra.europa.eu/en/publication/2014/violence-against-women-eu-wide-survey-results-glance.
61. Garcia-Moreno C, Riecher-Rössler A, editors. Violence against women and mental health. Basel: Karger; 2013.
62. Oram S, Khalifeh H, Howard LM. Violence against women and mental health. Lancet Psychiatry. 2017;4(2):159–70.
63. WHO. Global and regional estimates of violence against women. Prevalence and health effects of intimate partner violence and non-partner sexual violence. Geneva: World Health Organization; 2013. Available from: https://www.who.int/reproductivehealth/publications/violence/9789241564625/en/.
64. Devries K, Seguin M. Violence against women and suicidality: does violence cause suicidal behaviour? In: Garcia-Moreno C, Riecher-Rössler A, editors. Violence against women and mental health, vol. 178. Basel: Karger; 2013. p. 148–58.
65. Trevillion K, Oram S, Feder G, Howard LM. Experiences of domestic violence and mental disorders: a systematic review and meta-analysis. PLoS One. 2012;7(12):e51740.

66. Dworkin ER, Menon SV, Bystrynski J, Allen NE. Sexual assault victimization and psychopathology: a review and meta-analysis. Clin Psychol Rev. 2017;56:65–81.
67. MacMillan H, Wathen N. Child sexual abuse of girls. In: Garcia-Moreno C, Riecher-Rössler A, editors. Violence against women and mental health, vol. 178. Basel: Karger; 2013. p. 96–106.
68. Martin S, Parcesepe A. Sexual assault and women's mental health. In: Garcia-Moreno C, Riecher-Rössler A, editors. Violence against women and mental health, vol. 178. Basel: Karger; 2013. p. 86–95.
69. Hollwich S, Franke I, Riecher-Rössler A, Reiter-Theil S. Therapist-client sex in psychotherapy: attitudes of professionals and students towards ethical arguments. Swiss Med Wkly. 2015;145:w14099.
70. Tschan W. Abuse in doctor-patient relationships. In: Garcia-Moreno C, Riecher-Rössler A, editors. Violence against women and mental health, vol. 178. Basel: Karger; 2013. p. 129–38.
71. Franke I, Riecher-Rössler A. Professional sexual misconduct in psychiatry – a literature review on incidence, offender characteristics and interventions (in preparation).
72. Violence against women: the health sector responds 2017. Available from: http://apps.who.int/iris/bitstream/10665/82753/1/WHO_NMH_VIP_PVL_13.1_eng.pdf?ua=1.
73. Brückner B, Muheim F, Berger P, Riecher-Rössler A. Charakteristika von Suizidversuchen türkischer Migranten im Kanton Basel-Stadt. Resultate der WHO/EURO-Multizenterstudie. Nervenheilkunde. 2011;7:517–22.
74. Yilmaz TA, Riecher-Rössler A. Suizidversuche in der ersten und zweiten Generation der ImmigrantInnnen aus der Türkei. Neuropsychiatr. 2008;22(4):261–7.
75. Cortina L, Leskinen E. Workplace harassment based on sex: a risk factor for women's mental health problems. In: Garcia-Moreno C, Riecher-Rössler A, editors. Violence against women and mental health, vol. 178. Basel: Karger; 2013. p. 139–47.
76. Leskinen EA, Cortina LM, Kabat DB. Gender harassment: broadening our understanding of sex-based harassment at work. Law Hum Behav. 2011;35(1):25–39.
77. Borkenhagen A. Körperdysmorphe Störungen und kosmetische Chirurgie. In: Boothe B, Riecher-Rössler A, editors. Frauen in psychotherapie. Stuttgart: Schattauer; 2012. p. 172–9.
78. Orbach S. Weibliches Körperbild – ein Korsett für die Psyche? In: Wimmer-Puchinger B, Gutiérrez-Lobos K, Riecher-Rössler A, editors. Irrsinnig weiblich - Psychische Krisen im Frauenleben Hilfestellung für die Praxis. Berlin: Springer; 2016. p. 35–44.
79. Royal College of Obstetricians and Gynaecologists. Joint RCOG/BritSPAG release: issues surrounding women and girls undergoing female genital cosmetic surgery explored, 7. 2013. Available from: https://www.rcog.org.uk/en/news/joint-rcogbritspag-release-issues-surrounding-women-and-girls-undergoing-female-genital-cosmetic-surgery-explored/.
80. Goodman MP. Female genital cosmetic and plastic surgery: a review. J Sex Med. 2011;8(6):1813–25.
81. Rutz W, Klotz T. Healthy lifestyles and help-seeking in males--no improvement in sight. Psychiatr Prax. 2007;34(8):367–9.
82. Addis ME. Gender and depression in men. Clin Psychol Sci Pract. 2008;15(3):153–68.
83. Seidler ZE, Dawes AJ, Rice SM, Oliffe JL, Dhillon HM. The role of masculinity in men's help-seeking for depression: a systematic review. Clin Psychol Rev. 2016;49:106–18.
84. Sieverding M, Matterne U, Ciccarello L. What role do social norms play in the context of men's cancer screening intention and behavior? Application of an extended theory of planned behavior. Health Psychol. 2010;29(1):72–81.
85. Schrijvers DL, Bollen J, Sabbe BG. The gender paradox in suicidal behavior and its impact on the suicidal process. J Affect Disord. 2012;138(1-2):19–26.
86. Hegerl U. Prevention of suicidal behavior. Dialogues Clin Neurosci. 2016;18(2):183–90.
87. Howard LM, Ehrlich AM, Gamlen F, Oram S. Gender-neutral mental health research is sex and gender biased. Lancet Psychiatry. 2017;4(1):9–11.
88. EU.Reportonpromotinggenderequalityinmentalhealthandclinicalresearch(2016/2096(INI))bythe Committee on Women's Rights and Gender Equality. Available from: http://www.europarl.europa.eu/sides/getDoc.do?pubRef=-//EP//TEXT+REPORT+A8-2016-0380+0+DOC+XML+V0//EN.

89. Wittchen HU, Jacobi F, Rehm J, Gustavsson A, Svensson M, Jonsson B, et al. The size and burden of mental disorders and other disorders of the brain in Europe 2010. Eur Neuropsychopharmacol. 2011;21(9):655–79.

Suggested Reading

Chandra PS, Herman H, Riecher-Rössler A, Fisher J, editors. Mental health and illness worldwide. mental health and illness of women. Springer: in press.

Garcia-Moreno C, Riecher-Rössler A (volume editors). Violence against women and mental health. In: Riecher-Rössler A, Sartorius N (series editors) Key issues in mental health, vol. 178. Karger, Basel. 2013.

Kohen D, editor. Oxford textbook of women and mental health. Oxford: Oxford University Press; 2010.

Nolen-Hoeksema S. Emotion regulation and psychopathology: the role of gender. Annu Rev Clin Psychol. 2012;8:161–87.

Riecher-Rössler A, Steiner M (volume editors) Perinatal stress, mood and anxiety disorders - from bench to bedside. In: Riecher-Rössler A, Steiner M (series editors) Bibliotheca Psychiatrica, vol 173. Karger, Basel. 2005.

Riecher-Rössler A. Prospects for the classification of mental disorders in women. Eur Psychiatry. 2010;25:189–96.

Riecher-Rössler A. Oestrogens, prolactin, hypothalamic-pituitary-gonadal axis, and schizophrenic psychoses. Lancet Psychiatry. 2017;4:63–72.

Soares C, Warren M (volume editors.) The menopausal transition - interface between gynecology and psychiatry. In: Riecher-Rössler A, Steiner M (series editors) Key issues in mental health, formerly Bibliotheca Psychiatrica, vol. 175. Karger, Basel. 2009. (Key Issues in Mental Health, formerly Bibliotheca Psychiatrica).

Subotsky F, et al. Abuse of the doctor-patient relationship. London: RCPsych; 2010.

Sutter-Dallay AL, Glangeaud-Freudenthal NM-C, Guedeney A, Riecher-Rössler A, editors. Joint care of parents and infants in perinatal psychiatry. Berlin: Springer; 2016.

Website

EU Report on promoting gender equality in mental health and clinical research (2016/2096(INI)) by the Committee on Women's Rights and Gender Equality. Available from: http://www.europarl.europa.eu/sides/getDoc.do?pubRef=-//EP//TEXT+REPORT+A8-2016-0380+0+DOC+XML+V0//EN.

Gender, Genoma, and Health

6

Elena Bonora

Key Points

- Integration of sex and gender considerations into health research can strongly strengthen health research, facilitate specificity in health policies and planning, and contribute to reach health equity goals.
- In humans, sex is determined by the presence of the sex-specific chromosomes but also by epigenetic events that include DNA methylation, histone modifications, and microRNAs (miRNAs), acting on gene expression and regulation.
- These complex interplays are implicated in the molecular definition of sex differences. Disentangling these effects can help in understanding the phenotypic variations in health and disease, which could not exclusively be explained by genomic analyses.

Over the past few years, there has been an increasing awareness that the integration of sex and gender considerations into health research can strengthen the overall health evidence base, facilitate specificity in health policies and planning, guide clinicians to better tailor medical care to individuals, and contribute to reach health equity goals [1–3] (Fig. 6.1).

According to the World Health Organization, "sex refers to the genotypic, phenotypic and anatomical characteristics of a sexually reproducing organism, whereas 'gender' is a socio-cultural identity that is learned over time" [4]. "Sex" in health research is classified as either "female" or "male." The term "gender" refers to "socially constructed roles, behaviors, expressions and identities of girls, women, boys, men, and gender diverse people, including how people perceive themselves and each other, how they act and interact" [4]. The absence of sex- and

E. Bonora (✉)
Unit of Medical Genetics, Department of Medical and Surgical Sciences, University of Bologna, Bologna, Italy
e-mail: elena.bonora6@unibo.it

I. Tarricone, A. Riecher-Rössler (eds.), *Health and Gender*,
https://doi.org/10.1007/978-3-030-15038-9_6

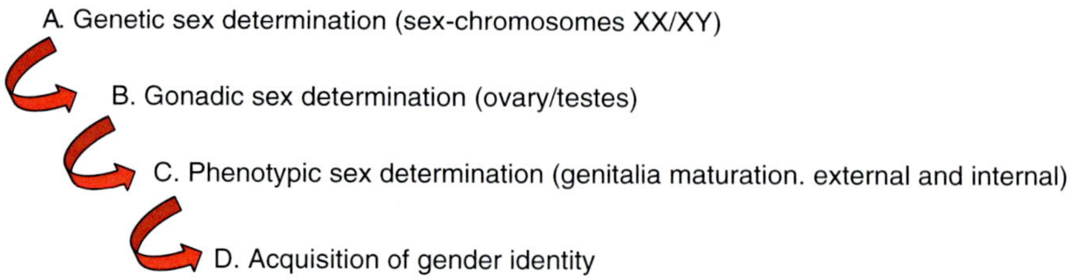

Fig. 6.1 Sequential events leading to sex and gender definition

gender-separated data in many health research findings is problematic for a full understanding of health-impairing events/causes and prevents ameliorating health inequities [5]. Many health outcomes are gendered, such as working conditions and access to sex-related health services [6, 7]. Gender and sex considerations are clinically relevant in pain, diabetes, heart diseases, mental health, and sexually transmitted diseases [1]. The Gendered Innovations project, an international collaboration of scientists formed in 2009, has highlighted the importance of sex and gender analysis in all phases of research and the severe implications of incorrectly deploying/completely ignoring the concepts of sex and gender [8]. In this framework, genomic studies in humans in health and disease have to take into account the inclusion of these parameters as important variables in data analysis.

6.1 Sex Is Genetically Determined

In humans, sex is determined by the presence of the sex-specific chromosome Y that stops recombination in order to maintain the genes encoding for sex-determining factors, whereas the remaining genes degenerate [9]. As a result, the sex-determining chromosome carries fewer genes than its recombining counterpart (in humans the X chromosome). The X chromosome has evolved regulatory mechanisms to maintain a balanced expression of X-linked genes [10]. Genetic differences between sexes originate therefore from the presence or absence of genes encoded on the Y chromosome, from X-chromosome-linked gene dosage and mosaicisms [11]. Early in gestation X-chromosome inactivation (XCI) determines which one of the X chromosomes is transcriptionally silenced in each somatic cell by the production of XIST, a long noncoding RNA transcribed from the X chromosome that will be inactivated [10]. In some tissues, paternally and maternally derived X chromosomes can be preferentially silenced, at least in mice [11]. However, the major random X-inactivation makes the female a functional mosaic of cells that express alleles by either X chromosome, leading to stochastic, female-specific functional diversity on different spatial scales [10]. Moreover, the variability of clinical manifestations in female carriers of X-linked diseases, such as in adrenoleukodystrophy and in X-linked intellectual disabilities as Christianson syndrome, can be ascribed to these events [12, 13].

The X chromosome contains a large number of genes encoding for proteins involved in nervous system development and synapse structure and function [14]. Due to random X-inactivation, females heterozygous at an X-linked locus can express the different alleles in different cells or tissues [10]. X-inactivation varies depending on tissue type and developmental stage, and some X-linked genes escape inactivation, referred to as "X escapees" [15].

The sex-determining region Y (SRY) gene on the Y chromosome is a master regulator of genes involved in male gonad development and determination [16]. In fact, an active process of masculinization occurs in order to make a male, and if anything is altered in this process, the fetus will develop with a female phenotype [17]. Several disorders of sex development derive from defects of SRY and related genes, with loss-of-function mutations leading to a female phenotype (sex reversal, Table 6.1, [18]). It is interesting to consider a potential role of SRY as a factor involved in the sexual dimorphism observed in human diseases [18]. One example is Hirschsprung's disease (HSCR) or congenital megacolon, characterized by a male-female ratio as high as 5:1 in patients [19]. A recent study identified that many of the HSCR disease susceptibility genes are targets for SRY, including the tyrosine kinase receptor RET, whose mutations account for half of the familial and a third of HSCR sporadic forms [19]. SRY competitively displaces activating transcription factors for RET expression, acting as a RET negative modifier [20].

Table 6.1 Examples of gene defects leading to abnormalities in sex development in humans

Gene	Locus	Phenotype (loss-of-function)	OMIM (Online Mendelian Inheritance in Man) accession number
SRY	Chromosome Yp11.2	Female XY (sex reversal)	480000
SOX9	Chromosome 17p24	Female XY (sex reversal)	608160
SF1	Chromosome 9q33	Female XY (sex reversal) Adrenocortical deficiency, premature ovarian failure, spermatogenic failure	184757
DMRT1	Chromosome 9q34	Female XY (sex reversal)	602424
WT1	Chromosome 11p13	Female XY (sex reversal) Renal defects, Wilms tumors	194070
DAX1	Chromosome Xp21.2	Congenital adrenal hypoplasia, with hypogonadotropic hypogonadism	300200
AR	Chromosome Xq12	Female XY, androgen insensitivity	313700

Numbers in OMIM (www.omim.org) are the gene identifiers with related clinical phenotypes

6.2 Effect of Sex-Regulated Tissue Expression: The Example of the Brain

Possession of a Y chromosome leads to SRY expression and causes testis development with the production of testosterone. One of the most interesting aspects of testosterone release can be observed in the brain, where it is transformed into estrogen and induces structural and organizational changes [21, 22]. In mice, female brains are protected from defeminization through the effect of alpha-fetoprotein (AFP), which binds estradiol and prevents it from entering the brain [22]. Female AFP−/− null mice show a masculinization of structure and sexual behavior [22].

The increasing studies of epigenetic events provide additional information of the sexual differentiation in the developing brain. Epigenetics is considered a "potentially heritable process that can permanently modify gene expression in absence of genome sequence variations" [23]. These processes include DNA methylation, histone modifications, and microRNAs (miRNAs), acting on gene expression and regulation both in gametes, which leads to transfer the phenotypic variation from one generation to another and in mitotic tissues, when modifications are transferred to the daughter cells [23].

DNA methylation due to covalently linking a methyl group to cytosine nucleotides is considered a transcriptional repression of the target gene. Cytosine hydroxymethylation, instead, activates transcription, indicating that DNA methylation is dynamically regulated [24].

Histones in the chromatin nucleosome are extensively modified at the N-terminal [23]. Based upon the type and positions of modifications, such changes can regulate chromatin accessibility [23]. miRNA, short (~20 nucleotide) noncoding RNAs, can regulate the transcription and translation of target genes by direct binding to the messenger RNAs [25].

DNA methylation of estrogen receptor alpha (ERα) has been linked to the expression of sexual behavior. In fact, females treated with a methylation inhibitor behaved sexually as males, when given a testosterone challenge in adulthood [26], one of the first evidence that ovary-independent brain feminization is an active process requiring DNA methylation. There is also a different methylation of the ERα gene in sex-related dimorphic brain regions such as the medial preoptic area, in the hypothalamus [22, 27]. Transient modification of histones in ERα promoter regions differs between male and female brain prenatally, epigenetically differentiating the developing brain in a sex-related way [27]. These modifications may be connected to anxiety: for example, specific nuclei related to threat-monitoring in the limbic region can be "masculinized" by combined testosterone exposure and H3 modification, in an early postnatal critical window [28].

Studies on the effects of the neonatal hormone rise reveal that they occur during critical development period and form the base for male and female phenotypic behaviors and physiology [26, 27]. These effects include sex-specific alterations in gene and protein expression, neuronal and glial development, neural cell death, and synaptic connectivity [27]. A second hormone surge at puberty is also necessary for the manifestation of many male- and female-typical behaviors in adulthood [29].

Taking into account these differences, it is not surprising that sex can influence manyfold the degree of susceptibility to diseases: for example, males show a higher propensity for some neurological diseases, including Parkinson's disease, schizophrenia, autism spectrum disorders, and addiction [30–32]. Females show higher susceptibility to neurodegenerative diseases, e.g., Alzheimer's disease and anxiety-related disorders and depression [33, 34]. Women are reported to have twice the lifetime risk of developing depression compared to men and with more symptoms, as determined by multiple depression scales [34].

Therefore, the effects of sex are important variables, and epigenetic mechanisms are now implicated in the molecular definition of sex differences in neural gene expression and function. Disentangling these effects can help in understanding the phenotypic variations in health and disease, which could not exclusively be explained by genomic analyses, considering that these regulatory mechanisms can integrate intrinsic and extrinsic signals onto the genome facilitating the organism adaptation to the environment [35].

References

1. Gahagan J, Kimberly Gray K, Whynacht A. Sex and gender matter in health research: addressing health inequities in health research reporting. Int J Equity Health. 2015;14:12. https://doi.org/10.1186/s12939-015-0144-4.
2. Miller V, Rice M, Schiebinger L, Jenkins M, Werbinski J, Nunez A, et al. Embedding concepts of sex and gender health differences into medical curricula. J Womens Health. 2013;22:194–202.
3. Miller V. Why are sex and gender important to basic physiology and translational and individualized medicine? Am J Physiol Heart Circ Physiol. 2014;306:H781–8.
4. World Health Organization (WHO). Human rights and gender equality in health sector strategies. Geneva: WHO; 2011. http://www.who.int/gender/documents/human_rights_tool/en/.
5. Pinn V. Sex and gender factors in medical studies: implications for health and clinical practice. JAMA. 2003;289:397–400.
6. Campos-Serna J, Ronda-Pérez E, Artazcoz L, Moen BE, Benavides FG. Gender inequalities in occupational health related to the unequal distribution of working and employment conditions: a systematic review. Int J Equity Health. 2013;12:57. https://doi.org/10.1186/1475-9276-12-57.
7. Brankovic I, Verdonk P, Klinge I. Applying a gender lens on human papillomavirus infection: cervical cancer screening, HPV DNA testing, and HPV vaccination. Int J Equity Health. 2013;12:14. https://doi.org/10.1186/1475-9276-12-14.
8. Gendered innovations in science. Health & Medicine, Engineering, and Environment. Sex and gender analysis policies of major granting agencies. 2014.
9. Hughes JF, Page DC. The biology and evolution of mammalian Y chromosomes. Annu Rev Genet. 2015;49:507–27. https://doi.org/10.1146/annurev-genet-112414-055311.
10. Sahakyan A, Plath K, Rougeulle C. Regulation of X-chromosome dosage compensation in human: mechanisms and model systems. Philos Trans R Soc Lond B Biol Sci. 2017;372:pii: 20160363. https://doi.org/10.1098/rstb.2016.0363.
11. Amakawa Y, Sakata Y, Hoki Y, Arata S, Shioda S, Fukagawa T, et al. A new Xist allele driven by a constitutively active promoter is dominated by Xist locus environment and exhibits the parent-of-origin effects. Development. 2015;142:4299–308. https://doi.org/10.1242/dev.128819.
12. Jangouk P, Zackowski KM, Naidu S, Raymond GV. Adrenoleukodystrophy in female heterozygotes: underrecognized and undertreated. Mol Genet Metab. 2012;105:180–5.

13. Morrow EM, Pescosolido MF. Christianson syndrome. In: Adam MP, et al., editors. GeneReviews. Seattle, WA: University of Washington; 2018. 1993–2018.
14. Bassani S, Zapata J, Gerosa L, Moretto E, Murru L, Passafaro M. The neurobiology of X-linked intellectual disability. Neuroscientist. 2013;19:541–52. https://doi.org/10.1177/1073858413493972.
15. Carrel L, Brown CJ. When the Lyon (ized chromosome) roars: ongoing expression from an inactive X chromosome. Philos Trans R Soc Lond B Biol Sci. 2017;372:pii: 20160355. https://doi.org/10.1098/rstb.2016.0355.
16. Jobling MA, Tyler-Smith C. Human Y-chromosome variation in the genome-sequencing era. Nat Rev Genet. 2017;18:485–97. https://doi.org/10.1038/nrg.2017.36.
17. Eggers S, Ohnesorg T, Sinclair A. Genetic regulation of mammalian gonad development. Nat Rev Endocrinol. 2014;10:673–83. https://doi.org/10.1038/nrendo.2014.163.
18. Fleming A, Vilain E. The endless quest for sex determination genes. Clin Genet. 2005;67:15–25.
19. Torroglosa A, Alves MM, Fernández RM, Antiñolo G, Hofstra RM, Borrego S. Epigenetics in ENS development and Hirschsprung disease. Dev Biol. 2016;417:209–16. https://doi.org/10.1016/j.ydbio.2016.06.017.
20. Li Y, Kido T, Garcia-Barcelo MM, Tam PK, Tabatabai ZL, Lau YF. SRY interference of normal regulation of the RET gene suggests a potential role of the Y-chromosome gene in sexual dimorphism in Hirschsprung disease. Hum Mol Genet. 2015;24:685–97. https://doi.org/10.1093/hmg/ddu488.
21. Simerly RB. Wired for reproduction: organization and development of sexually dimorphic circuits in the mammalian forebrain. Annu Rev Neurosci. 2002;25:507–36. 22.
22. McCarthy MM. Estradiol and the developing brain. Physiol Rev. 2008;88:91–124.
23. D'Urso A, Brickner JH. Mechanisms of epigenetic memory. Trends Genet. 2014;30:230–6. https://doi.org/10.1016/j.tig.2014.04.004.
24. Moore LD, Le T, Fan G. DNA methylation and its basic function. Neuropsychopharmacology. 2013;38:23–38. https://doi.org/10.1038/npp.2012.112.
25. Morgan CP, Bale TL. Sex differences in microRNA regulation of gene expression: no smoke, just miRs. Biol Sex Differ. 2012;3:22.
26. Nugent BM, Wright CL, Shetty AC, Hodes GE, Lenz KM, Mahurkar A, et al. Brain feminization requires active repression of masculinization via DNA methylation. Nat Neurosci. 2015;18:690.
27. MM MC, Auger AP, Bale TL, De Vries GJ, Dunn GA, Forger NG, et al. The epigenetics of sex differences in the brain. J Neurosci. 2009;29:12815–23.
28. Somerville LH, Whalen PJ, Kelley WM. Human bed nucleus of the stria terminalis indexes hypervigilant threat monitoring. Biol Psychiatry. 2010;68:416–24.
29. Sisk CL. Hormone-dependent adolescent organization of socio-sexual behaviors in mammals. Curr Opin Neurobiol. 2016;38:63–8.
30. Baba Y, Putzke JD, Whaley NR, Wszolek ZK, Uitti RJ. Gender and the Parkinson's disease phenotype. J Neurol. 2005;252:1201–5.
31. Satterthwaite TD, Wolf DH, Roalf DR, Ruparel K, Erus G, Vandekar S, et al. Linked sex differences in cognition and functional connectivity in youth. Cereb Cortex. 2015;25:2383–94.
32. Mitra I, Tsang K, Ladd-Acosta C, Croen LA, Aldinger KA, Hendren RL, et al. Pleiotropic mechanisms indicated for sex differences in autism. PLoS Genet. 2016;12:e1006425. https://doi.org/10.1371/journal.pgen.1006425.
33. Andersen K, Launer LJ, Dewey ME, Letenneur L, Ott A, Copeland JR, et al. Gender differences in the incidence of AD and vascular dementia: the EURODEM studies. EURODEM incidence research group. Neurology. 1999;53:1992–7.
34. Breslau N, Schultz L, Peterson E. Sex differences in depression: a role for preexisting anxiety. Psychiatry Res. 1995;58:1–12.
35. Ratnu VS, Emami MR, Bredy TW. Genetic and epigenetic factors underlying sex differences in the regulation of gene expression in the brain. J Neurosci Res. 2017;95:301–10. https://doi.org/10.1002/jnr.23886.

Women at Work

7

Dina Guglielmi and Elena Luppi

Key Points

- Studies on women participation in the workforce show inequalities and distinguish vertical and horizontal segregation. Despite their progress in education and training, the gender pay gap and glass ceiling phenomenon persist.
- Women's labour force participation rates have increased in the last decade, but nevertheless women earn less than men and are more likely to work part-time than men and to obtain career advancement and representation in political and business leadership positions.
- Unequal distribution of family duties could hindrance female presence in labour market leading to situations of work-family conflict (WFC), which represents one of the main psychosocial risk factors leading to poorer health and reduced psychological well-being.
- Considering the increase in the studies that confirm the health implications of work-family conflict, it is important to shift attention to the positive side of work-family relationship. Work and family could benefit from each other rather than being conceptualized as conflicting.
- In order to promote good work-family role conciliation, scholars and practitioners could purpose interventions both at individual and organizational levels.

Despite the increase of women participation in workforce over the last few decades, their presence still remains affected by numerous hindrances and mechanisms of segregation. As stated by the last OECD report [1], gender gap persists in all areas of social and economic life, even if the size of this gap has often changed.

D. Guglielmi (✉) · E. Luppi
Department of Education Studies, University of Bologna, Bologna, Italy
e-mail: dina.guglielmi@unibo.it

I. Tarricone, A. Riecher-Rössler (eds.), *Health and Gender*,
https://doi.org/10.1007/978-3-030-15038-9_7

The cultural, social and demographic studies on gender inequalities distinguish two kinds of segregation:

- Vertical segregation, corresponding to the scarce presence of women at the top positions of organizations, institutions and workplaces in general; this is also called "hierarchical segregation" ([2], p. 32). This form of segregation is described through the metaphor of "glass ceiling phenomenon" an invisible obstacle inhibiting or blocking women to the access of power and decision-making roles.
- Horizontal segregation is the unbalanced distributions of women and men workers in certain sectors [2]: in all OECD countries women are more likely to be present in work fields related with care or education and are underrepresented in the STEM (Science Technology, Engineering and Mathematics) sectors.

These mechanisms of segregation also explain another phenomenon of gender segregation in labour market: the gender pay gap, the differences in salaries of women and men occupying the same position in the same organizations [3].

The data published in the last OECD [1] report make very evident that gender segregations still persist even if young women in almost every country now get more years of schooling than young men (see Graphic 7.1). Despite their good results at school, girls are much less likely to study in the STEM fields. Women's labour force participation rates have increased in the last decade, but nevertheless women earn less than men and are more likely to work part-time than men and to obtain career advancement and representation in political and business leadership positions.

The report underlines a few progresses made in crucial policy areas, such as the paternal leaves: OECD countries increased the incentives for fathers, considering this male commitment in unpaid work as an essential mean for the increase of father's and mother's well-being and to combat gender stereotypes. Moreover, about two thirds of OECD countries have introduced since 2013 new pay equity initiatives and measure such as gender quotas to increase the number of women in political and private sector leadership [1].

In the document "Strategy for equality between women and men—2010–2015", the European Commission [5] also put into evidence the two opposite trends: the increase of women on the labour market and their progresses in education and training and the persistence of gender pay gap, gender horizontal and vertical segregation and glass ceiling phenomenon. According to the analysis provided by the European Commission, parenthood and the unequal division of unpaid domestic work are the first cause of gender segregation in the labour market as you can observe in the following graph (Graphic 7.2).

In line with this, it could be useful to go deeper with the relationship between family and work roles. Beyond the fact that unequal distribution of family duties could hindrance female presence in labour market, this could also lead to situations of work-family conflict (WFC), namely, a form of inter-role conflict in which work and family roles are in some cases incompatible [6], especially for female workers. As outlined by Hagqvist et al. [7] even when working force is sustained by equality policies and anti-discrimination laws promoting women participation in labour

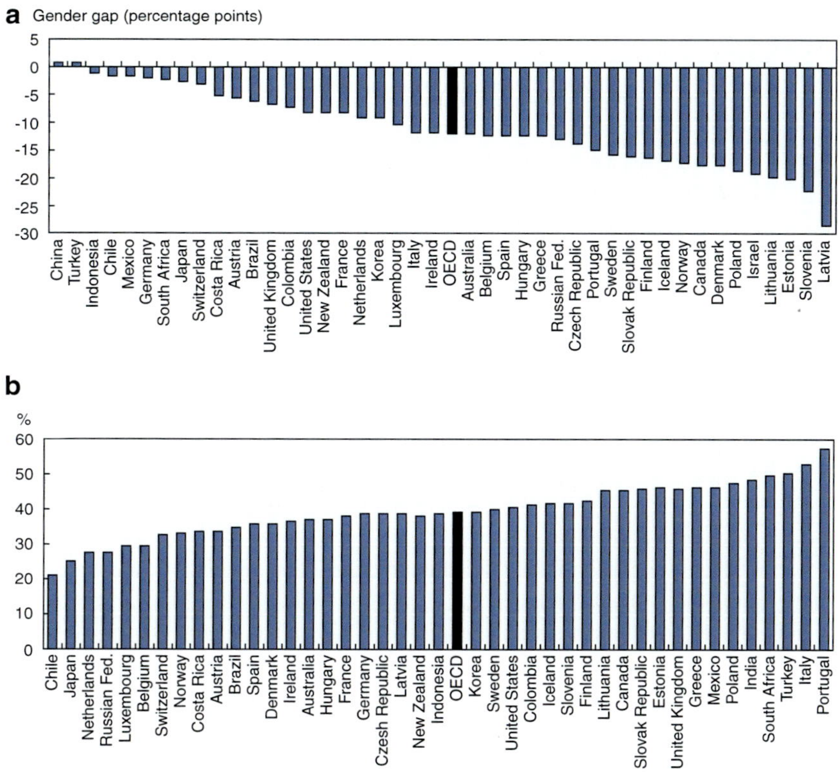

Graphic 7.1 Gender gap. Source: OECD [4], OECD Education at a Glance 2016: OECD Indicators, OECD Publishing, Paris. Panel **a**: Gender gap (male minus female) in the share of the population that has attained tertiary education, 25–34 year-olds, 2015 or latest available year[a]. Panel **b**: Female share (%) of tertiary graduates in science, mathematics and computing, 2014 or latest available year[b]

market, female workers are still more expected to carry out family duties than men, thus experiencing stronger negative relationships between WFC and well-being. Interference between family and work responsibilities represents one of the main psychosocial risk factors leading to poorer health, reduced psychological well-being and negative organizational outcomes.

According to the Sixth European Working Conditions Survey, women have a greater amount of paid (working) and unpaid (nonworking) hours than men, resulting in more exposed work-family interferences and its negative outcomes such as lower life and family satisfaction, psychological strain as well as lower levels of engagement, commitment and job satisfaction [8].

Therefore it also seems important to shift attention to the positive side of work-family relationship and to many theoretical constructs, such as positive spillover, work-family enrichment, work-family facilitation and work-family enhancement reflecting the idea that work and family could benefit from each other rather than

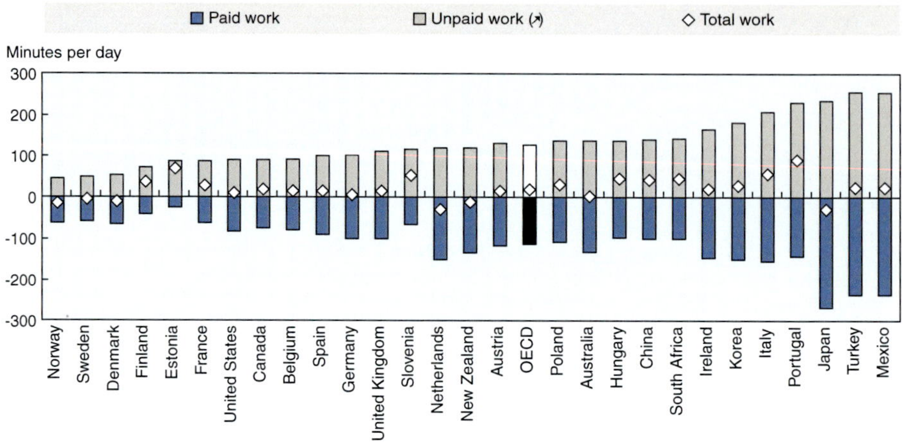

Graphic 7.2 Gender gap in minutes spent per day on paid and unpaid work, female minus male, 15–64 year-olds. Source: OECD Gender Data Portal, http://www.oecd.org/gender/data/

being conceptualized as conflicting. This change in perspective could be useful for scholars and practitioners in understanding how workers (and women with family caring duties in particular) could be facilitated to balance their working and nonworking lives and the interventions to be carried out both at individual and organizational levels for good work-family role conciliation. Such interventions could allow women workers to invest the resources gained in one role to enhance performance in the other role. Considering the increase in the studies that confirm the health implications of work-family conflict, these interventions, at the same time, could lead to an improvement of the health of working women managing work-family interaction.

On the organizational level, companies could offer many resources in order to balance working and nonworking roles beyond classic work arrangements such as flexitime. For example, as reported by Morganson et al. [9], managers and supervisor with a positive leadership style may inspire, by means of positive communication, their employees to reflect how job-related resources and skills (e.g. perseverance, pressure-coping skills) could help them to cope with nonworking demands and duties. Moreover, positive leaders could act as a role model for their employees by transmitting them practices in effective management of work-family commitments and by encouraging them to carry out such practices. Leadership training could be included in organizational family-work culture development interventions such as family-supportive supervisor behaviour (FSSB) training, aimed to foster, among others, role modelling behaviours through examples and exercises about positive strategies and experiences in facing work-family conflict and fostering work-family conciliation and enrichment. Odle-Dusseau et al. [10] found out that FSSB training had positive effects on employees' job satisfaction, turnover intention and supervisor-evaluated employee performance.

At an individual level, Morganson et al. [9] suggested that psychological capital, a multidimensional positive mental state combining self-efficacy, optimism, hope and resiliency, may be beneficial to cope with, among others, work-family interface demands. Psychological capital could counteract WFCs, by enhancing confidence to handle them, optimism to reframe them as temporary, hope to set up different strategies to face them and resilience to mobilize one's resources to come over setbacks and failure in conciliating his own commitments. Therefore, authors indicated psychological capital intervention (PCI, developed by [11]) as a useful intervention boost. In an enrichment/spillover perspective, increasing psychological capital in order to cope with WFC could be useful even to gain better health and well-being seeing the relationship between psychological capital and health.

References

1. OECD. The pursuit of gender equality: an uphill battle. Paris: OECD Publishing; 2017.
2. Bettio F, Verashchagina A. Gender segregation in the labour market: root causes, implications and policy responses in the EU. Luxembourg: Publications Office of the European Union; 2009.
3. Blackburn R, Jarman J. Gendered occupations: exploring the relationship between gender segregation and inequality. GeNet ESRC gender equality network, University of Cambridge Working Paper No 5. 2005.
4. OECD. OECD education at a glance 2016: OECD indicators. Paris: OECD Publishing; 2016. https://doi.org/10.1787/eag-2016-en.
5. European Commission. Strategy for equality between women and men — 2010-2015. Luxembourg: Publications Office of the European Union; 2011.
6. Greenhaus JH, Beutell NJ. Sources of conflict between work and family roles. Acad Manag Rev. 1985;10(1):76–88.
7. Hagqvist E, Gådin KG, Nordenmark M. Work–family conflict and well-being across Europe: the role of gender context. Soc Indicat Res. 2017;132(2):785–97.
8. Eurofound. Sixth European working conditions survey – overview report. Luxemburg: Publication Office of the European Union; 2017.
9. Morganson VJ, Litano ML, O'neill SK. Promoting work–family balance through positive psychology: a practical review of the literature. Psychol Manag J. 2014;17(4):221.
10. Odle-Dusseau HN, Hammer LB, Crain TL, Bodner TE. The influence of family-supportive supervisor training on employee job performance and attitudes: an organizational work–family intervention. J Occup Health Psychol. 2016;21(3):296.
11. Luthans F, Avey JB, Avolio BJ, Norman SM, Combs GM. Psychological capital development: toward a micro-intervention. J Organiz Behav. 2006;27:387–93.

Suggested Reading

European Agency for Safety and Health at Work. European Risk Observatory report, Expert forecast on emerging psychosocial risks related to occupational safety and health. Luxembourg. https://osha.europa.eu/en/tools-and-publications/publications/reports/7807118.: Office for Official Publications of the European Communities; 2007.

Greenhaus JH, Powell GN. When work and family are allies: a theory of work-family enrichment. Acad Manage Rev. 2006;31(1):77–92.

Grönlund A, Öun I. In search of family-friendly careers? professional strategies, work conditions and gender differences in work–family conflict. Community Work Fam. 2018;21(1):87–105.

Kan D, Yu X. Occupational stress, work-family conflict and depressive symptoms among Chinese bank employees: the role of psychological capital. Int J Environ Res Public Health. 2016;13(1):pii: E134.

Payne S, Doyal L. Older women, work and health. Occup Med. 2010;60(3):172–7.

Rajadhyaksha U, Korabik K, Aycan Z. Gender, gender-role ideology, and the work-family interface: a cross-cultural analysis. In: Gender and the work-family experience: an intersection of two domains. Cham: Springer International Publishing; 2015. p. 99–117.

Women, Migration and Social Environment

8

Meryam Schouler-Ocak, Ilaria Tarricone, C. Bignardi, and D. Berardi

Key Points

- The number of immigrants in the world has more than doubled since 1975.
- Women comprise slightly less than half of all international migrants.
- Immigrants are heterogeneous and diverse in regard to their country of origin, reasons for migration, experiences and stress-related risk factors during the stages of premigration, migration and post-migration.
- In the hosting countries, social support, social exclusion, a lack of familiarity with rights, entitlements, gaps in health literacy and discrimination are risk factors for poor mental health.
- In the post-migration phase, individual psychological resources, social support, a successful acculturation processes, cultural variations and time since relocation are identified as statistically significant protective factors.

M. Schouler-Ocak (✉)
Psychiatric University Clinic of Charité at St. Hedwig Hospital, Berlin, Germany
e-mail: meryam.schouler-ocak@charite.de

I. Tarricone
Bologna Transcultural Psychosomatic Team (BoTPT), Department of Medical and Surgical Sciences, Alma Mater Studiorum, University of Bologna, Bologna, Italy

C. Bignardi
Pace Now – Pace Adesso Onlus, Bologna, Italy

D. Berardi
Dipartimento di Scienze Biomediche e Neuromotorie, DIBINEM, Università di Bologna, Bologna, Italy

I. Tarricone, A. Riecher-Rössler (eds.), *Health and Gender*,
https://doi.org/10.1007/978-3-030-15038-9_8

8.1 Introduction

Global migration and the increasing number of immigrant diversities influence the needs in the psychosocial and health-care system. Migration is a process during which a person moves from one cultural setting to another in order to settle for a longer period of time or permanently [1]. A ‘migrant’ is any person who has crossed an international border, regardless of the length of their stay. Immigrants may move en masse or singularly. Many people can be viewed both as ‘immigrants’ and as ‘members of ethnic minorities’. The latter covers groups that do not belong to the category ‘migrant’. For instance, the offspring of immigrants, especially the so-called second and third generation, are not immigrants themselves but may nevertheless be affected by many of the same issues as the first generation, including cultural, linguistic or biological factors, as well as social factors like acceptance or rejection as well as acculturation stress factors by the majority. Immigrants are a heterogeneous group in regard to their country of origin, reasons for migration, experience during the migration and legal status. Migration takes many forms, including forced and voluntary movement even if it is difficult to distinguish between forced and voluntary migration; the reasons for migration often include both. Immigrants experience stress-related risk factors during the stages of premigration, migration and post-migration. The number of immigrants in the world has more than doubled since 1975. In January 2015, the number of people living in the EU-28 who were citizens of non-member countries was at 19.8 million, the number of people living in the EU-28 who had been born outside of the EU was at 34.3 million, and all together 54.1 million immigrants were living in Europe [2]. The composition of immigration by countries is very different. In 2015 the main hosting countries were Germany (7.5 million persons), the United Kingdom (5.4 million), Italy (5.0 million), Spain (4.5 million) and France (4.4 million). These five Member States collectively hosted 76% of all immigrants in EU. The same five Member States had a 63% share of the EU-28’s population [2]. Women comprise slightly less than half of all international migrants. The share of female migrants fell from 49% in 2000 to 48% in 2017. Female migrants outnumber male migrants in Europe, Northern America, Oceania and Latin America and the Caribbean, while in Africa and Asia, particularly Western Asia, migrants are predominantly men [3].

At the national level, social rights are largely dependent on the right to reside and the individual conditions attached to one’s permit. Migration or residence status is consistently cited as one of the most significant factors determining access to affordable and adequate health services for immigrants in a country [3] in a clear example of how migration and health intersect to influence the underlying conditions of health [4]. According to Gonzales et al. [5], the linking of social rights to residence status means that people with precarious status tend to live in precarious living conditions, which has significant consequences for the health of individuals as well as for the well-being of their families and communities. Gonzales et al. [5] reported that there is growing evidence that precarious residence status is itself a risk factor for poor mental health and that more secure status can have a positive impact on mental health and well-being [5].

8.2 Social Factors

According to Bhugra et al. [6, 7], factors such as poverty, persecution or violence may play a main role in the process of migration, in which moving from one cultural and social setting to another for an extended period of times is involved and the loss of the familiar language attitudes, values, social structures and support networks may be also involved [6, 7]. Eisenbruch [8] terms it as loss 'cultural bereavement'. Many authors underline that the cultural bereavement may be misdiagnosed because of linguistic and cultural misunderstandings and because of the use of Western diagnostic criteria in non-Western people [6, 7, 9–11]. Social factors including cultural bereavement, culture shock, social defeat, as well as a discrepancy between expectations and achievement, and acceptance by the hosting country can also affect adjustment [6, 7, 11, 12]. These experiences, along with related factors such as acculturation stress, limited or loss of social networks and social isolation, language and cultural barriers, unemployment, low socioeconomic status and lack of or barriers to access to mental health-care services, have negative effects on immigrants' mental health [13, 14]. According to some researchers, the role of gender was identified in relation to immigrant settlement and mental health [15, 16]. Sword et al. reported that immigrant women are significantly more likely to have low levels of social support, unmet health literacy needs and low family incomes and require financial assistance in comparing with Canadian-born women [17].

Several authors pointed out that lack of social networks and support has been associated with increased risk for distress and mental illness [18–20]. In some cases, the same relationship or social network can provide positive support while being a source of contention or disaccord [21]. Furthermore, social support may be provided by formal or informal sources with expectations of reciprocity that may create stress to individuals due to feelings of obligation [21].

Additionally, Butler et al. [22] underlined that individual psychological resources, social support, the acculturation process, cultural variations and time since relocation are identified as statistically significant protective factors against the development of common mental disorder among immigrants.

8.3 Social Support and Mental Health Outcomes

Several authors documented the relationship between lack of social support and depression among immigrant women well [17, 23–26]. According to Stewart et al. [27], pregnant new immigrants who experienced violence also had inadequate levels of social support and reported more depression, anxiety, somatization and post-traumatic stress disorder on standardized tests. Furthermore, Ahmed et al. [28] could identify that social isolation is one of the main reasons for the depressive symptoms presented by women who have been in Canada less than 5 years. Moreover, Zelkowitz et al. [29] pointed out that pregnant immigrant women who are depressed had poorer functional status and somatic symptoms, lacked social support, experienced more stressful life events and exhibited 'poor marital adjustment'.

In line with these authors, several other studies underlined that poor social support was identified as one of the key risk factors for postpartum depression among immigrant women [16, 30–32]. Other authors [33] found that immigrant women with depressive symptoms had significantly lower social support scores than nonimmigrant women. Further, Zelkowitz et al. [34] reported that marital quality of life was the best predictor for postpartum depression among immigrant women, particularly because they may lack social support from the family they might otherwise have relied on after giving birth. In another study [24] it was found that immigrant mothers receiving weak spousal support had higher prevalence rates of depression compared with nonimmigrant mothers. The authors highlighted that there are positive effects of social support on immigrant mental health [24]. Furthermore, some studies suggested that social support can improve mental health and/or alleviate the negative effects of mental illnesses [35, 36]. Interestingly, Dennis et al. [37] found that providing emotional and informational support by telephone was effective in preventing postpartum depression among 'high-risk women'. Miszkurka et al. ([38], p. 359) pointed out that social support in form of 'favouring integration and poverty reduction interventions could reduce the risk of antenatal depression'. In a study of Black women in Montreal, Whitley and Green [39] could found that social support from the extended family was a key variable that helped buffer psychosocial stressors.

Within the EU, huge differences exist in national asylum policy standards and practices [40], e.g. undocumented immigrants are particularly vulnerable groups, many being likely to be exposed to further trauma in the host country; certain groups such as trafficked women may be kept under highly degrading and traumatizing circumstances [41] with any kind or social support. Mladovsky et al. [42] pointed out that a lack of familiarity with rights, entitlements, gaps in health literacy, social exclusion and direct and indirect discrimination are risk factors for bad mental health outcomes of immigrants.

8.4 Social Support, Social Conflict and Mental Health Service Use

According to Guruge et al. [43], the literature is limited about the role of social conflict and reciprocity within informal social networks, which play an important role in shaping the access and use of mental health services among immigrant women. The literature underlines that immigrants are more likely to underutilize the sources of social support. The reasons are unawareness of these services or inability to access them [7, 17, 28, 44], transportation problems or mobility issues [45, 46] and a lack of culturally safe [47, 48] as well as linguistically appropriate services [11, 48, 49]. Additionally, reasons are also that a part from the staff may be faced with significant language difficulties, negative stereotypes and expectations of treatment that cannot be fulfilled [50], so that there is lack of cultural competence, which involves professional values which must include sensitivity, non-discrimination and responsiveness to the psychiatric needs of any patient [11]. Furthermore, stigma, which plays an important role, is associated with seeking help, particularly for mental health issues [51, 52]. Additionally, intercultural and institutional barriers should be mentioned [11]. De Jong [53] used the term 'interculturalization' and defines it as the adaptation of mental health services to suit patients from different cultures. He developed a model to promote and assess interculturalization of mental health-care services in Western multicultural societies. He suggested four contexts in which changes are necessary: (1) the relationships between the immigrant patient and the health-care workers and the treatment team; (2) organizational adaptations required in the treatment context of the mental health-care facility; (3) the relationship between the mental health facility and the ethnic communities; and (4) the relationship between the mental health-care system, other facilities and society at large [53]. According to De Jong [53], this model is designed to negotiate the barriers mentioned above and increase the usage of the health-care services.

8.5 Social Support Interventions

Guruge et al. [43] underlined the need for social support interventions, programmes and services for immigrant women to improve their mental health and well-being. In this review Guruge et al. [43] also revealed the need to develop practice and policy mechanisms to address the social support needs of immigrant women. According to Dennis et al. [37], one important way to improve social support for immigrant women is to meet their informational needs. As mentioned by George and Chaze [54], both informal and formal sources of support can play a crucial role in meeting these needs. As reported in several studies, most of the stress faced by immigrants in the settlement period is caused by financial uncertainties, and formal and informal sources of support can play an important role in helping immigrants to build social networks that can facilitate finding employment [17] and managing the stressful processes. MacDonnell et al. [55] pointed out that it is also important to advocate for supportive work environment and fair wage as well as social inclusion of immigrants into the larger society.

In particular, services could be made more accessible through means such as providing cultural competency which is at the heart of good clinical practice. It is as relevant to majority of mental health practitioners dealing with minority patients as it is for minority dealing with majority patients. Cultural competence involves professional values which must include sensitivity, non-discrimination and responsiveness to the psychiatric needs of any patient [11]. There are different models available for cultural competency training, and these should be regularly used and also evaluated and properly adjusted if necessary. Cultural competency is 'everyone's business', and in order to provide services which are adequate for immigrant patients and their families, mental health practitioners must take the lead in terms of both receiving cultural competence training and putting it into practice [11]. Cultural competence is a multi-faceted skill. It is essential that a thorough evaluation of cultural competence training and cost-benefit analysis of the method be carried out in varying settings. This will enable the professionals to learn how many resources can be saved and how much better patient engagement is. An exploration of idioms of distress, explanatory models and the use of other therapies such as complementary and alternative medicine can then be used to improve and provide efficient and efficacious services for minority groups [11].

Additionally, mental health practitioners must also encourage the creation, funding and evaluation of programmes for newcomers to reduce isolation and facilitate the social inclusion. These programmes should also increase immigrant women's awareness of, and knowledge about, the social, psychological and physical correlates of mental health and illness [43]. Furthermore, policies and programmes are needed to provide culturally safe support and intersectoral collaboration to provide appropriate and timely informational, financial, emotional, instrumental and appraisal support for immigrant women. Alvi et al. [56] and Guruge et al. [57] underlined that it is also important to ensure that service responses are appropriate through evaluative research. According to Guruge et al. [43], researchers need to continue to evaluate the relationships between social support, social conflict and mental health among immigrant women and to introduce health interventions to ensure that the needs of this population are being addressed effectively.

8.6 Perceived Social Support

Drogendijk et al. [58] and Haber et al. [59] reported that perceived social support is a term encompassing a variety of characteristics of an individual's social world and the relationship between the individual and the social environment. Social support could be defined as those social interactions that provide individuals, and embed them into, a network of social relationships perceived to be caring and readily available in times of need. According to Hobfoll [60], the role of perceived social support has been examined in post-traumatic responses following traumatic events. Brewin and Holmes [61] pointed out that the subjective perception of social support is an influential factor in recovery. Studies undertaken after disasters have shown that social support has a stress-buffering effect for post-traumatic problems [62, 63]. Additionally, in different studies, perceived lack of social support systems and perceived lack of sharing of emotions have been found to be risk factors for post-disaster mental health disorders [64, 65]. Matsumoto [66] underlined that with regard to non-Western ethnic minorities, two rather contrasting phenomena are existing. On the one hand, certain groups of non-Western ethnic minorities are considered to live in collectivistic communities, and in these communities 'the self' is defined as part of a larger group such as the family [67, 68]. In collectivistic societies, providing social support is more of a compelling duty than a free and voluntary act it is expected. Their members sacrifice their personal interests to benefit the collective, for example, the extended family, so that affected members of these communities are likely to receive more social support after disasters or in case of illness than affected Western persons, especially in the long term [67, 69]. It is well known that in collectivistic societies gender has an impact on social support. Often, males receive more social support because of their gender. However, Salinero-Fort et al. [70] pointed out that the proportion of the global perception of social support among immigrants and natives was 79.2% and 94.2%, respectively. The lack of global social support showed a significant association with being male among others. For the dimensions of lack of social support, the higher association was being an immigrant and suffering stress. Norris and Alegria [71] reported that disaster victims who were members of ethnic minority groups in Western countries received less emotional support than their affected counterparts who were members of ethnic majority groups. Furthermore, Norris et al. [72] and Dirkzwager et al. [73] found that empirical studies have shown that they were indeed more at risk than Western person of developing mental health problems (such as post-traumatic stress disorder (PTSD)) after disasters in the short, intermediate and long term [74]. Kaniasty and Norris [75] underlined that the lack of social support in the long term is a consequence of mental health problems following a disaster. They highlighted as a result of more disaster-related problems faced by affected ethnic minorities that they are less likely to receive social support than affected natives.

In a study [76] it was reported that men had significantly higher health-related quality of life compared to women. The findings demonstrated that being married in both genders and lower age in men were significantly associated with higher level of perceived social support. Obviously, gender plays a role in perceived social support.

8.7 Social Exclusion, Stigma and Discrimination

Other risk factors, e.g. social exclusion, stigma and discrimination, can affect the mental health of immigrants too. In this line, Cantor-Graee and Selten [77] put forward the hypotheses of chronic experience of social defeat related to poor mental health and risk of psychosis in immigrants. Bhui et al. [78], Küey [52] and Lederbogen et al. [79] pointed out that stigma and social exclusion commonly affect a person's recovery process as well as opportunities for societal participation. Küey [52] underlined that stigmatization and discrimination which are often faced by the immigrants in the host country are also emphasized as strong influencing factors of the mental health consequences of migration. Racist assaults, whether physical or verbal, constitute a breeding ground for fear, uncertainty and mistrust and, in particular, can lead to the reactivation of previously experienced traumatic events; in turn, this can lead to the exacerbation of mental health symptoms and disorders. An extensive body of literature shows that perceived discrimination is associated with health problems, including depressive symptoms [80], psychiatric disorders [78, 81–84] and general poor self-rated health [85]. Studies found that perceived discrimination is associated with underutilization of care in general [86, 87], medical care delays and non-adherence to treatment [88, 89], pharmacy prescription delays and medical tests delays [90, 91] or substituting alternative health care to conventional health care [92]. It is easily understandable that there is an association between perceived discrimination within health-care settings and underutilization in situations where patients avoid disagreeable medical encounters. One explanation might be, e.g. that women are more likely to experience traumatic events in the course of their lives. Women's stronger tendency to develop PTSD may also be related to the fact that the types of traumas to which they are more frequently exposed (e.g. sexual assault and rape) are socially stigmatized, and so they do not therefore receive sufficient social support [93]. Ideologies, which consider the family unit as sacred and do not approve of interference with domestic violence because it is regarded as an aspect of 'family privacy', also contribute to women being deprived of adequate support and to higher rates of trauma-related problems. Lamkaddem et al. [94] reported that the relation between perceived discrimination outside health-care settings and underutilization of health care is less easy to explain, because studies focussing on underlying mechanisms are scarce. According to Lamkaddem et al. [94], some answers were formulated, for which empirical testing lacks until now. Burgess et al. [87] found evidence for an independent effect of perceived discrimination outside health-care settings on health-care underutilization. The authors suggested that experiences of perceived discrimination outside health-care settings might lead individuals to avoid dominant culture institutions. According to the authors [87], these include the health-care system, in which discrimination might occur as well. Perez et al. [95] could find that there is an association between perceived discrimination outside health-care settings and perceived quality of care, so that perceived impaired quality of care is able to affect utilization of health care. Lamkaddem et al. [94] discussed that the effect of perceived discrimination outside health-care settings on health-care utilization would therefore be mediated by perceived quality of care. Consequently, perceived discrimination may also have impact on health-care-seeking behaviour. Bazargan et al. [92] pointed out that discrimination feelings are strongly related to alternative health-care use. For example, immigrants of Turkish and Moroccan origin also report high levels of perceived discrimination in The Netherlands [96]. According to Lamkaddem et al. [94], in The Netherlands, it is common for some immigrant groups to spend holidays in the countries of origin. According to a Dutch report [97], on health and well-being of elderly immigrants, 63% of the Turkish elderly who spent a holiday in the country of origin also visited a health-care provider there (42% for the Moroccan group). Lamkaddem et al. [94] could not find any studies examining the effect of perceived discrimination on the use of health care in the country of origin. The authors [94] studied perceived discrimination in relation to health-care utilization within the Turkish and Moroccan groups in The Netherlands. They found that perceived discrimination outside health-care settings influences the non-attendance of ethnic minorities to the GP. Additionally, they pointed out that a lasting discrimination feeling is related to a persistent non-attendance to the GP among ethnic minorities in the longitudinal perspective [94]. Furthermore, the authors found that the use of health care in the country of origin is not a substitution to the health care in the host country and that the implication in the context of the Dutch gatekeeping system is that GP non-attendance might jeopardize health of the concerned groups, seen the little alternatives for GP care. According to the authors [94], it might also put unnecessary pressure on emergency care.

8.8 Influence of Acculturation Strategies

Numerous studies investigated the associations between acculturation strategies and various health-related outcomes [98]. Berry developed the conceptual framework of acculturation strategies, which contains four types of attitudes/strategies 'integration, assimilation, separation and marginalization' that individuals may adopt when encountering foreign cultural environments [98]. The associations between these strategies and mental health are moderated by the characteristics of the cultural groups and the host societies. In multicultural societies the integration strategy is usually inversely associated with mental ill health, while the marginalization strategy has a positive association with mental ill health. According to Berry [99] and Ward [100], the assimilation and separation strategies usually have less predictive power. In numerous studies it was found that poor social support, economic difficulties, female gender, unemployment, poor sociocultural adaptation, adverse life events after arrival and premigration traumatic episodes are associated with mental ill health [101–103]. Furthermore, a high level of perceived ethnic discrimination has also been shown to predict mental illness among immigrants [104]. Most of these studies have been based on small non-representative samples of fairly recently arrived refugees originating from a single country. Tinghög et al. [105] examined whether the immigrants' acculturation strategies are independently associated with mental ill health when adjusting for traumatic episodes. Several factors were schematically divided into three groups: (1) nonimmigrant-specific risk factors of persistent character (e.g. unfavourable socioeconomic situation); (2) nonimmigrant-specific risk factors of sudden and traumatic character (e.g. specific types of traumatic episodes, number of traumatic episodes experienced); and (3) immigrant-specific risk factors (e.g. ethnic discrimination, poor sociocultural adaptation) [105].

It is well known that in the field of cross-cultural psychiatry and anthropology, the ways of expressing and perceiving mental distress vary between cultures [106]. It is also known that culture plays an important role in the symptom presentation of distress and illness and, moreover, that cultural factors have quite an impact on the diagnostic process and the treatment strategies in all populations [7]. The main aim of the study of Tinghög et al. [105] was to investigate how nonimmigrant-specific factors (i.e. traumatic episodes, level of education, economic situation, marital status, status incongruence, employment status) and certain immigrant-specific factors (i.e. perceived ethnic discrimination, sociocultural adaptation, acculturation strategies) were associated with mental ill health among immigrants. Their second objective was to test whether these potential risk factors added up could satisfactorily explain the supposed difference in mental health status between people originating from Iran and Iraq in comparison to Finns. These three immigrant groups are all quite large in Sweden [105]. The authors found that unemployment, being a woman, low level of sociocultural adaptation, poor economic situation, being divorced/widow/widower and a high number of types of traumatic episode were associated with mental ill health. These findings were in accordance with previous research on refugees/immigrants [101–103]. They found also that a high level of commitment to the separation strategy was directly associated with symptom levels of depression/

anxiety. Adjustment made for traumatic experiences was a new finding. The authors could not find that commitment level to an integration or assimilation strategy was associated with mental ill health. Additionally, Tinghög et al. [105] pointed out that the risk factors detected were the same regardless of whether mental ill health was considered in terms of low subjective well-being or a high symptom level. The authors underlined that the suggestion that traumatic premigration experiences, in combination with strains in exile, elevate the risk for poor mental health, which has been advocated elsewhere [101, 107], was not supported in their study. They could not find a significant interaction effects between number of types of trauma and immigrant- or persistent nonimmigrant-specific factors.

Beyond all these facts, Butler et al. [22] highlighted that individual psychological resources, social support, a successful acculturation processes, cultural variations and time since relocation are identified as statistically significant protective factors against the development of common mental disorders among immigrants. Butler et al. [22] found new enlightening points including the significant impact of varying patterns of psychological distress, which is the most adverse for common mental disorder [22].

In this line, van Bergen, van Balkom, Smit and Saharso [108] investigated the origins of suicidal behaviour among female immigrants. In a case file study, in at least half of the cases, Turkish, South Asian and Moroccan women experienced specific stressful life events related to their family honour. In life story interviews with South Asian-Surinamese, Turkish and Moroccan immigrant young women who had attempted suicide, suicidal behaviour was influenced by the ability and right to act autonomously with regard to strategic life choices (e.g. choice of spouse, decision to file for a divorce, enrolment in education), as well as by the questioning of cultural values of self-sacrifice and protection of honour.

8.9 Mental Health in Refugee, Asylum Seeker and Immigrant Patients

Migration is one of the risk factors for developing mental disorders, in particular, that traumatized immigrants may face psychological distress. They have been exposed to adverse conditions before, during and after migration [6, 7, 12, 22]. In all these steps of migration, immigrants may have been exposed to deprivation, persecution, violence, imprisonment and human rights violation, including sexual harassment and even torture [7, 12]. According to Bourque et al. [109], data from studies on risk for psychosis showed that stress factors in the post-migratory stage overall have more impact on mental health than those in the premigratory stage [109]. Other authors reported [110–113] that the loss of loved ones/caregivers and/or livelihood, the destruction of property, deprivation, persecution, insecure living conditions, war, torture, imprisonment, terrorist attacks, abuse and sexualized violence are traumatic experiences of refugees and asylum seekers. The decision to flee is followed by the journey itself, which in the case of people arriving to Europe can last several years [114]. The flight generally includes travel by land and sea under harrowing conditions, extensive physical and psychological stress experience frequently leading to a number of health consequences [115]. Refugees experience bodily injuries and illness, mostly related to the travel and housing conditions along the way, but also frequent psychological trauma. Once they reach their destination, acute physical concerns are treated, yet psychological issues are frequently ignored due to logistic and capacity limitations [116–118].

Gender-specific reasons for fleeing were primarily expressed by women from Afghanistan and Somalia, who most frequently mentioned fear of forced marriage and honour killings. Women of all countries of origin expressed fear of sexual violence as reason for fleeing, yet fear of genital mutilation was mentioned by 10% of the women from Somalia [119]. This somewhat low number compared to the widely spread practice of female genital mutilation (FGM) in the region [120, 121] is surprising. In the study of Jesuthasan et al. [119] due to either social acceptance or resignation, 12% of the women reported sexual contacts as minors. This might reflect a high incidence of child marriages but could also include experiences of sexual coercion. The clear distinction between these two phenomena was beyond the scope of the study yet warrants further exploration especially in consideration of its relevance to self-perception. In fact, having had sexual contacts as a minor negatively correlated with self-satisfaction in the study sample. The negative impact of non-consensual sexual actions, especially in minors, on self-respect and self-image has been described before and could be at the root of the observations [122].

According to Heeren et al. [123], experiences, e.g. defencelessness and disorientation, conditions of cold or heat, hunger and thirst, lack of medical care, robbery, assault and discrimination, during the process of flight are often. Furthermore, many women may be subjected to different kinds of sexual assaults and violations [124, 125].

According to Jesuthasan et al. [119], the interviewed female refugees subjectively defined their quality of life of as average; however, different patterns in different domains emerged. Satisfaction with personal relationships was elevated, pointing at the role of social support and social cohesion as important factors for well-being [126]. Women with lower educational status appeared slightly less affected, yet the overall perception was predominantly negative. This might directly associate with the conditions of scarcity and overcrowding experienced by the women, as well as the lack of privacy and comfort due to shelter conditions in the wake of the 2015 mass migration to Germany. Next to the direct dissatisfaction with current housing conditions, the apprehension of being unable to secure a private apartment for one's family in the short and medium term might increase this disappointment. However, housing problems also represent a tangible issue amenable of potential solutions and might have been mentioned more frequently than other relevant problems, which cannot be solved directly, e.g. end of the conflict in their home country or family reunion.

Lindert et al. [127] highlighted that the rate of mental disorders was twice as high among refugees than among economic immigrants in Europe. While 44% of the refugees and asylum seekers suffered from depression, 40% suffered from anxiety disorders and 36% from PTSD. Gerritsen et al. [128] found that among refugees and asylum seekers, 56% suffered from depression, 56% from anxiety disorders and 21% from PTSD. Other studies reported that the rate of PTSD among asylum seekers and refugees as being ten times higher than in the general population [129, 130]. Additionally, Frommberger et al. [131] pointed out that especially in chronic cases, refugees and asylum seekers who suffer from PTSD also develop other illnesses. It was emphasized that seven out of ten people suffering from PTSD also suffer from another psychiatric disorder, e.g. anxiety disorders, depression, somatization disorders and addiction. Several studies have the focus on the psychiatric morbidity among different types of immigrants in different countries. Priebe et al. [132] published in a report for WHO that in general, the rates of psychotic, mood and substance use disorders in groups of refugees and asylum seekers appear similar to those found in host countries. Additionally, they found that post-traumatic stress disorder (PTSD) is more common in refugees and asylum seekers [132].

Heeren et al. [133] underlined in a Swiss study that illegal immigrants, asylum seekers and refugees had higher psychiatric morbidity compared with native groups and that about half of the asylum seekers and refugees fulfilled PTSD criteria [134]. In a systematic review and meta-analysis, Steel et al. [115] pointed out that an average for PTSD in refugees and asylum seekers was between 13% and 25%. Hassan et al. [134] underlined that some forcibly displaced people are at particularly higher risk for mental disorders: women in female-headed households; adolescents; the elderly; those lacking documentation; persons with disabilities or pre-existing health or mental health issues; survivors of various forms of violence; and those in extreme poverty [134]. Similarly, to Heeren et al. [123], and unlike to Laban et al. [135], Winkler et al. [136] found no significant relationship between the other mental illnesses and the length of stay. Obviously, this is because their samples had a relatively short stay in Germany.

8.10 Case Study: Prevention Has No Colour 2.0 Bologna (Italy)

Prevention has no colour 2.0 is a project started in 2012 in the metropolitan area of Bologna (Italy), and it promotes social inclusion, with a strong focus on women and their communities. The aim of the project is to spread among foreign communities the culture of oncological prevention, in particular of breast and cervix cancer. The logic behind the intervention is to create opportunities of encounter to meet women and their families and to explain the importance of participating to Pap test and mammography national campaigns. The applicant organization, Pace Adesso Peace Now (an ONLUS founded in 2000), works in partnership with the National Health Department (AUSL-IRCCS Bologna). One relevant action is to understand, through focus groups, the representations of illness and cancer in different cultures, in order to be more effective in spreading the message on the importance of oncological prevention. Furthermore, extensive work in this field has shown that migrants face most of the difficulties once on the hosting country, which can impact their mental health hindering their possibility to integrate in the local society if not addressed in due time. Given Italy's strategic and central position in European politics concerning the reception of refugees and migrants, this project represents a valuable and fundamental action that needs to be implemented.

Since 2015 the partnership with the National Health Department has been enforced through the collaboration with the Mutual Self Help Group (Department of Mental Health and Pathological Addictions, Local Health Authority) and the Bologna Transcultural Psychosomatic Team (BoTPT)—Department of Medical and Surgical Sciences (DIMEC), University of Bologna.

The BoTPT is a multidisciplinary study and research centre of the Department of Medical and Surgical Sciences—University of Bologna. The team provides consultations in partnership with the Department of Mental Health of Bologna designed to identify the mental and psychosocial needs of migrants and to direct them to appropriate services. The consultation includes psychiatrists, researchers, psychologists, medical doctors, students, psychiatrists, registrars and medical anthropologists, and if needed, a cultural mediator joins the team [137]. In addition, the BoTPT delivers training and support activities to informal carers, general practitioners, psychiatrists and mental health operators, social workers, medical students and psychiatric trainees. Training is specially directed to social and voluntary workers working with asylum seekers and traumatized immigrants [138–140].

The intent of this joint work is to answer the needs of migrants through an approach that is respectful and mindful of their different cultural backgrounds. An important point of this work is the presence of linguistic mediation, necessarily not only to translate the languages but also to mediate the different vision and codes, behind the own culture.

The team has created groups of discussion for refugees and asylum seekers led by professionals from different disciplines (social operators, counsellors, psychotherapists and psychiatrist). This initiative intends to offer to professionals the opportunity to understand how to taunt in on the life histories of migrants while, at the same time, giving them tools to help them to recover their balance and come to terms with their traumatic life experiences.

Narration is the most effective tool that migrants possess; it is an instrument to give a sense to their past and to overcome the dimension of fatalism and impotence that often afflicts them. The experience of asylum seekers and refugees, often characterized by shocking events such as wars, violence, abuses and natural disasters, deeply impacts the migratory process, which is no longer perceived as a free choice but as a life-saving necessity.

The possibility to talk about their own life and share it with other migrants and professionals represents a valuable approach to contextualize and socialize one's own experience. Starting from a proverb or a philosophical consideration, the participants had the opportunity to engage with and think critically about taken for granted aspects of their own cultural background and compare it with those of the other participants. This activity allows to solicit a more creative and assertive way of thinking, helping the person to overcome the negative experience and regain the capacity to hope and plan for a better future.

For professionals, listening to the stories of migration is an important step to enforce their cultural skills. Furthermore, the experience of listening in a group setting helps to solicit dynamics of mirroring and existential comparison. On the level of the therapeutic relationship, a professional has the opportunity to learn the importance of the 'stay of proceeding' (*epoché* by Edmund Husserl [141]) and to acquire a different vision of life, with different cultural concepts, in order to develop respect and the empathy.

8.11 Conclusion

According to Laban et al. [102], post-migration factors have a high impact on the development of psychiatric disorders. Social exclusion and social defeat seam to play an important role in causing mental disorders among migrants, particularly among women, since they are more often passive migrants, migrated for family reunion purpose, bordered into the household to care children and without access to work and social activities.

Furthermore, it is well known that social support, social conflicts, social exclusion, a lack of familiarity with rights, entitlements, gaps in health literacy and direct and indirect discrimination are risk factors for poor mental health outcomes. Individual psychological resources, social support, a successful acculturation processes, cultural variations and time since relocation are identified as statistically significant protective factors against the development of common mental disorders among immigrants, men and women.

According to Laban and Dijk [135], quantitative epidemiological studies still dominate. Little anthropological research with qualitative methodologies and an 'experience-near' approach has been conducted [13]. This approch could be more successful in understanding mental and physical illness causation among migrant women, as well as the use of nonbiomedical health care, health-seeking behaviour, cultural identity and mental health, and patient-therapist interaction, which are some of the more relevant factors that influence physical and mental health promotion and care among migrants, especially those migrant groups less integrated in the host society, as migrant women very often are. Further research in these fields is urgently needed.

References

1. https://www.un.org/esa/population/publications/ReplMig.
2. https://ec.europa.eu/eurostat/statistics-explained/index.php?title=Migration_and_migrant_population_statistics.
3. UN. International migration report 2017. New York, NY: United Nations; 2017.
4. Hannigan A, et al. How do variations in the definitions of 'migrant' and their application influence the access of migrants to health care services? Geneva: WHO; 2016.
5. Tobias M. Social rank: a risk factor whose time has come? Lancet. 2017;389:1172.
6. Gonzales RG, Brant K. Analysis: DACA boosts young immigrants' well-being, mental health. NBC News, June 15, 2017. https://www.nbcnews.com/news/latino/analysis-daca-boosts-young-immigrants-well-being-mental-health-n772431.

7. Bhugra D, Gupta S, Bhui K, Craig T, Dogra N, Ingleby JD, et al. WPA guidance on mental health and mental health care in migrants. World Psychiatry. 2011;10(1):2–10.
8. Bhugra D, Gupta S, Schouler-Ocak M, Graef-Calliess I, Deakin NA, Qureshi A, Dales J, Moussaoui D, Kastrup M, Tarricone I, Till A, Bassi M, Carta M. EPA Guidance mental health care of migrants. Eur Psychiatry. 2014;29(2):107–15.
9. Eisenbruch M. From post-traumatic stress disorder to cultural bereavement: diagnosis of Southeast Asian refugees. Soc Sci Med. 1991;33:673–80.
10. Heinz A, Deserno L, Reininghaus U. Urbanicity, social adversity and psychosis. World Psychiatry. 2013;12(3):187–97.
11. Schouler-Ocak M, Graef-Calliess IT, Tarricone I, Qureshi A, Kastrup M, Bhugra D. EPA guidance on cultural competence training. Eur Psychiatry. 2015;30(3):431–40.
12. Bhugra D. Migration and mental health. Acta Psychiatr Scand. 2004;109(4):243–58.
13. Guruge S, Collins E. Working with women: issues and strategies for mental health professionals. Toronto, ON: Centre for addiction and mental health (CAMH); 2008.
14. Reitmanova S, Gustafson DL. 'They can't understand it': maternity healthcare needs of immigrant Muslim women in St. John's, New foundland. Matern Child Health J. 2008;12:101.
15. Guruge S, Humphreys J. Barriers affecting access to and use of formal social supports among abused immigrant women. Can J Nurs Res. 2009;41:64–84.
16. O'Mahony JM, Donnelly TT. How does gender influence immigrant and refugee women's postpartum depression help-seeking experiences? J Psychiatr Ment Health Nurs. 2013;20:714–25.
17. Sword W, Watt S, Krueger P. Postpartum health, service needs, and access to care experiences of immigrant and Canadian-born women. J Obstet Gynecol Neonatal Nurs. 2006;35:717–27.
18. Tang TN, Oatley K, Toner BB. Impact of life events and difficulties on the mental health of Chinese immigrant women. J Immigr Minor Health. 2007;9:281–90.
19. Puyat JH. Is the influence of social support on mental health the same for immigrants and non-immigrants? J Immigr Minor Health. 2013;15:598–605.
20. Sethi B. Newcomers health in Brantford and the counties of Brant, Haldimand and Norfolk: perspectives of newcomers and service providers. J Immigr Minor Health. 2013;15:925–31.
21. Tilden VP, Galyen RD. Cost and conflict the darker side of social support. W J Nurs Res. 1987;9:9–18.
22. Butler M, Warfa N, Khatib Y, Bhui K. Migration and common mental disorder: an improvement in mental health over time? Int Rev Psychiatry. 2015;27(1):51–63.
23. Dennis C-L, Ross LE, Grigoriadis S. Psychosocial and psychological interventions for treating antenatal depression. Cochrane Database Syst Rev. 2007;3
24. Mechakra-Tahiri S, Zunzunegui MV. Self-rated health and postnatal depressive symptoms among immigrant mothers in Québec. Women Health. 2007;45:1–17.
25. O'Mahony JM, Donnelly TT, Este D, et al. Using critical ethnography to explore issues among immigrant and refugee women seeking help for postpartum depression. Issues Ment Health Nurs. 2012a;33:735–42.
26. O'Mahony JM, Donnelly TT, Bouchal SR, et al. Barriers and facilitators of social supports for immigrant and refugee women coping with postpartum depression. Adv Nurs Sci. 2012b;35:E42–56.
27. Stewart DE, Gagnon AJ, Merry LA, et al. Risk factors and health profiles of recent migrant women who experienced violence associated with pregnancy. J Womens Health. 2012;21:1100–6.
28. Ahmed A, Stewart DE, Teng L, et al. Experiences of immigrant new mothers with symptoms of depression. Arch Womens Ment Health. 2008;11:295–303.
29. Zelkowitz P, Schinazi J, Katofsky L, et al. Factors associated with depression in pregnant immigrant women. Transcult Psychiatry. 2004;41:445–64.
30. Logsdon CM, Birkimer JC, Simpson T, et al. Postpartum depression and social support in adolescents. J Obstet Gynecol Neonatal Nurs. 2005;34:46–54.
31. Dennis CL, Ross LE. Depressive symptomology in the immediate postnatal period. Can J Psychiatry. 2006a;51:265–73.

32. Dennis C-L, Ross LE. Women's perceptions of partner support and conflict in the development of postpartum depressive symptoms. J Adv Nurs. 2006b;56:588–99.
33. Stewart DE, Gagnon A, Saucier J-F, et al. Postpartum depression symptoms in newcomers. Can J Psychiatry. 2008;53:121–4.
34. Zelkowitz P, Saucier J-F, Wong T, et al. Stability and hange in depressive symptoms from pregnancy to two months postpartum in childbearing immigrant women. Arch Womens Ment Health. 2008;11:1–11.
35. Coker AL, Smith PH, Thompson MP, et al. Social support protects against the negative effects of partner violence on mental health. J Womens Health Gender Based Med. 2002;11:465–76.
36. Gibney S, McGovern M. Social support networks and mental health: evidences from share. J Epidemiol Community Health. 2011;65:1–431.
37. Dennis C-L, Hodnett E, Reisman M, et al. Effect of peer support on prevention of postnatal depression among high risk women: multisite randomized controlled trial. Br Med J. 2009;338:a3064.
38. Miszkurka M, Goulet L, Zunzunegui MV. Immigrant status, antenatal depressive symptoms, and frequency and source of violence: what's the relationship? Arch Womens Ment Health. 2012;15:387–96.
39. Whitley R, Green S. Psychosocial stressors and buffers affecting black women in Montreal. Can J Commun Ment Health. 2008;27:37–48.
40. Rechel IB, Mladovsky P, Ingleby D, Mackenbach JP, McKee M. Migration and health in an increasingly diverse Europe. Lancet. 2013;381:1235–45.
41. Schouler-Ocak M, Kastrup MC. Refugees and asylum seekers in Europe. Die Psychiatrie. 2015;12:241–6.
42. Mladovsky P, Ingleby D, McKee M, Rechel B. Responding to diversity: an exploratory study of migrant health policies in Europe. Health Policy. 2012;105:1–9.
43. Guruge S, Thomson MS, George U, Chaze F. Social support, social conflict, and immigrant women's mental health in a Canadian context: a scoping review. J Psychiatr Ment Health Nurs. 2015;22(9):655–67.
44. Donnelly TT, Hwang JJ, Este D, et al. If I was going to kill myself, I wouldn't be calling you. I am asking for help: challenges influencing immigrant and refugee women's mental health. Issues Ment Health Nurs. 2011;32:279–90.
45. Chiu L, Ganesan S, Clark N, et al. Spirituality and treatment choices by South and East Asian women with serious mental illness. Transcult Psychiatry. 2005;42:630–56.
46. Stewart M, Shizha E, Makwarimba E, et al. Challenges and barriers to services for immigrant seniors in Canada: 'you are among others but you feel alone'. Int J Migr Health Soc Care. 2011;7:16–32.
47. Lai DWL, Surood S. Predictors of depression in aging South Asian Canadians. J Cross Cult Gerontol. 2008;23:57–75.
48. DWL L, Surood S. Types and factor structure of barriers to utilization of health services among aging South Asians in Calgary, Canada. Can J Aging. 2010;29:249–58.
49. Taylor LE, Taylor-Henley S, Doan L. Older immigrants: language competencies and mental health. Can J Commun Ment Health. 2005;24:23–33.
50. Tseng W-S. A clinician's guide to cultural psychiatry. London: Academic Press; 2003.
51. Ryder AG, Alden LE, Paulhus DL. Is acculturation unidimensional or bidimensional? A head-to-head comparison in the prediction of personality, self-identity, and adjustment. J Pers Soc Psychol. 2000;79:49–65.
52. Küey L. Trauma and migration: the role of stigma. In: Meryam S-O, editor. Trauma and migration. New York, NY: Springer; 2015. p. 57–69.
53. De Jong JT, Van Ommeren M. Mental health services in a multicultural society: interculturalization and its quality surveillance. Transcult Psychiatry. 2005;42(3):437–56.
54. George U, Chaze F. Tell me what I need to know: South Asian Women, social capital and settlement. J Int Migr Integr. 2009;10:265–82.
55. MacDonnell JA, Dastjerdi M, Bokore N, et al. Becoming resilient: promoting the mental health and wellbeing of immigrant women in a Canadian context. Nurs Res Pract. 2012;4:1–10.

56. Alvi S, Zaidi A, Ammar N, et al. A comparative and exploratory analysis of socio-cultural factors and immigrant women's mental health in a Canadian context. J Immigr Minor Health. 2012;14:420–32.
57. Guruge S, Ford-Gilboe M, Samuel-Dennis J, et al. Rethinking social support and conflict: lessons from a study of women who have separated from abusive partners. Nurs Res Pract. 2012;12:1–10.
58. Drogendijk AN, van der Velden PG, Gersons BPR, Kleber RJ. Lack of perceived social support among immigrants after a disaster: comparative study. Br J Psychiatry. 2011;198:317–22. https://doi.org/10.1192/bjp.bp.110.077644.
59. Haber MG, Cohen JL, Lucas T, Baltes BB. The relationship between selfreported received and perceived social support: a meta-analytic review. Am J Community Psychol. 2007;39:133–44.
60. Hobfoll SE. Stress, culture, and community. The psychology and philosophy of stress. New York, NY: Plenum Press; 1998.
61. Brewin CR, Holmes EA. Psychological theories of posttraumatic stress disorder. Clin Psychol Rev. 2003;23:339–76.
62. Kaniasty K. Social support and traumatic stress. PTSD Res Quart. 2005;16:1–8.
63. Chen ACC, Keith VM, Leong KJ, Airriess C, Li W, Chung KY, et al. Hurricane Katrina: prior trauma, poverty and health among Vietnamese-American survivors. Int Nurs Rev. 2007;54:324–31.
64. Adams RE, Boscarino JA. Predictors of PTSD and delayed PTSD after disaster. The impact of exposure and psychosocial resources. J Nerv Ment Dis. 2006;194:485–93.
65. Guay S, Billette V, Marchand A. Exploring the links between posttraumatic stress disorder and social support: processes and potential research avenues. J Trauma Stress. 2006;19:327–38.
66. Matsumoto D. Mapping expressive differences around the world. The relationship between emotional display rules and individualism versus collectivism. J Cross Cult Psychol. 2008;39:55–74.
67. Bhugra D. Cultural identities and cultural congruency: a new model for evaluating mental distress in immigrants. Acta Psychiatr Scand. 2005;111:84–93.
68. Almeida J, Molnar BE, Kawachi I, Subramanian SV. Ethnicity and native status as determinants of perceived social support: testing the concept of familism. Soc Sci Med. 2009;68:1852–8.
69. Drogendijk AN, Van der Velden PG, Boeije H, Kleber RJ, Gersons BPR. 'De ramp heeft ons leven verwoest': de psychosociale weerslag van de vuurwerkramp Enschede op Turkse getroffenen. ['The disaster ruined our lives': the psychosocial impact of the Enschede Fireworks disaster on Dutch/Turkish victims.]. Med Antropol. 2005;17:217–32.
70. Salinero-Fort MÁ, del Otero-Sanz L, Martín-Madrazo C, de Burgos-Lunar C, Chico-Moraleja RM, Rodés-Soldevila B, Jiménez-García R, Gómez-Campelo P, HEALTH & MIGRATION Group. The relationship between social support and self-reported health status in immigrants: an adjusted analysis in the Madrid Cross Sectional Study. BMC Fam Pract. 2011;12:46.
71. Norris FH, Alegria M. Promoting disaster recovery in ethnic-minority individuals and communities. In: Marsella AJ, Johnson JL, Watson P, Gryczynski J, editors. Ethnocultural perspectives on disasters and trauma. foundations, issues and applications. New York, NY: Springer; 2008. p. 15–35.
72. Norris FH, Friedman MJ, Watson PJ, Byrne CM, Diaz E, Kaniasty K. 60,000 Disater victims speak: Part I. An empirical review of the empirical literature, 1981–2001. Psychiatry. 2002;3:207–39.
73. Dirkzwager AJE, Grievink L, Van der Velden PG, Yzermans CJ. Risk factors for psychological and physical health problems after a man-made disaster. Prospective study. Br J Psychiatry. 2006;189:144–9.
74. DiGrande L, Perrin MA, Thorpe LE, Thalji L, Murphy J, Wu D, et al. Posttraumatic stress symptoms, PTSD, and risk factors among lower Manhattan Residents 2–3 year after the September 11, 2001 terrorist attacks. J Trauma Stress. 2008;21:264–73.
75. Kaniasty K, Norris FH. Longitudinal linkages between perceived social support and posttraumatic stress symptoms: sequential roles of social causation and social selection. J Trauma Stress. 2008;21:274–81.

76. Jalali-Farahani S, Amiri P, Karimi M, Vahedi-Notash G, Amirshekari G, Azizi F. Perceived social support and health-related quality of life (HRQoL) in Tehranian adults: Tehran lipid and glucose study. Health Qual Life Outcomes. 2018;16(1):90.
77. Cantor-Graae E, Selten JP. Schizophrenia and migration: a meta-analysis and review. Am J Psychiatry. 2005;162(1):12–24.
78. Bhui K, Stansfeld S, McKenzie K, et al. Racial/ethnic discrimination and common mental disorders among workers: findings from the EMPIRIC Study of ethnic minority groups in the United Kingdom. Am J Public Health. 2005;95:496–501.
79. Lederbogen F, et al. City living and urban upbringing affect neural social stress processing in humans. Nature. 2011;474:498–501.
80. van Dijk TK, Agyemang C, de Wit M, Hosper K. The relationship between perceived discrimination and depressive symptoms among young Turkish-Dutch and Moroccan-Dutch. Eur J Public Health. 2011;21:477–83.
81. Noh S, Kaspar V. Perceived discrimination and depression: moderating effects of coping, acculturation, and ethnic support. Am J Public Health. 2003;93:232–8.
82. Veling W, Selten JP, Susser E, et al. Discrimination and the incidence of psychotic disorders among ethnic minorities in The Netherlands. Int J Epidemiol. 2007;3:761–8.
83. Veling W, Susser E, van Os J, et al. Ethnic density of neighborhoods and incidence of psychotic disorders among immigrants. Am J Psychiatry. 2008;165:66–73.
84. Williams DR, Neighbors HW, Jackson JS. Racial/ethnic discrimination and health: findings from community studies. Am J Public Health. 2003;93:200–8.
85. Harris R, Tobias M, Jeffreys M, et al. Racism and health: the relationship between experience of racial discrimination and health in New Zealand. Soc Sci Med. 2006;63:1428–41.
86. Borrell C, Muntaner C, Gil-Gonzalez D, et al. Perceived discrimination and health by gender, social class, and country of birth in a Southern European country. Prev Med. 2010;50:86–92.
87. Burgess DJ, Ding Y, Hargreaves M, et al. The association between perceived discrimination and underutilization of needed medical and mental health care in a multi-ethnic community sample. J Health Care Poor Underserved. 2008;19:894–911.
88. Casagrande SS, Gary TL, LaVeist TA, et al. Perceived discrimination and adherence to medical care in a racially integrated community. J Gen Intern Med. 2007;22:389–95.
89. Thrasher AD, Earp JA, Golin CE, et al. Discrimination, distrust, and racial/ethnic disparities in antiretroviral therapy adherence among a national sample of HIV-infected patients. J Acquir Immune Defic Syndr. 2008;9:84–93.
90. Mouton CP, Carter-Nolan PL, Makambi KH, et al. Impact of perceived racial discrimination on health screening in black women. J Health Care Poor Underserved. 2010;21:287–300.
91. Van Houtven CH, Voils CI, Oddone EZ, et al. Perceived discrimination and reported delay of pharmacy prescriptions and medical tests. J Gen Intern Med. 2005;20:578–83.
92. Bazargan M, Norris K, Bazargan-Hejazi S, et al. Alternative healthcare use in the under-served population. Ethn Dis. 2005;15:531–9.
93. Nolen-Hoeksema S. Abnormal psychology. New York, NY: McGraw-Hill; 2011.
94. Lamkaddem M, Essink-Bot M-L, Devillé W, Foets M, Stronks K. Perceived discrimination outside health care settings and health care utilization of Turkish and Moroccan GP patients in The Netherlands. Eur J Public Health. 2012;22(4):473–8.
95. Perez D, Sribney WM, Rodriguez MA. Perceived discrimination and self-reported quality of care among Latinos in the United States. J Gen Intern Med. 2009;24(Suppl 3):548–54.
96. Netherlands Institute for Social Research. Disciminatiemonitor niet-westerse allochtonen opde arbeidsmarkt. The Hague: Netherlands Institute of Social Research (SCP); 2007.
97. Institute for Social Research. Gezondheid en welzijn van allochtone ouderen. The Hague: Netherlands Institute for Social Research (SCP); 2004.
98. Berry JW, Sam D. Acculturation and adaptation. In: Berry JW, Segall MH, Kagitcibasi C, editors. Handbook of cross-cultural psychology, Social behavior and applications, vol. 3. Boston, MA: Allyn and Bacon; 1997.
99. Berry JW. Acculturation and health: theory and research. In: Kazarian SS, Evans DR, editors. Cultural clinical psychology: theory, research and practice. Oxford; New York, NY: Oxford University Press; 1998.

100. Ward C. Acculturation. In: Landis D, Bhagat R, editors. Handbook of intercultural training. 2nd ed. Thousand Oaks, CA: Sage Publications; 1996.
101. Knipscheer JW, Kleber RJ. The relative contribution of post-traumatic and acculturative stress to subjective mental health among Bosnian refugees. J Clin Psychol. 2006;62:339–53.
102. Laban CJ, Gernaat HBPE, Komproe IH, Schreuders GA, De Jong JTVM. Impact of a long asylum procedure on the prevalence of psychiatric disorders in Iraqi asylum seekers in the Netherlands. J Nerv Ment Dis. 2004;192:843–52.
103. Schweitzer R, Melville F, Steel Z, Lacherez P. Trauma, post-migration living difficulties and social support as predictors of psychological adjustment in resettled Sudanese refugees. Aust N Z J Psychiatry. 2006;40:179–87.
104. Noh S, Beiser M, Kaspar V, Hou F, Rummens J. Perceived racial discrimination, depression and coping: a study of Southeast Asian refugees in Canada. J Health Soc Behav. 1999;40:193–207.
105. Tinghög P, Al-Saffar S, Castensen J, Nordenfelt L. The association of immigrant- and non-immigrant specific factors with mental ill health among immigrants in Sweden. Int J Soc Psychiatry. 2010;56(1):74–93.
106. Good B, Kleinman A. Culture and depression: studies in the anthropology and cross-cultural psychiatry of affect and disorder. Berkeley, CA: University of California Press; 1985.
107. Silove D, Sinnerbrink I, Field A, Manicavasagar V, Steel Z. Anxiety, depression and PTSD in asylum seekers: associations with pre-migration trauma and post-migration stressors. Br J Psychiatry. 1997;170:351–7.
108. Van Bergen DD, van Balkom AJ, Smit JH, Saharso S. "I felt so hurt and lonely": suicidal behaviour in South Asian – Surinamese, Turkish, and Moroccan women in Netherlands. Transcult Psychiatry. 2012;49(1):69–86.
109. Bourque F, van der Ven E, Malla A. A meta-analysis of the risk for psychotic disorders among first- and second-generation immigrants. Psychol Med. 2011;41(5):897–910.
110. Rasmussen A, Nguyen L, Wilkinson J, Raghavan S, Vundla S, Miller KE, et al. Rates and impact of trauma and current stressors among Darfuri refugees in eastern Chad. Am J Orthopsychiatry. 2010;80(2):227–36.
111. Neuner F, Schauer M, Karunakara U, Klaschik C, Robert C, Elbert T. Psychological trauma and evidence for enhanced vulnerability for posttraumatic stress disorder through previous trauma among West Nile refugees. Biomed Central Soc. 2004;4:34–40.
112. Roberts B, Browne J. A systematic review of factors influencing the psychological health of conflict-affected populations in low- and middle-income countries. Glob Public Health. 2011;6(8):814–29.
113. Mazur VM, Chahraoui K, Bissler L. [Psychopathology of asylum seekers in Europe, trauma and defensive functioning]. [Article in French]. Encéphale 2015;41(3):221–228.
114. UNHCR. Global trends. Forced displacement in 2016.
115. Steel Z, Chey T, Silove D, Marnane C, Bryant RA, van Ommeren M. Association of torture and other potentially traumatic events with mental health outcomes among populations exposed to mass conflict and displacement: a systematic review and meta-analysis. JAMA. 2009;302(5):537–49.
116. Zimmerman C, Kiss L, Hossain M. Migration and health: a framework for 21st century policy-making. PLoS Med. 2011;8(5):e1001034.
117. Bozorgmehr K, Razum O. Refugees in Germany—untenable restrictions to health care. Lancet. 2016;388(10058):2351–2.
118. Doocy S, Lyles E, Akhu-Zaheya L, Burton A, Burnham G. Health service access and utilization among Syrian refugees in Jordan. Int J Equity Health. 2016;15(1):108.
119. Jesuthasan J, Sönmez E, Abels I, Kurmeyer C, et al. Near-death experiences, attacks by family members and absence of health care in their home countries affect the quality of life of refugee women in Germany – a multi-region cross-sectional gender-sensitive study. BMC Med. 2018;16:15.
120. Squires A, Aiken LH, van den Heede K, Sermeus W, Bruyneel L, Lindqvist R, Schoonhoven L, Stromseng I, Busse R, Brzostek T, et al. A systematic survey instrument translation process for multi-country, comparative health workforce studies. Int J Nurs Stud. 2013;50(2):264–73.

121. Schmidt S, Muhlan H, Power M. The EUROHIS-QOL 8-item index: psychometric results of a cross-cultural field study. Eur J Public Health. 2006;16(4):420–8.
122. Mitike G, Deressa W. Prevalence and associated factors of female genital mutilation among Somali refugees in eastern Ethiopia: a cross-sectional study. BMC Public Health. 2009;9:264.
123. Heeren M, Mueller J, Ehlert U, Schnyder U, Copiery N, Maier T. Mental health of asylum seekers: a cross-sectional study of psychiatric disorders. BMC Psychiatry. 2012;12:114.
124. Arcel L, Kastrup M. War, women and health. NORA. 2004;12:40–7.
125. Helweg-Larsen K, Kastrup MC. Consequences of collective violence with particular focus on the gender perspective--secondary publication. Dan Med Bull. 2007;54(2):155–6.
126. Female Refugees in Germany: Language, Education and Employment. 2017. http://www.bamf.de/SharedDocs/Anlagen/EN/Publikationen/Kurzanalysen/kurzanalyse7_gefluchetete-frauen.pdf;jsessionid=B2ACC1BBA55118115EF063972A25AF77.2_cid359?__blob=publicationFile. Accessed 11 Jan 2018.
127. Lindert J, Ehrenstein OS, Priebe S, Mielck A, Brähler E. Depression and anxiety in labour migrants and refugees. Soc Sci Med. 2009;69:246–57.
128. Gerritsen AAM, Bramsen I, Devillé W, Van Willigen LHM, Hovens JE, Van der Ploeg HM. Use of health care services by Afghan, Iranian, and Somali refugees and asylum seekers living in The Netherlands. Eur J Public Health. 2006;16(4):394–9.
129. Fazel M, Wheeler J, Danesh J. Prevalence of serious mental disorder in 7000 refugees resettled in western countries: a systematic review. Lancet. 2005;365(9467):1309–14.
130. Crumlish N, O'Rouke K. A systematic review of treatments for post-traumatic stress disorder among refugees and asylum-seekers. J Nerv Ment Dis. 2010;198(4):237–51.
131. Frommberger U, Angenendt J, Berger M. Posttraumatische Belastungsstörung – eine diagnostische und therapeutische Herausforderung. Deutsches Ärzteblatt. 2014;11(5):59–66.
132. Priebe S, Giacco D, El-Nagib R. Public health aspects of mental health among migrants and refugees: a review of the evidence on mental health care for refugees, asylum seekers and irregular migrants in the WHO European Region. Copenhagen: WHO Regional Office for Europe; 2016. (Health Evidence Network (HEN) Synthesis Report 47).
133. Heeren M, Wittmann L, Ehlert U, Schnyder U, Maier T, Müller J. Psychopathology and resident status - comparing asylum seekers, refugees, illegal migrants, labor migrants, and residents. Compr Psychiatry. 2014;55(4):818–25.
134. Hassan G, Ventevogel P, Jefee-Bahloul H, Barkil-Oteo A, Kirmayer LJ. Mental health and psychosocial wellbeing of Syrians affected by armed conflict. Epidemiol Psychiatr Sci. 2016;25(2):129–41.
135. Laban CJ, van Dijk R. Main topics in transcultural psychiatric research in the Netherlands during the past decade. Transcult Psychiatry. 2013;50(6):792–816.
136. Winkler JG, Brandl EJ, Bretz HJ, Heinz A, Schouler-Ocak M. [The influence of residence status on psychiatric symptom load of asylum seekers in Germany]. [Article in German; Abstract available in German from the publisher]. Psychiatr Prax. 2019;46(4):191–9.
137. Tarricone I, Atti AR, Braca M, Pompei G, Morri M, Poggi F, et al. Migrants referring to the Bologna Transcultural Psychiatric Team: reasons for drop-out. Int J Soc Psychiatry. 2011;57(6):627–30.
138. Tarricone I, Atti AR, Salvatori F, Braca M, Ferrari S, Malmusi D, Berardi D. Psychotic symptoms and general health in a socially disadvantaged migrant community in Bologna. Int J Soc Psychiatry. 2009;55(3):203–13.
139. Tarricone I, Mimmi S, Paparelli A, Rossi E, Mori E, Panigada S, Carchia G, Bandieri V, Michetti R, Minenna G, Boydell J, Morgan C, Berardi D. First-episode psychosis at the West Bologna Community Mental Health Centre: results of an 8-year prospective study. Psychol Med. 2012;42(11):2255–64.
140. Braca M, Berardi D, Mencacci E, Murri MB, Mimmi S, Allegri F, et al. Understanding psychopathology in migrants: a mixed categorical-dimensional approach. Int J Soc Psychiatry. 2014;60(3):243–53.
141. Husserl E. Introduction to transcendental phenomenology. Translation of lecture delivered at the Sorbonne, Feb. 23 and 25, 1929. Sackville, NB: Atcost Press; 2003. https://www.mta.ca/uploadedFiles/Community/Bios/Cyril_Welch/Husserl.pdf.

For Media, "Women's Health" Often Stands for "Beauty"

9

Roberta Villa

> **Key Points**
> - Media often address health communication to women, but contents are mainly focused on wellness and on the impact of health issues on physical appearance.
> - Great attention is given to a low body weight as proxy of health, much more than when addressing men.
> - Another main subject is breast cancer, but also in this case, written and visual communication highlights positive outcomes, while it overlooks negative or controversial issues.
> - The objective is to catch the public's eye, reassuring.
> - The current crisis of traditional media is supposed to worsen the trend of identifying women's health with beauty.

In most cultures, women are supposed to have a pivotal *role* as wives, mothers or adult daughters in performing *health*-related activities for *family* members. Despite a growing gender equality in housework, women are still often the main responsible for grocery shopping and cooking, planning doctor visits and check-ups, taking care of ill members and so on, in most families, even in developed countries.

Women are also well known for being very interested in issues related to health and wellbeing. They are therefore favourite **targets of health information, communication and promotion** on media outlets: so, by addressing women, they can get more audience/readers/views for media and more targeted information for advertisers. Health issues of any kind, even if not strictly related to women's health, are consequently much more common in women's magazines and TV shows than in general outlets (Table 9.1).

R. Villa (✉)
Università Ca' Foscari, Venezia, Italy
e-mail: robertaida.villa@unive.it

I. Tarricone, A. Riecher-Rössler (eds.), *Health and Gender*,
https://doi.org/10.1007/978-3-030-15038-9_9

Table 9.1 Interest in scientific news by gender, age and education (% of US adults interested in each science news topic)

	Health and medicine	Food and nutrition	Technology	Energy and environment	Mind and brain	Space and astronomy	Evolution
US adults %	70	61	57	50	50	40	26
Men	62	50	69	54	45	50	28
Women	78	71	45	47	54	30	25

Modified from "Science news and information today" survey, by Pew Research Center. USA, 2017

When looking at messages directly targeted to women themselves, anyway, a peculiarity stands out: most issues concern their maternal role (pregnancy or childcare) or have some esthetical implications, reflecting old-fashioned gender identities, when the main interest of women was being attractive, in order to get married and to give his husband nice, healthy and strong children. This approach tends to be still prevalent in media and advertising, even if in real life this attitude is overcome, at least partially, by nowadays culture, in which women can be fulfilled, even without kids and despite their physical appearance.

Research performed on health communication focused to women is scarce: a PubMed search by relevance performed in October 2017, with "women" + "media" + "health" as entries, shows that **most studies concerning health information are somehow related to beauty and physical appearance**. Among the first 40 papers found, excluding papers related to very local experiences, only one regards the communication on magazines about elective caesarean delivery [1], one is about skin cancer early detection [2], and another is a mass media campaign to raise women's awareness of the link between alcohol and cancer [3].

9.1 Breast Cancer

The only other health relevant issue not directly related to appearance is **breast cancer**, as emerged by a study on cancer and the media published on the *Archives of Internal Medicine* in 2010 [4]. After analysing 436 articles, among 2228 related to cancer and published in 2 years by 15 main US magazines and newspapers, authors showed that breast cancer is overall the favourite cancer subject by printed media in the USA.

Communication on breast cancer, anyway, is often incorrect: it is usually presented as a disease more frequent in young women than it is, an optimistic view about its prognosis is offered, and the advantages of screening and early diagnosis are emphasised.

A more recent analysis of breast cancer coverage in magazine advertisement showed that "while ads offered minimal informative content about the disease or about ways by which sales will contribute to the breast cancer cause, they integrated 'breast cancer appeals', such as the colour pink, the pink ribbon, and mostly positive depictions of survivorship and hope, into the ads. Breast cancer thus took centre stage in the persuasive content of the ads, but a back seat when it came to their informative content" [5].

For instance, in this wide communication effort about breast cancer and the importance of screening and early diagnosis by mammography, little room is dedicated to explain the risks of overdiagnosis [6], which is a difficult, but an essential, point for women to understand.

On the same subject, a Canadian study shows that articles on breast cancer in fashion magazines are usually illustrated by smiling young, Caucasian, attractive women with intact breasts [7]. Authors compared content, tone and themes in about 90 images related to 30 articles in 6 Canadian women's and fashion magazines published between 2005 and 2010. About half of the articles had both positive and negative tones, while almost 88% of women in the photos had positive facial expressions. Eight out of ten portrayed women were Caucasian and young; more than 90% had a healthy body type, and all of them appeared attractive and with intact breasts (100%). Both screening and treatment were seldom represented in pictures (5.5%) as well as rare was a visual impact of the disease or of the treatment on the body of a woman, who cannot therefore imagine how she will look after surgery (4.4%). While the articles focused on medical issues, images were mainly about beauty or fashion, potentially misleading women.

These divergent messages, which can have great impact on breast cancer education, depend on the media's need to catch the eye of the reader, which is easier with beautiful, young breast than with surgery scars. But it also reflects the idea of women' role that keeps being prevalent in our society: a role strictly related to maternity and beauty.

9.2 Body Weight

Most other studies focusing on women's health in media therefore reflect the favourite topics targeted to women: health as a means to pursue wellness and beauty.

In this scenario, the greatest focus is given to body weight, considered as the main health indicator for women.

A content analysis performed by researchers from Ohio University examined about 5000 magazine pages published in top-selling US women's health and fitness magazines in 2010. Body shaping and weight loss contributed to roughly one-fifth of all editorial content in these magazines, being a major issue in them. In these articles, the findings show an overemphasis on appearance over health and on exercise over caloric reduction and the combination of both behaviours, going so against public health recommendations [8].

Actually, obesity and overweight are undoubtedly very serious risk factor for many common chronic diseases (cancer, diabetes, hypertension, cardiovascular diseases) [9]. Perception of healthy weight, though, is not always consistent with attractiveness, which is often associated with lower than healthy body mass index, especially in women [10]. One cannot find the same insistence on weight when talking about men, whose belly is often regarded with a smile.

On the other hand, many other modifiable risk factors depending on lifestyles are not less relevant than body weight. For instance, smoking, which was once more common in men, is now changing the epidemiology of lung cancer, which used to be very rare in women, while now its incidence is skyscraping among them.

Nevertheless, when talking to women, media never focus on risk of death or other severe diseases caused by cigarettes, as they do with men. They rather tend to mention aesthetic or relational consequences, such as yellow fingers, old-looking skin or bad smell of smokers, as if the main objective of a woman should still always be being pleasant to others. This is not the case for men, whose health seems to be a value in itself.

9.3 The Media Revolution

In the last years, information about health, more than being searched on Google, has been delivered directly to people, mainly by new social media. Belonging to Facebook groups or following opinion leaders on Twitter or other platforms, women, as well as men, are daily overwhelmed by waves of correct and incorrect contents about risks and/or recommendations about their health: exams that should be done, supplements that should be taken, weird diets to follow and so on.

The current crisis of mainstream media risks worsening all of this. In order to catch more attention by the public, health and wellbeing contents are increasingly merging, with the second often overwhelming the first.

The main victims of this communication strategy, aimed at conquering a larger audience, could end up to be women, ideal target of an aggressive health guerrilla marketing and more and more often convinced that they need to be beautiful much more than healthy.

References

1. Campo-Engelstein L, Howland LE, Parker WM, Burcher P. Scheduling the stork: media portrayals of women's and physicians' reasons for elective cesarean delivery. Birth. 2015;42:181–8.
2. Basch CH, Ethan D, Hillyer GC, Berdnik A. Skin cancer prevention coverage in popular US women's health and fitness magazines: an analysis of advertisements and articles. Global J Health Sci. 2014;6:42–8.
3. Dixon HG, Pratt IS, Scully ML, Miller JR, Patterson C, Hood R, Slevin TJ. Using a mass media campaign to raise women's awareness of the link between alcohol and cancer: cross-sectional pre-intervention and post-intervention evaluation surveys. BMJ Open. 2015;5:e006511.
4. Fishman J, Ten Have T, Casarett D. Cancer and the Media. How does the news report on treatment and outcomes? Arch Intern Med. 2010;170:515–8.
5. AbiGhannam N, Chilek LA, Koh EE. Three pink decades: breast cancer coverage in magazine advertisements. Health Commun. 2017;2:1–7.
6. Overdiagnosis implies that, in order to save one single life, many more women are diagnosed with breast cancer and consequently treated, without any impact on their life expectancy.

7. McWhirter JE, Hoffman-Goetz L, Clarke JN. Can you see what they are saying? Breast cancer images and text in Canadian women's and fashion magazines. J Cancer Educ. 2012;27:383–91.
8. Willis LE, Knobloch-Westerwick S. Weighing women down: messages on weight loss and body shaping in editorial content in popular women's health and fitness magazines. Health Commun. 2014;29:323–31.
9. World Health Organization. Obesity and overweight factsheet. Geneva: WHO; 2018. http://www.who.int/mediacentre/factsheets/fs311/en/.
10. Brierley ME, Brooks KR, Mond J, Stevenson RJ, Stephen ID. The body and the beautiful: health, attractiveness and body composition in men's and women's bodies. PLoS One. 2016;11:e0156722.

Suggested Reading

Gamble TK, Gamble M. Gender communication and health. In: The gender communication connection. New York, NY: Routledge; 2014.
Liuccio M. Gender, health, and communication. J Comm Healthcare. 2015;8:5–6.
Wakefield MA, Loken B, Hornik RC. Use of mass media campaigns to change health behavior. Lancet. 2010;376:1261–71.
Zaman F, Underwood C. The gender guide for health communication programs. Baltimore, MD: Johns Hopkins Bloomberg School of Public Health/Center for Communication Programs; 2003.

Health and Gender in Movies

10

Barbara Tarricone

Key Points

- Gender and disease in movies
- Portrayal of the sick person in Hollywood films
- Mental illness and blockbusters
- Bias toward sick women in mainstream films
- The female body in mainstream films

A widely spread saying in Hollywood goes that portraying a mentally or physically disabled person bears more chances for an Oscar nomination that any other role, and it is true that 16% of the Oscar winners between 1927 and 2012 were in fact for performances that involved disease or disability.[1] But what's that portrayal like in relation to the gender of the sick person? Is it unbiased or is it different based on sex? Without any pretense of being exhaustive of such a massive subject, I would like to offer an overview of what seems to be the main recurrent themes in Oscar-winning movies and blockbusters centered around a disease or a disability. I will, in short, focus on some of the pictures that contribute the most to shape our collective image of what disease and disability look like in men and women. All of the following considerations need to be placed in a wider context: movies with female leads (healthy or otherwise) are overall significantly less than movies with male main characters. The Center for the Study of Women in Television and Film found in fact that women led only 29% of the top 100 grossing films of 2016.[2] With that in mind, we will see

[1] http://www.bbc.com/news/entertainment-arts-16932374.

[2] http://www.digitalspy.com/movies/news/a821818/females-leading-roles-in-hollywood-reach-all-time-high-still-only-29-percent/.

B. Tarricone (✉)
Sky TV, Milan, Italy
barbara.tarricone.cons@sky.it

I. Tarricone, A. Riecher-Rössler (eds.), *Health and Gender*,
https://doi.org/10.1007/978-3-030-15038-9_10

how Hollywood differs in portraying sick men and women and, with the exception of the mentally ill, does not chose to represent sick women as strong leads.

The most important words in the English language are not "I love you" but "It's benign." So quipped Harry Block, Woody Allen in his 1997 Academy Award-nominated movie "Deconstructing Harry"—certainly the pervasiveness of cancer in our society has made it into a favorite subject for movies so much as to constitute its own genre: the so-called cancer movies. From "Love Story" (1970, six Oscar nominations and one win) to "The Fault in our Stars" (2014, 307 million dollars grossed at the box office), to "Terms of Endearment" (1983, five Oscars including best picture, best actress, and best actor), to "P.S. I Love You" (2007, 156 million dollars grossed at the box office), to "The Bucket List" (2007, 157 million dollars grossed at the box office), the intrusion of cancer in the life of a couple, or the doomed lovers, and the renewed zest for life infused by the knowledge that a terminal disease is cutting time short are all favorites in movies. Most likely shying away from the more realistic aspects of the disease to romanticize it, cancer is a guaranteed tear-jerker and box office draw. It's worth noticing how the emphasis on the vulnerability of the oncological patient is placed especially on the woman, beautifully lit and dying, while stoic and courageous traits are more likely connected to the sick man. In "P.S. I Love You," for example, the terminally ill and extremely romantic Gerard Butler won't cave in to despair; instead he will write ten love letters to support his wife after his death. In "The Bucket List," the equally terminally ill but more rampant Jack Nicholson and Morgan Freeman will escape the hospital to go on a road trip together to fully savor life.

Heroics are also Tom Hanks and Matthew McConaughey in the AIDS themed and based on true events "Philadelphia" (1993, two Academy Awards) and "The Dallas Buyers Club" (2014, three Oscars). The fight against all odds in the wake of a huge blow (Hanks as an unjustly fired HIV-positive gay lawyer suing his colossal law firm and receiving compensation on his death bed, McConaughey as a HIV-positive straight cowboy tricking big pharma) granted each of the two actors an Oscar. Philadelphia is also widely recognized for having brought to the forefront HIV and AIDS in 1993, the apex of the contagion, humanizing the disease and possibly helping antidemonize the homosexual community. Based in 1985, "The Dallas Buyers Club" gained its three Oscars in 2013.

The year before and the year after the Academy Awards paid tribute to two movies that deal with similar conditions: "Amour" (best foreign film in 2012) and "Still Alice" (best actress for Julianne Moore in 2014). In both movies a woman is affected by a degenerative disease. In "Amour" it's a stroke that impairs the cognitive and motive skills of the wife of an elderly couple (wonderful Emmanuel Riva and Jean Louis Trintignant). In "Still Alice" the character portrayed by Julianne Moore is affected by Alzheimer with an early onset shaking the foundations of her marriage and family life. It seems to me how these cases once more underline how Hollywood seems more at ease with having women passively affected by a disabling condition, leaving it to the men to be the fighters or the unlikely heroes.

Let's take a look at some of the many movies that deal with yet again extraordinary men (not women) that despite a severely handicapping condition were able to be successful in their careers and/or lead an exemplary life. "My Left Foot: The Story of Christy Brown" is a 1989 biographical drama that brought an Academy Award for Best Actor to Daniel Day Lewis for portraying the life of a man born with cerebral palsy and only able to use his left foot. The "Theory of Everything" is a 2014 intimate portrayal of Stephen Hawking's life beyond his contributions to theoretical physics. Stephen Hawking (portrayed by Eddie Redmayne, that won an Oscar for the role) is affected by ALS and, the movie seems to tell us, braved the courage to face his disease, thanks to his bond with his (now ex) wife Jane. This, of the unwavering supporting role of women, seems to be somewhat of a recurring theme. The recent "Breathe" (starring Andrew Garfield and Claire Foy) tells us the story of Robin Cavendish, who became paralyzed from the neck down by polio at age 28 but didn't give up on life (and moved on to become a pioneer for the severely disabled), mainly thanks to the unwavering support and love of his wife. "The Diving Bell and the Butterfly" is inspired by the true story of Elle editor Jean Dominique Bauby, who is affected by locked-in syndrome after a stroke. His body cannot move, and his mind cannot sit still; the results are four Oscar nominations that, once again, conspire to let us be comfortable with a disabled man whose mind is undefeated. Pedro Almodovar, on the other hand, centered his 2002 Oscar-winning "Talk to Her" around two comatose women. But their presence is, in the film only that of beautiful still lives, objects of desire for the men that took care of them.

While we still have to see a blockbuster movie that has a physically disabled or diseased female character as a strong lead, taking a look at films that deal with mental illness, we seem to appreciate a more unbiased representation. In 2010 we watched two entirely fictional movies with two main characters affected by what we can conclude to be schizophrenia: a man, Leonardo DiCaprio in "Shutter Island," and a woman, Natalie Portman (who won an Oscar for the part) for "The Black Swan." They're equally strong leads, fascinating and center of the action. In 1988 we sympathized with Dustin Hoffman stealing the scene to Tom Cruise in his Oscar-winning performance as an autistic man in "Rain Man." It is the role for a sociopathic woman in the 1999 "Girl, Interrupted" that brought Angelina Jolie her only Oscar. The Academy Awards applauded the performance of murderous Charlize Theron as real-life serial killer Aileen Wuornos in the 2003 drama "Monster" as it did with Anthony Hopkins cannibal and serial killer in the 1991 thriller "Silence of the Lambs" or with murderous Kathy Bates in the 1990 "Misery." Leaving it to a different place to judge whether these movies are accurate representation of mental disease, I would like to underline here what it seems to be a preference in Hollywood movies: to portray mentally ill people, regardless of their sex, as strong leads, positive or negative, succumbing to their conditions or overcoming it, in all cases actively carrying the action throughout the movie. The same as we saw cannot be said for physically disabled or diseased women.

Why is this form of representation so biased is up for discussion. My opinion is that our cinematographic mass culture is not yet able to disassociate vulnerability and passiveness with sick women and conversely is not comfortable with men being vulnerable and passive carriers of disease. And why does this not hold true for mentally ill women? I think it stems from how Hollywood choses to look at the female body. That culture has still a very strong taboo in watching an unattractive (under conventional standards) female lead that is not a villain. The female body needs to be young and healthy or else can be left fading in the background. A mentally ill woman can still be seen as attractive, but a physically ill woman cannot. A man can be paralyzed from the neck down and the audience will focus on his dreams and on his mind, but the same cannot yet happen, in movies, to a woman: under the same circumstances, the focus will still remain on her body.

Suggested Reading

Altenloh E. A sociology of the cinema; the audience (1914). Screen. 2001;42(3):249–93.

Barron L. An actress compelled to act: Angelina Jolie's "Notes from My Travels" as celebrity activists/travel narrative. Postcolon Stud. 2009;12(2):221–8.

Beauchamp C. Without lying down. Frances Marion and the powerful women of hollywood. Berkeley, CA: University of California Press; 1997.

Galbiati G. La pazza gioia:cinema, donne e malattia mentale, magazine3D.it. 2017.

Haskell M. From reverence to rape The treatment of women in the movies. Chicago, IL: The University of Chicago Press; 1987.

Kassenbrock R. 9 Oscar nominated movies that got disease and disability (almost right). 2015. Themighty.com.

Montini F. 'Cancer movies', quando la malattia è protagonista del film, Repubblica.it. 2016.

Pradavelli V. Le donne del cinema, Dive, registe, spettatrici. Bari: Editori Laterza; 2014.

Tramonte M, Stagnitta S. Cinema, psicologia, psicoanalisi e sofferenza mentale:Rassegna filmografica, funzionegamma.it.

Women in Music: The Case of Italian Opera

11

Giuseppina La Face

Key Points

- Art music in the Western tradition can express feelings and depict moods and psychic processes. Musical works of art can stage conflicts and passions which, although belonging to the past, still affect our lives today.
- Of all musical genres, opera displays the power to plastically represent the countless aspects of the passions, through definite, perceivable forms. In this way it functions as a kind of deep-reaching, albeit unconscious, "school of feelings."
- Within a well-organized formal structure, a soprano aria like that of Elvira in Verdi's *Ernani* allows women listeners to experience her anguished feelings and simultaneously observe them with the "involved" detachment afforded by a work of art.
- In his *Macbeth* Verdi has shown how far female *hybris* can push, what physical metamorphosis it can induce, and even just how powerful a woman's influence on a man can be.
- Violetta's aria in the third act of Verdi's *La traviata*, through the clarity of its form, gives a sublime musical and theatrical representation of the "loneliness of the dying."

Art music in the Western tradition, be it exclusively instrumental or associated with a verbal text, can express feelings and depict moods and psychic processes, even dysfunctional ones.[1] In this respect it can be a powerful vehicle of emotional education,

[1] In the monograph *La casa del mugnaio: ascolto e interpretazione della "Schöne Müllerin,"* Florence, Leo S. Olschki, 2013 (German edition *Das Haus des Müllers: zur Interpretation von*

G. La Face (✉)
Art Department, Alma Mater Studiorum - Bologna University, Bologna, Italy
e-mail: Giuseppina.laface@unibo.it

I. Tarricone, A. Riecher-Rössler (eds.), *Health and Gender*,
https://doi.org/10.1007/978-3-030-15038-9_11

for the young and less young, women and men.[2] But that is not all. Musical works of art, even from distant epochs, can stage conflicts and passions which, although belonging to the past, still affect our lives today: a conscious, thoughtful discussion, prepared by a guided listening of the music piece, allows to better analyze, understand, and interiorize them.[3]

In this process, a major role is played by two factors. The first is that music "presentifies" feelings and emotions, as if they were taking place before our very eyes, or even *within* us. The second is that it does this through definite, perceivable forms. Both factors allow listeners, on the one hand, to identify with the feeling represented by the sounds and, on the other hand, to become aware of it, by distancing themselves from it and observing it with detachment.

Of all musical genres, opera displays this power in the most evident way, by closely connecting word, music, and scene. The fact that opera theater has existed for four centuries and still shows no signs of decline may have to do with its ability to plastically and vividly represent the countless aspects of the passions and the infinite nuances of the psyche: this is why it played, and still plays, the role of a deep-reaching, albeit unconscious, "school of feelings."[4] Let us now look at three eloquent examples of this, drawn from operas by Giuseppe Verdi (1813–1901).

First of all, I would like to discuss *Ernani* (1844), a masterpiece which the composer, in collaboration with librettist Francesco Maria Piave, drew from the Romantic drama *Hernani ou L'honneur castillan* by Victor Hugo (1830). The plot is set in sixteenth-century Spain, an epoch as remote from Verdi as it is for us today. In this mid-nineteenth-century Italian opera, the blooming of a feeling is formalized into a structure, referred to by musicologists as *la solita forma* (the usual form), which describes the inner organization of the "numbers" that make up an opera. As a rule, the *solita forma* comprises four movements: Scena, Cantabile (or Adagio), Tempo di mezzo, and Cabaletta. In duets and trios, between the Scena and the Cantabile, a so-called Tempo d'attacco is interpolated.[5] The *solita forma* has both a

Franz Schuberts Liedzyklus "Die schöne Müllerin," Vienna, Praesens, 2013), I attempted to carry out a cross-disciplinary analysis (musicological and psychopathological) of a work of poetry and music, whose subject is the representation of a depressive process that leads to suicide.

[2] On the importance of emotional literacy, I am referring primarily to Massimo Baldacci, *La dimensione emozionale del curricolo: l'educazione affettiva razionale nella scuola*, Milan, Franco Angeli, 2008; see also *I profili emozionali dei modelli didattici: come integrare istruzione e affettività*, edited by Massimo Baldacci, Milan, Franco Angeli, 2009.

[3] I will not go into the vast psychiatric and philosophical literature on emotions, which are postulated to be universal entities having a biological basis or, according to other authors, phenomena that are co-determined by their historical and cultural context.

[4] See Lorenzo Bianconi, "La forma musicale come scuola dei sentimenti," in *Educazione musicale e formazione*, edited by Giuseppina La Face and Franco Frabboni, Milan, Franco Angeli, 2008, pp. 85–120.

[5] The expression is only found once in period sources, in a book by the initiator of Verdi criticism: Abramo Basevi, *Studio sulle opere di Verdi*, Florence, Tofani, 1859, p. 194 ("… la solita forma de' duetti, … che vuole un *tempo d'attacco*, l'*adagio*, il *tempo di mezzo*, e la *Cabaletta*,") translated by Edward Schneider and Stefano Castelvecchi: "This piece … shows that there is no loss of effect in departing from the usual form for duets, which requires a *tempo d'attacco*, an adagio, a *tempo di mezzo*, and a cabaletta," in A. Basevi, *The Operas of Verdi*, Chicago - London, University of

musical and theatrical significance: it alternates between moments when the action is carried forward and others in which it stands still, to allow for the expression of "affections," or feelings.[6]

I will now examine the entrance aria, which the female protagonist of *Ernani*, Elvira, sings when she first appears on stage. The young Castilian noblewoman, in love with an outlaw, Ernani, is waiting in anguish for the decrepit aristocrat Silva, her betrothed, in whose castle she is staying as a guest. The recited monologue of Elvira builds the Scena, the section in which we learn about the circumstances of the plot ("Surta è la notte, e Silva non ritorna … | Ah non tornasse ei più! …," Night time is here, and Silva has not yet come back. Ah, I wish he would never come back!). The singing takes off in the Cantabile, when Elvira thinks about Ernani and cries out for him as if he were physically present ("Ernani!… Ernani, involami | all'abborrito amplesso," Ernani! Take me away from the loathed embrace): here the action is suspended, and feeling prevails in a broad, passionate melodic phrase. Once the Cantabile is over, the Tempo di mezzo introduces the maids as they bring the wedding gifts of Elvira's suitor ("Quante d'Iberia giovani | te invidieran, signora!", My Lady, you will be envied by so many young Iberian women!). This new situation interrupts Elvira's train of thoughts: the meeting with Silva approaches threateningly. Elvira again pours out her soul, this time in an impetuous Cabaletta, a swift, lively movement in which she gushes her love for the outlaw ("(Tutto sprezzo che d'Ernani | non favella a questo core)" I despise everything that does not talk to my heart about Ernani). Although her feeling is private, and Elvira expresses it *to herself*, the anxiety of the reluctant bride is noticed by the maids, who also make comments aside, *a parte* ("(Sarà sposa, non amante, | se non mostra giubilar)" She does not appear to rejoice, so she will be a bride, not a lover). The Cabaletta heightens and emphasizes this tension, amplifying the force of passion and eliciting applause. The individual movements of "solita forma" are neatly sculpted here, perfectly identified and distinct in their musical character and dramatic content. The anguish that torments Elvira both in solitude and during the rituals of court life is tangible.

The story and the feeling embodied in this aria from *Ernani* through its "solita forma," although obviously set in the sixteenth-century Spain, would certainly not be out of place in the nineteenth-century Italy.[7] They apparently look very distant from our time. Yet a simple consideration is enough to modify this initial impression: even today, in many parts of the world, many women still experience a similar condition to that of Elvira—they are forced to marry a man they do not love, possibly much older, just because their family, social conventions, or traditions demand

Chicago Press, 2013, p. 167.—Harold Powers, "'La solita forma' and 'The Uses of Convention'," in *Acta Musicologica*, 59 (1987), pp. 65–90, produced evidence that Basevi's description applies to most of the pieces that make up an early nineteenth-century Italian opera.

[6] In modern English, the word "affection" describes the feeling of tenderness that connects two individuals. In the sixteenth-/seventeenth-century psychology, the same word meant "affection of the soul," an emotion or disturbance caused by a positive or negative factor: a "passion," be it sad or joyful, suffered by the individual.

[7] A memorable representation of the male obsession with bossing women around can be seen in *Lucia di Lammermoor*, by Salvadore Cammarano and Gaetano Donizetti (1835, from Walter Scott's *The Bride of Lammermoor*).

so. But even in the Western world today, it is far from uncommon for women to be subjected to pressure from their authoritarian fathers and brothers, which harm their physical and mental health. Within the well-organized structure of the "solita forma," the soprano aria in *Ernani* allows women to identify with Elvira (who becomes the emblem of so many abused human beings), to experience her feelings and simultaneously observe them with the sense of "involved" detachment produced by a work of art. And it indirectly allows men to grasp the vicious mechanisms of coercion typical of a male-dominated society.

In another masterpiece, Verdi perfectly succeeds in adapting the "solita forma" to depict a deeply upsetting female character: Lady Macbeth. Here the musician draws from a sublime model, Shakespeare's tragedy *Macbeth*. The same-titled Verdi opera was performed in 1847 in Florence and then reworked for the Paris production of 1865, with a libretto by the abovementioned Piave, which also includes substantial contributions by poet Andrea Maffei. In the Italian composer's opera, the history of the Scottish nobleman and of his spouse who, out of thirst for power, do not hesitate to murder a king, reaches appalling heights of violence and cruelty.

One example will suffice. Let us reread the first monologue of Lady Macbeth in Shakespeare (act I, scene v): it expresses all the fierceness of this arrogant character who, in her euphoria, already sees herself on the throne and plans the killing of the king, who is a guest at their castle. In a macabre hymn to the night, Lady Macbeth calls upon the spirits to deprive her of her sex ("unsex me here"), annihilate the female virtues of mercy and love in her, and fill her with terrible cruelty ("And fill me from the crown to the toe, top-full | Of direst cruelty"), thicken her blood ("Make thick my blood"), and turn the milk in her breasts into gall ("Come to my woman's breasts | And take my milk for gall"), so that she may be more successful in pushing her husband to commit murder.

It is a blood-curdling soliloquy. Verdi's libretto omits such cruel verbal imagery. The task of giving substance to this terrible character is assigned to singing, in her entrance aria (act I, scene v, number 3). This is achieved through an imperious, whiplash-like gesture in the Scena (after the reading of her husband's letter, "Nel dì della vittoria io le incontrai…," I met them on the day of victory …), which becomes even more aggressive in the Cantabile, "Vieni! t'affretta! accendere | vo' quel tuo freddo core!" (Come! Hurry up! I want to light that cold heart of yours!), and finally through the frenzied excitement and bragging virtuosity of the Cabaletta, "Or tutti sorgete, ministri infernali" (Rise ye all, infernal ministers), immediately after the Tempo di mezzo (a march that provides the soundtrack for the servant's dispatch: King Duncan is about to arrive at the castle). Tackling this impossibly demanding aria right off, with her voice still cold, is a challenge for the singer. Verdi knew it well: but he did not want a soprano with a "figura bella, buona" (who looked good, lovely), who could sing flawlessly, "alla perfezione"; he was looking for a Lady "brutta e cattiva" (ugly, evil), who would not sing, "non cantasse," "una voce aspra, soffocata, cupa" (a harsh, muffled, dull voice), which had to sound somewhat diabolical, "avesse del diabolico."[8] These words show that the musician

[8] These rather unusual demands were expressed by Verdi in a letter dated November 21, 1848, in preparation for a revival of *Macbeth* at the San Carlo Theater in Naples. In Florence, in 1847, Verdi

had fully grasped the extraordinary nature of the staged events and of the words of Shakespeare. Above all he showed to have realized how far female *hybris* can push, what physical metamorphosis it can induce, and even (this becomes evident in the rest of the opera) just how powerful a woman's influence on a man can be, enough to weave a cocoon of euphoria around him, throw him into raving madness, and, finally, lead him to annihilation.

In this case, too, the literary text and the musical work are distant from our age. But the themes of passion for power and unrestrained ambition are always relevant, and neither men nor women are immune from it. A legitimate drive to succeed should always be brought in harmony with our deep humanity. Women in particular should be aware of just how powerful their influence on the innermost feelings of men is, for good or for bad. While *Ernani* offers us a portrait of male violence, *Macbeth* visualizes a story of extreme misuse of power by a woman, which fuels the couple's delusion of grandeur and leads to the collapse of their psyche.

While the structure of "solita forma," which I have identified here in two famous arias, is one of the fundamental formal devices in Italian opera, it is not the only one. There are other models of musical form that are used for representing situations and feelings with sounds: what is never absent is, indeed, the constructive role of form. This is clearly perceivable even to untrained listeners, who, without realizing it, let themselves be carried away by it: opera theater is conceived to immediately produce a strong impression, and a distinctly recognizable form is instrumental in achieving this purpose.

My last example is drawn from one of the universally known masterpieces of Verdi, *La traviata* (1853), from the novel *La dame aux camélias* by Alexandre Dumas *fils* (1848). First let me make a short introduction. In Romantic opera, the hero or heroine usually dies. Whether it occurs in the presence of the other, dismayed characters[9] or face to face with a distraught relative,[10] the event of death generates a mournful echo in those present. In *La traviata* Violetta dies of consumption *chez soi*, in front of a few friends who have rushed to her bedside.[11] Before the end, in the third act, we witness a moment of vertiginous emotion, "Addio del passato bei sogni ridenti" (Farewell you beautiful, cheerful dreams of the past). Over a subdued "tremolo" in the strings, Violetta, alone, is reading (not singing!) the letter she has

had found an ideal performer in Marianna Barbieri Nini, who left a direct account of her rehearsals (extracts, with English parallel text, in *Verdi's Macbeth: A Sourcebook*, edited by David Rosen and Andrew Porter, Cambridge, Cambridge University Press, 1984, pp. 49–53).

[9]As is the case in *Simon Boccanegra* (1857, revised version 1881) and *Un ballo in maschera* (1859).

[10]As in *Rigoletto* (1851). An illuminating essay is in David Rosen, *How Verdi's Serious Operas End*, in *Atti del XIV Congresso della Società internazionale di Musicologia: Trasmissione e recezione delle forme di cultura musicale*, edited by Angelo Pompilio et al., Turin, EDT, 1990, III, pp. 443–450.

[11]In the nineteenth century, before the introduction of antibiotics, consumption and syphilis were incurable, fatal illnesses. From its earliest symptoms until death, consumption normally progressed over the course of 10–12 months. In the libretto of *La traviata* (by F. M. Piave), "il primo atto succede in agosto, il secondo in gennaio, il terzo in febbraio" (the first act takes place in August, the second in January, the third in February).

received from Monsieur Germont, the father of her lover ("Teneste la promessa … La disfida | ebbe luogo," You kept your promise … The duel did take place): her Alfredo will come to her, to ask for forgiveness and to be reunited with her. Throughout this short melodrama,[12] the violins whisper the love theme, which in the first act had been sung in full voice. It is as if sound turned into a memory and spoke to us softly of an endless, lost love. The woman looks at herself in the mirror and sees the pangs of illness on her face. Joy and sorrow are about to end; the grave is where we are all bound to. She then bids farewell to life in a simple form: two *couplets*,[13] or stanzas, with the same meter (six double hexasyllables plus a final hexasyllable functioning as a refrain: "Or tutto finì," It is all over now) and the same music. Both stanzas are introduced successively by the aching chant of an oboe, like an *alter ego* of the mind as it contemplates a vanished past.

Violetta thinks that she, a high-class courtesan, both desired and rejected, will receive neither flowers nor a cross. She prays God that he may accept her soul. The first couplet in each stanza has a dirge-like melody, a sort of slow waltz that livens up and expands in the third and fourth verses. Her supplication to the Lord is vibrant, urgent: "Ah della Traviata sorridi al desio; | a lei, deh perdona; tu accoglila, o Dio!" (Ah, smile at this lost woman's yearning; alas, forgive her; accept her, o God!). Eventually the singing slumps down—con "un fil di voce," in a whisper, writes Verdi—above the final refrain, "Or tutto finì!" (It is all over, now!). This look at the past, expressed in the melodrama and expanded in the aria, especially through the clarity of its form, gives us a picture of a very young person who, with clarity of mind, disillusion, and sadness, looks back at her life and prepares for imminent death. It is an existential and emotional situation which many young women still experience today, despite the impressive progress of medical science. "Addio del passato" is the sublime musical and theatrical representation of the "loneliness of the dying."[14] This is why we are moved by it even after the umpteenth listening.

In conclusion, I have presented three pieces from Verdi's theater, although I could have selected any other great composer. What I have written aims at showing how Western art music, if transmitted and understood correctly, can help us reflect on ourselves, develop our relationships ethically, and even become aware of how we relate to the crucial moments of existence. In other words, it can benefit our mental health.

---

[12] A "melodrama" is a theatrical technique, popular between the eighteenth and nineteenth century in France and Germany but rather unusual in Italy (where it was dubbed *melologo*), which combines the spoken recitation of dramatic dialogue with an orchestral accompaniment.

[13] This is the term used by Abramo Basevi in his chapter on *La traviata* in the already mentioned *Studio sulle opere di Verdi* (engl. trans. p. 196: "and there are a good number of arias that are repeated in the manner of *couplets*"), to underscore the French-like quality of this work.

[14] The phrase is drawn from the title of an essay by Norbert Elias, *Über die Einsamkeit der Sterbenden in unseren Tagen* (Frankfurt a.M., Suhrkamp, 1982; Engl. trans.: *The Loneliness of the Dying and Humana conditio*, Dublin, University College Dublin Press, 2010).

Appendix 11.1: Francesco Maria Piave—Giuseppe Verdi, *Ernani* (Venice, La Fenice, 1844)

Atto I, scena III

Ricche stanze di Elvira nel castello di Silva. È notte.

ELVIRA

Surta è la notte, e Silva non ritorna!... [Scena]
Ah non tornasse ei più!...
Questo odiato veglio,
che quale immondo spettro ognor m'insegue,
col favellar d'amore
più sempre Ernani mi configge in core.

Ernani!... Ernani, involami *Andantino piuttosto vivo* [Cantabile]
all'abborrito amplesso.
Fuggiam... Se teco vivere
mi sia d'amor concesso,
per antri e lande inospite
ti seguirà il mio piè.
Un Eden di delizia
saran quegli antri a me.

Scena IV

Detta ed Ancelle, che entrano portando ricchi doni di nozze.

ANCELLE

Quante d'Iberia giovani *Allegretto* [Tempo di mezzo]
te invidieran, signora!
Quante ambirieno il talamo
di Silva che t'adora!
Questi monili splendidi
lo sposo ti destina,
tu sembrerai regina
per gemme e per beltà.
Sposa domani in giubilo
te ognun saluterà.

ELVIRA		
M'è dolce il voto ingenuo		
che il vostro cor mi fa.		
(Tutto sprezzo che d'Ernani	***Allegro con brio***	[Cabaletta]
non favella a questo core,		
non v'ha gemma che in amore		
possa l'odio tramutar.		
Vola, o tempo, e presto reca		
di mia fuga il lieto istante;		
vola, o tempo, al core amante		
è supplizio l'indugiar.)		
ANCELLE		
(Sarà sposa, non amante,		
se non mostra giubilar.) *(partono.)*		

Appendix 11.2: Francesco Maria Piave/Andrea Maffei—Giuseppe Verdi, *Macbeth* (Florence, La Pergola, 1847)

Atto I, scena V

Atrio nel castello di Macbeth, che mette in altre stanze.

LADY MACBETH, *leggendo una lettera.*	***Allegro***	[Scena]
"Nel dì della vittoria io le incontrai…	[declamato]	
"Stupito io n'era per le udite cose,		
"quando i nunzj del Re mi salutaro		
"Sir di Caudore, vaticinio uscito		
"dalle veggenti stesse		
"che predissero un serto al capo mio.		
"Racchiudi in cor questo segreto. Addio."		
Ambizïoso spirto	[recitativo]	
tu sei, Macbetto,… alla grandezza aneli,		
ma sarai tu malvagio?		
Pien di misfatti è il calle		
della potenza, e mal per lui che il piede		
dubitoso vi pone e retrocede!		
Vieni! t'affretta! accendere	***Andantino***	[Cantabile]
vo' quel tuo freddo core!		
L'audace impresa a compiere		

io ti darò valore;
di Scozia a te promettono
le profetesse il trono…
Che tardi? accetta il dono,
ascendivi a regnar.

Scena VI

Un servo, e la precedente.

SERVO *Allegro* [Tempo di mezzo]

Al cader della sera il Re qui giunge.

LADY

Che di'? Macbetto è seco?

SERVO Ei l'accompagna.

La nuova, o donna, è certa.

LADY

Trovi accoglienza, quale un Re si merta.

Scena VII

LADY MACBETH *sola.*

Duncano sarà qui?... qui? qui la notte?...

Or tutti sorgete, — ministri infernali, *Allegro maestoso* [Cabaletta]
che al sangue incorate — spingete i mortali!
Tu notte ne avvolgi — di tènebra immota;
qual petto percota — non vegga il pugnal.

Appendix 11.3: Francesco Maria Piave—Giuseppe Verdi, *La Traviata* (Venice, La Fenice, 1853)

Atto III, scena I
Camera da letto di Violetta. Nel fondo è un letto con cortine mezzo tirate; una finestra chiusa da imposte interne; presso il letto uno sgabello su cui una bottiglia d'acqua, una tazza di cristallo, diverse medicine. A metà della scena una toilette, *vicino un canapè; più distante un altro mobile su cui arde un lume da notte, varie sedie ed altri mobili. La porta è a sinistra; di fronte v'è un caminetto con fuoco acceso.*

[…]

Scena IV

VIOLETTA *che trae dal seno una lettera e legge.*

"Teneste la promessa… La disfida	***Andantino***	[Scena: melologo]
"ebbe luogo; il barone fu ferito,		
"però migliora,… Alfredo		
"è in stranio suolo; il vostro sagrifizio		
"io stesso gli ho svelato.		
"Egli a voi tornerà pel suo perdono;		
"io pur verrò… Curatevi… mertate		
"un avvenir migliore;		
"Giorgio Germont"… È tardi!... *(desolata)*		[Scena: recitativo]
Attendo, attendo… né a me giungon mai!...		
Oh come son mutata!... *(si guarda nello specchio)*		
Ma il Dottore a sperar pure m'esorta!...		
Ah con tal morbo ogni speranza è morta!...		
Addio del passato bei sogni ridenti!...	***Andante mosso***	[Couplet 1]
le rose del volto già sono pallenti;		
l'amore d'Alfredo pur esso mi manca,		
conforto, sostegno dell'anima stanca…		
Ah della Traviata sorridi al desio;		
a lei deh perdona! tu accoglila, o Dio.		
Or tutto finì.		
Le gioie, i dolori fra poco avran fine;		[Couplet 2]
la tomba ai mortali di tutto è confine!...		
Non lacrima o fiore avrà la mia fossa,		
non croce col nome che copra quest'ossa!		
Ah della Traviata sorridi al desio,		
a lei deh perdona! tu accoglila, o Dio.		
Or tutto finì. *(siede)*		

Suggested Reading

Basevi A. *Studio sulle opere di Verdi*. Florence: Tofani; 1859. (English edition: *The Operas of Verdi*, ed. by Edward Schneider and Stefano Castelvecchi, Chicago–London: University of Chicago Press, 2013, p. 167).

Bianconi La Face G. *La casa del mugnaio: ascolto e interpretazione della "Schöne Müllerin"*. Florence: Leo S. Olschki; 2003. (German edition *Das Haus des Müllers: zur Interpretation von Franz Schuberts Liedzyklus "Die schöne Müllerin"*, Vienna: Praesens, 2013).

Bianconi L. "La forma musicale come scuola dei sentimenti." In: La Face G, Frabboni F, editors. *Educazione musicale e formazione*. Milan: Franco Angeli; 2008. p. 85–120.

Budden J. *The operas of Verdi*, 3 vols., Oxford: Oxford University Press, 1973–1981. (and subsequent editions).

Hepokoski J. A. *Genre and content in mid-century Verdi: 'Addio, del passato' ("La traviata", Act III)*. Cambridge Opera Journal. 1989;1:249–76.

Hutcheon L, Hutcheon M. *Opera: desire, disease, death*, Lincoln–London: University of Nebraska Press; 1996.

Hutcheon L, Hutcheon M. *Opera: the art of dying*. Cambridge, MA: Harvard University Press; 2004.

Kerman J. *Opera as drama*, new and revised edition. Berkeley, CA: University of California Press; 1988.

Powers H. La solita forma and The uses of convention. *Acta Musicologica*. 1987;59:65–90.

Rosen D. How Verdi's serious operas end. In: Pompilio A, et al., editors. *Atti del XIV Congresso della Società internazionale di Musicologia: Trasmissione e recezione delle forme di cultura musicale*, vol. 3. Turin: EDT; 1990. p. 443–450.

Rosen D, Porter A, editors. *Verdi's 'Macbeth': a sourcebook*. Cambridge: Cambridge University Press; 1984.

12 Sport and Gender

Franco Trevisani and Francesco Della Villa

Key Points

- Due to anatomical, physiological and hormonal differences, women are more prone to develop some exercise-related diseases, such as *musculo-skeletal*, *hormonal* and *haematological* disorders.
- The female athlete triad is a connection between *low energy availability*, *functional hypothalamic amenorrhoea* and *osteopenia/osteoporosis*. This model may explain several disorders of women practising sports at a competitive level.
- Women are more likely to suffer from knee ligament injuries, namely, *anterior cruciate ligament (ACL) injuries* and *patellofemoral pain (PFP)*, than men.
- *Iron deficiency* frequently occurs in sporting women, with a prevalence up to 50% in sporting adolescents. The main consequence of this deficiency is anaemia that adversely affects performance and quality of life.
- Preventative measures consisting in *exercise-based interventions*, *training adaptation* and *dietary optimisation* can efficiently prevent (and treat) exercise-related hormonal and haematological disorders and musculoskeletal injures in women practising sports.

12.1 Introduction: Women, Sport and Medicine

There is a rapidly mounting interest in defining the differences between male and female adaptations to physical activity and sport demands, largely because the history of women and sport is much younger than that of men. For example, the first

F. Trevisani (✉) · F. D. Villa
Department of Medical and Surgical Science, School of Sport and Physical Exercise Medicine, Alma Mater Studiorum - University of Bologna, Bologna, Italy
e-mail: franco.trevisani@unibo.it

I. Tarricone, A. Riecher-Rössler (eds.), *Health and Gender*,
https://doi.org/10.1007/978-3-030-15038-9_12

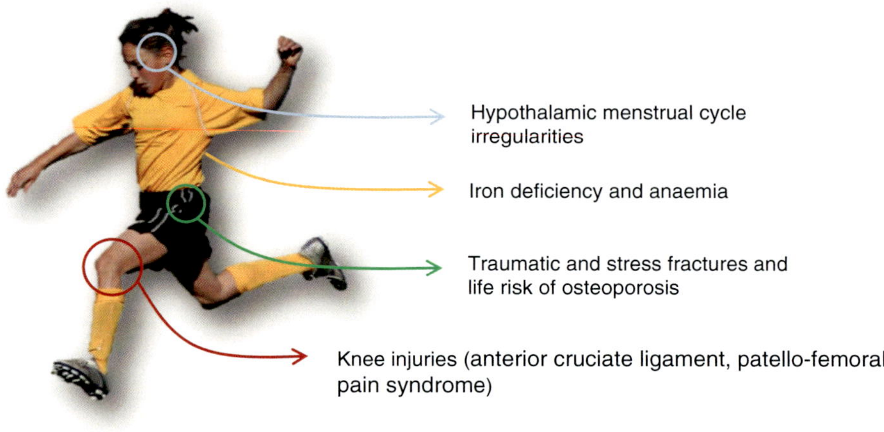

Fig. 12.1 Sport-related clinical conditions that are specific or more common in women than in men

women's Olympic marathon was held in 1984, nearly 90 years after the first modern male Olympic marathon. Therefore, studies on women's health/diseases in relation to physical activity and sport represent a relatively new branch of medicine.

The increasing number of female athletes all over the world, some of them involved in high-impact sports such as football (nearly 30 million women worldwide practise football) [1], is a strong drive to study and apply evidence-based practices to female practising sports.

Due to anatomical, physiological and hormonal differences between genders, women are more prone to develop some acute and chronic pathologic conditions related to sport demands. For instance, women have an increased likelihood of developing sport-related anaemia and of suffering from osteo-articular injuries, particularly of the legs (Fig. 12.1).

This chapter gives an overview of the most frequent sport-related disorders threatening women's health and provides information about the prevention of these conditions and the management of female athletes through their whole live.

12.2 Musculoskeletal and Ligament Injuries

Women are predisposed to certain types of sport-related musculoskeletal injuries, especially to knee-related damage. Two musculoskeletal conditions (one chronic and one acute condition) have been widely studied in female athletes. The *patellofemoral pain (PFP)* is a chronic functional disease presenting with anterior knee pain. It is caused by a dynamic malalignment of the patellofemoral joint, which is more frequent in women than in men [2]. PFP is particularly common among female runners and female athletes involved in jumping and pivoting sports (e.g. volleyball, basketball). PFP has a multifactorial origin, where quadriceps muscle function and strength, hip and core muscles strength and dysfunctional biomechanics play a role [3]. PFP is generally an exacerbating clinical condition, with multiple presentations over the years and should be addressed promptly by the sports medicine specialist. In the presence of anterior knee pain, a rapid workout aimed at excluding all potential organic causes (i.e. patellofemoral osteoarthritis, extensor apparatus osteochondritis) should be done. Thereafter, an appropriate exercise intervention has to be implemented. A recent consensus statement indicates that a programme of strength exercises involving knee and hip muscles (in combination) is the most valuable option for treatment and prevention of PFP [4].

Women participating in pivoting, cutting and jumping sports, like soccer, basketball and volleyball, are more predisposed than men to undergo acute noncontact (without direct contact of an opponent) knee ligament injuries. For instance, the risk of a lesion of the *anterior cruciate ligament* (ACL) is 2–4 times greater in female athletes compared with male athletes with the same exposure [5]. This is particularly true for teenage soccer players, in whom the reported ACL injury rate is 11.7 per 100,000 female athletes versus 4.7 for the male counterpart [6]. The ACL injury is a serious and potentially career-threatening injury and may predispose to early onset of knee osteoarthritis. Therefore, athletic and team trainers, athletes and sports medicine doctors must be aware of such a gender-related predisposition, in order to take preventative measures addressing modifiable risk factors and decreasing the likelihood of this serious lesion.

The greater risk for female athletes of sustaining an ACL injury is related to several factors. The first one relies on the inner diversity of the musculoskeletal system, especially at the lower limb, where women present with a different static alignment, wider pelvis and greater Q angle, a narrower knee intercondylar notch and smaller ligaments [7].

The second one is due to hormonal factors. Indeed, the early ovulatory phase of the menstrual cycle is associated with the greatest risk of ACL injury [8]. On this respect, Zazulack et al. documented an impact of the menstrual cycle phase on tensile properties of the ACL, likely due to an effect of oestrogens at ACL level that has specific receptors for these hormones [9].

The third, and probably most relevant factor, is the dysfunctional neuromuscular control and biomechanical profiles shown by women during complex movement patterns. Women were found to perform cutting and landing tasks with less knee flexion, greater knee valgus and higher external knee valgus moment [10–12] that are known risk factors for ACL injuries (Fig. 12.2). A possible explanation of this motion attitude relies on a greater dominance of quadriceps muscles over hamstring and gluteus muscles in women than in men [12–14]. Consequently, women rely more on the anterior muscular kinetic chain than on the posterior one. Another aspect to be taken into account may be the static alignment of women, who generally present a wider pelvis and a greater Q angle [15]. These three biomechanical patterns place the knee ligaments at a greater risk of overload and injury. In particular, teenage female athletes should be considered "at-risk" individuals, as the increase in height and mass of the growth spurt occurring in this period of life also alters the neuromuscular control while increasing the load on static structures. The best strategy to reduce the risk of ACL injuries seems to address the neuromuscular control through specific intervention. Neuromuscular training (NMT) programmes, developed since the 1990s, consist of a series of specific exercises to complete

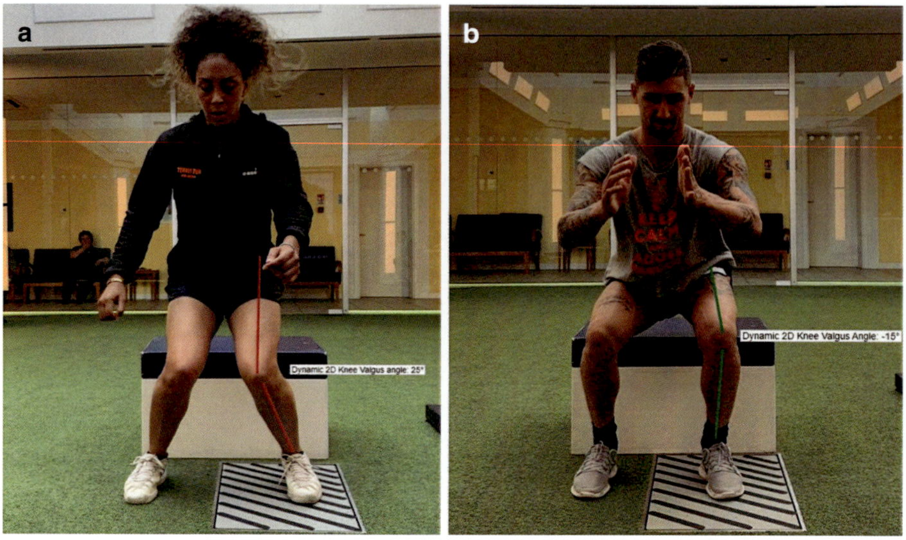
a
Dynamic 2D Knee Valgus angle: 25°
b
Dynamic 2D Knee Valgus Angle: -15°

Fig. 12.2 Different frontal plane movement profiles of a woman and a man during a double-leg drop vertical jump. (**a**) The woman shows a bilateral *dynamic knee valgus* alignment with knee in knocked position, using the static stabilisers (bones and ligaments) to absorb ground reaction forces. This motion pattern increases the risk of knee injuries and indicates a poor neuromuscular control. (**b**) The man controls very well the leg movement, with minimum frontal plane knee motion absorbing dynamic forces through the eccentric muscles contraction

during training and before competitions [16]. Prospective trials have shown the effectiveness of these programmes, leading to a pooled reduction in ACL injuries of 73% in female sports [17]. The completion of NMT programmes at least three times a week is therefore suggested to female athletes participating in high-impact sports to reduce the risk of injury.

12.3 Iron Deficiency and Anaemia

Iron deficiency (ID) and the related anaemia are frequently encountered in young female athletes. ID prevalence in the general population of menstruating women has been reported to be up to 22% [18], but in athletes, this figure is distinctly higher, reaching 52% in adolescent athletes. It is also argued that this condition may more often occur in endurance sports (distance running) and disciplines with a high prevalence of eating disorders (gymnastics, classic dance) [18, 19]. The predisposing effect to ID of physical activity has a multifactorial origin. Any type of exercise causes a transient pro-inflammatory status, and many steps of the complex iron metabolism can be affected from this condition [20]. Secondly, an intensive exertion increases hepcidin production [20], which reduces iron absorption and disrupts its transfer from macrophages to erythroblasts, thus favouring the development of the ID-induced anaemia. The higher rate of ID and anaemia in female compared to male athletes may be explained by the additional effect on iron loss of menses.

As a key component of haemoglobin (Hb), iron plays a crucial role in setting aerobic capacity and performance because of Hb being the main oxygen transporter to working muscles [21]. In addition, iron is a key component of the enzymatic system of the respiratory chain [20]. Hence, it is not surprising that ID adversely and greatly affects the performance and the training capacity of athletes.

ID can progress through three stages: non-anaemic ID (NAID) → ID with microcytosis and/or hypochromia (IDMH) → ID with anaemia (IDA). NAID indicates a condition characterised by a small reduction of iron store not affecting haematopoiesis. If a negative iron balance remains in place, the haematopoiesis will be affected, and the young red cells will become small and pale (microcytic and hypochromic anaemia), with a progressive reduction of mean cellular volume (MCV) and mean cellular haemoglobin (MCH). At this stage, serum ferritin is <30 mg/L, and when it crosses the threshold of 12 mg/L, also haemoglobin level starts to decrease, leading to the occurrence of the IDA. This ID evolution, frequently observed in female endurance athletes, must be distinguished from another condition that can occur in athletes, that is, the dilutional *pseudo-anaemia*, defined as low haematocrit and haemoglobin levels owing to an expanded plasma volume despite the presence of normal red cell mass and total haemoglobin mass. This condition is particularly frequent among high-level endurance athletes (prevalence of 10–15%) and can be easily distinguished for IDA as MCV and MCH remain within the normal range.

In order to prevent the development of ID during training, a regular check of blood parameters (haemoglobin level, MCV, MCH and ferritin) is warranted, especially in endurance female athletes.

When an ID is diagnosed, a proper workout is mandatory in order to exclude systemic causes (i.e. insufficient iron intake with the diet, malabsorption syndromes such as celiac disease, chronic blood loss from the gastrointestinal tract or metrorrhagia). When systemic conditions have been excluded, the first line of therapy for sport-related ID relies on *nutritional counselling*, including sufficient energy intake and five times/week intake of foods containing the haemoglobin-iron complex (i.e. fish and seafood) with the addition of legumes (i.e. breakfast cereals) and green vegetables. This should be combined with an oral iron supplementation (generally, 40–60 mg of elemental iron/day is appropriate). In order to increase the intestinal absorption, the physician should consider the use of enhancers (vitamin C) and suggest limiting the intake of inhibitors of iron uptake (coffee, black tea). In nonresponders or in the case of intolerance to oral therapy, intravenous iron supplementation should be considered. Athletes with persistently low iron values may benefit from a chronic oral supplementation, but caution should be payed as an iron overload can increase oxidative stress and induce secondary hemochromatosis (hemosiderosis). Therefore, long-term oral iron intake in the presence of normal ferritin values is not recommended and may be harmful [18].

12.4 Menstrual Cycle Irregularities

Another clinical problem of women practicing sports are menstrual cycle irregularities (MCI), especially during the early adolescence that can be prolonged in athletes, particularly in the presence of an eating disorder. As a theoretical pathological continuum, three distinct conditions of MCI have been correlated to sport: luteal phase defects, oligomenorrhoea and amenorrhoea.

Luteal phase defects (LPD) refer to a shortening of the luteal phase of the menstrual cycle, which is difficult to be diagnosed because the cycle remains regular and generally has a proper length (28 days). There seems to be a direct relationship between the amount of exercise and the likelihood of luteal phase defect development [22]. As already mentioned, LPD may precede other menstrual cycle irregularities and is related to a 2–4% bone loss per year in active sporting women [23].

Oligomenorrhoea (irregular menstrual cycle, with 3–6 menses per year) and *amenorrhoea* (absent menstruations or <3 cycle/year or no menses in the past 6 months) are more frequent in sport women than in the general female population. Their prevalence is indeed 10–20% in sport women compared to 5% of the general population, and it can be as high as 50% in competitive distance runners [24, 25]. The *primum movens* of these disorders would be an "energy drain" by physical exercise, leading to a negative energy balance. An increased energy expenditure due to strenuous and prolonged exertion, associated with suboptimal energy intake, stimulates compensatory mechanisms aimed at conserving the energy for vital functions [26]. This, in turn, causes a central suppression of reproductive function signals through the disruption of the hypothalamic-pituitary-ovarian axis which leads to a low-amplitude and irregular pulsatility of pituitary hormones and lowers the oestrogen and progesterone production. Moreover, the exercise-driven increase in corticotrophin releasing factor and corticotrophin inhibits the secretion of luteinizing hormone by the pituitary gland. Lastly, the exercise-driven increase in prolactin serum concentration may also be considered in the pathophysiology of MCI, although the exercise intensity must cross a certain threshold to cause an overproduction of this hormone [27]. The sport-related amenorrhoea is therefore a "hypothalamic amenorrhoea" and may be associated with other neuroendocrine disorders, such as thyroid dysfunction. A low fat mass is another factor which should be monitored to prevent the MCI occurrence, being both a potential risk factor (in thin athletes) for MCI development and a marker of chronic negative energy balance.

Infertility and abnormal bone mass loss (see the next paragraph) are potential consequences of MCI. As a matter of fact, fertility is generally reduced in competitive female athletes. The optimisation of both training intensity and energy intake, increasing the body fat content, is beneficial for these patients. Therefore, when a sporting woman presents with MCI, complete information on her clinical history, training volume and intensity and dietary intake should be collected. The patient must be carefully examined and her hormonal profile checked.

When the menstrual disorder is attributable to excessive exercise or an energetic imbalance, the first approach should rely on regaining a positive energetic balance by reducing the exercise volume and/or intensity and increasing/optimizing the dietary intake in order to recover the nutritional status [28]. The same principles of optimizing nutrition and training practices should also be adopted as a preventative measure, especially in high-risk sports such as long-distance running and ballet.

The second line of treatment, nowadays broadly utilised by athletes, is the intake of oral contraceptive pills (OCP) which can reduce both cycle irregularities and ID linked to abundant/irregular menses [29]. The prescription of this medication has to be preceded by a specific screening for cardiovascular risk factors and counselling regarding the lack of clear evidence that OCP alters performance, a frequent misconception of female athletes.

12.5 Bone Health and Osteoporosis

A correct physical exercise increases the bone mass peak and reduces the bone density loss occurring in adult and elderly people. On the contrary, an energy imbalance, due to poor nutrition and high activity output, and the consequent menstrual cycle irregularities have deleterious effects on life-long bone health, as heralded by the 4% yearly loss in bone density observed during the first 2/3 years of sport-related amenorrhoea. In order to establish a pathophysiological link between these potential problems of female athletes, the American College of Sports Medicine has proposed a triad including *low energy availability* (eating disorders and suboptimal energy intake), *hypothalamic menstrual disorder* (amenorrhoea) and *low bone mineral density* (osteopenia, osteoporosis) as interrelated factors [30] (Fig. 12.3).

The relationship between bone loss and menstrual disorders is multifactorial in nature. One cause is hypoestrogenism, but the pattern of bone remodelling in amenorrheic sporting women is atypical if compared to the postmenopausal one. Amenorrheic sporting women show *reduced* bone turnover with a reduction of bone formation [31], while postmenopausal women present with an *increased* turnover

Fig. 12.3 Female athlete pathological triad proposed by the American College of Sports Medicine

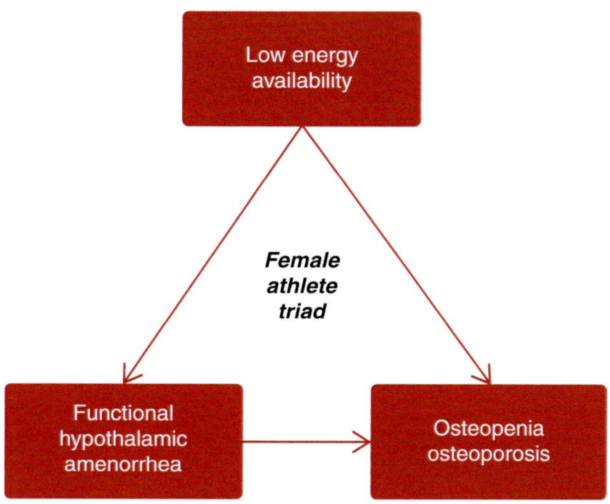

and bone resorption [32]. So, other pathogenic factors, such as a suboptimal energy intake, should be considered. Also, typical at-risk athletes, like distance runners, may have additional risk factors such as low calcium intake and greater training load [33].

Bone mass reduction in sporting women is responsible for two adverse events: (1) an increased risk of *stress fractures* during sporting or active life [34] and (2) the development of *osteoporosis* as long-term consequence.

The maintenance of the bone mass peak is crucial to prevent postmenopausal osteoporosis in former sporting women. Menstrual cycle irregularities in athletes are associated with a long-term reduction of bone mass compared with regularly menstruating athletes [35]. Proper preventative measures and treatments for the female athlete triad can annul or reduce the risk of bone mass impoverishment. Therefore, the optimisation of energy intake and expenditure, together with the intake of a well-balanced diet, should always be pursued by female athletes under the supervision of sports medicine physicians. Finally, as a low total bone mineral density (BMD) predicts stress fractures in runners [36], a pre-participation screening in female athletes at risk (i.e. long-distance runners, low-body fat athletes) may be useful to target subsequent interventions.

12.6 Conclusions

Female athletes have dysfunctional anatomical and physiological features predisposing to a number of different pathological events. The clinician should be aware of the origin and nature of these problems and should implement preventative measures consisting of exercise-based intervention, training and dietary optimisation. A proper treatment of sport-related injuries and disorders is also crucial to avoid long-term consequences.

References

1. FIFA Communication Division. FIFA big count: 270 million people active in football. 2006. http://www.fifa.com/mm/document/fifafacts/bcoffsurv/bigcount.statspackage_7024.pdf.
2. Wilson T. The measurement of patellar alignment in patellofemoral pain syndrome: are we confusing assumptions with evidence? J Orthop Sports Phys Ther. 2007;37:330–41. https://doi.org/10.2519/jospt.2007.2281.
3. Crossley KM, Stefanik JJ, Selfe J, Collins NJ, Davis IS, Powers CM, McConnell J, Vicenzino B, Bazett-Jones DM, Esculier JF, Morrissey D, Callaghan MJ. Patellofemoral pain consensus statement from the 4th International Patellofemoral Pain Research Retreat, Manchester. Part 1: Terminology, definitions, clinical examination, natural history, patellofemoral osteoarthritis and patient-reported outcome measures. Br J Sports Med. 2016;50:839–43. https://doi.org/10.1136/bjsports-2016-096384.
4. Crossley KM, van Middelkoop M, Callaghan MJ, Collins NJ, Rathleff MS, Barton CJ. Patellofemoral pain consensus statement from the 4th International Patellofemoral Pain Research Retreat, Manchester. Part 2: recommended physical interventions. Br J Sports Med. 2016;50:844–52. https://doi.org/10.1136/bjsports-2016-096268.

5. Arendt E, Dick R. Knee injury patterns among men and women in collegiate basketball and soccer. NCAA data and review of the literature. Am J Sports Med. 1995;23:694–701. https://doi.org/10.1177/036354659502300611.
6. Darrow CJ, Collins CL, Yard EE, Comstock RD. Epidemiology of severe injuries among United States high school athletes: 2005-2007. Am J Sports Med. 2009;37:1798–805. https://doi.org/10.1177/0363546509333015.
7. Laible C, Sherman OH. Risk factors and prevention strategies of non-contact anterior cruciate ligament injuries. Bull Hosp Jt Dis. 2013;72:70–5.
8. Wojtys EM, Huston LJ, Boynton MD. The effect of the menstrual cycle on anterior cruciate ligament injuries in women as determined by hormone levels. Am J Sports Med. 2002;30:182–8. https://doi.org/10.1177/03635465020300020601.
9. Zazulak BT, Paterno M, Myer GD, Hewett TE. The effects of menstrual cycle on anterior knee laxity; a systematic review. Sports Med. 2006;36:847–62. https://doi.org/10.2165/00007256-200636100-00004.
10. Malinzak RA, Colby SM, Kirkendall DT, Yu B, Garrett WE. A comparison of knee joint motion patterns between men and women in selected athletic tasks. Clin Biomech. 2001;16:438–45. https://doi.org/10.1016/S0268-0033(01)00019-5.
11. McLean SG, Neal RJ, Myers PT, Walters MR. Knee joint kinematics during the sidestep cutting maneuver: potential for injury in women. Med Sci Sports Exerc. 1999;31:959–68. https://doi.org/10.1097/00005768-199907000-00007.
12. Pollard CD, Sigward SM, Powers CM. Gender differences in hip joint kinematics and kinetics during side-step cutting maneuver. Clin J Sport Med. 2007;17:38–42. https://doi.org/10.1097/JSM.0b013e3180305de8.
13. Sigward SM, Powers CM. The influence of gender on knee kinematics, kinetics and muscle activation patterns during side-step cutting. Clin Biomech. 2006;21:41–8. https://doi.org/10.1016/j.clinbiomech.2005.08.001.
14. Sigward SM, Pollard CD, Havens KL, Powers CM. Influence of sex and maturation on knee mechanics during side-step cutting. Med Sci Sports Exerc. 2012;44:1497–503. https://doi.org/10.1249/MSS.0b013e31824e8813.
15. Alentorn-Geli E, Myer GD, Silvers HJ, Samitier G, Romero D, Lázaro-Haro C, Cugat R. Prevention of non-contact anterior cruciate ligament injuries in soccer players. Part 1: Mechanisms of injury and underlying risk factors. Knee Surg Sports Traumatol Arthrosc. 2009;17:705–29. https://doi.org/10.1007/s00167-009-0813-1.
16. Soligard T, Myklebust G, Steffen K, Holme I, Silvers H, Bizzini M, Junge A, Dvorak J, Bahr R, Andersen TE. Comprehensive warm-up programme to prevent injuries in young female footballers: cluster randomised controlled trial. BMJ. 2008;337:2469. https://doi.org/10.1136/bmj.a2469.
17. Sugimoto D, Myer GD, Barber Foss KD, Hewett TE. Specific exercise effects of preventive neuromuscular training intervention on anterior cruciate ligament injury risk reduction in young females: meta-analysis and subgroup analysis. Br J Sports Med. 2015;49:282–9. https://doi.org/10.1136/bjsports-2014-093461.
18. Clénin GE, Cordesa M, Huberb A, Schumacherc YO, Noackd P, Scalese J, Kriemlerf S. Iron deficiency in sports definition, influence on performance and therapy. Consensus Statement of the Swiss Society of Sports Medicine. Swiss Sports Exer Med. 2016;64:6–18. https://doi.org/10.4414/smw.2015.14196.
19. Sandström G, Börjesson M, Rödjer S. Iron deficiency in adolescent female athletes – is iron status affected by regular sporting activity? Clin J Sport Med. 2012;22:495–500. https://doi.org/10.1097/JSM.0b013e3182639522.
20. Latunde-Dada GO. Iron metabolism in athletes- achieving a gold standard. Eur J Haematol. 2013;90:10–5. https://doi.org/10.1111/ejh.12026.
21. Shah YM, Xie L. Hypoxia-inducible factors link iron homeostasis and erythropoiesis. Gastroenterology. 2014;146:630–42. https://doi.org/10.1053/j.gastro.2013.12.031.
22. Prior JC, Vigna YM. Ovulation disturbances and exercise training. Clin Obstet Gynecol. 1991;34:180–90.

23. Petit MA, Prior JC, Barr SI. Running and ovulation positively change cancellous bone in premenopausal women. Med Sci Sports Exerc. 1999;31:780–7. https://doi.org/10.1097/00005768-199906000-00004.
24. Nattiv A, Puffer JC, Green GA. Lifestyles and health risks of collegiate athletes: a multicenter study. Clin J Sport Med. 1997;7:262–72. https://doi.org/10.1097/00042752-199710000-00004.
25. Kaiserauer S, Snyder AC, Sleeper M. Nutritional, physiological, and menstrual status of distance runners. Med Sci Sports Exerc. 1989;21:120–5.
26. De Souza MJ, Williams NI. Beyond hypoestrogenism in amenorrheic athletes: energy deficiency as a contributing factor for bone loss. Curr Sports Med Rep. 2005;4:38–44. https://doi.org/10.1007/s11932-005-0029-1.
27. Chang FE, Dodds WG, Sullivan M, Kim MH, Malarkey WB. The acute effects of exercise on prolactin and growth hormone secretion: comparison between sedentary women and women runners with normal and abnormal menstrual cycles. J Clin Endocrinol Metab. 1986;62:551–6. https://doi.org/10.1210/jcem-62-3-551.
28. Alleyne J, Bennell K. Women and activity-related issues across the lifespan. In: Brukner K, editor. Clinical sports medicine. 4th ed. Sydney, NSW: McGraw-Hill; 2012. p. 910–35.
29. Frankovich RJ, Lebrun CM. Menstrual cycle, contraception and performance. In: Brukner K, editor. Clinical sports medicine. 4th ed. Sydney, NSW: McGraw-Hill; 2012. p. 251–71.
30. Nattiv A, Loucks AB, Manore MM. American College of Sports Medicine position stand. The female athlete triad. Med Sci Sports Exerc. 2007;39:1867–82. https://doi.org/10.1249/mss.0b013e318149f111.
31. Zanker CL, Swaine IL. Bone turnover in amenorrhoeic and eumenorrhoeic women distance runners. Scand J Med Sci Sports. 1998;8:20–6. https://doi.org/10.1111/j.1600-0838.1998.tb00224.x.
32. Prince RL, Dick I, Devine A. The effects of menopause and age on calcitropic hormones: a cross-sectional study of 655 healthy women aged 35 to 90. J Bone Miner Res. 1995;10:835–42. https://doi.org/10.1002/jbmr.5650100602.
33. Korpelainen R, Orava S, Karpakka J, Siira P, Hulkko A. Risk factors for recurrent stress fractures in athletes. Am J Sports Med. 2001;29:304–10. https://doi.org/10.1177/03635465010290030901.
34. Bennell KL, Malcolm SA, Thomas SA. Risk factors for stress fractures in track and field athletes. A twelve months prospective study. Am J Sports Med. 1996;24:810–8. https://doi.org/10.1177/036354659602400617.
35. Keen AD, Drinkwater BL. Irreversible bone loss in former amenorrheic athletes. JAMA. 1986;256:380–2. https://doi.org/10.1007/BF01623770.
36. Wentz L, Liu PY, Ilich JZ, Haymes EM. Dietary and training predictors of stress fractures in female runners. Int J Sport Nutr Exerc Metab. 2012;22:374–82. https://doi.org/10.1123/ijsnem.22.5.374.

Suggested Reading

Alaunyte I, Stojceska V, Plunkett A. Iron and the female athlete: a review of dietary treatment methods for improving iron status and exercise performance. J Int Soc Sports Nutr. 2015;6:12–38. https://doi.org/10.1186/s12970-015-0099-2.

Barrack MT, Gibbs JC, De Souza MJ, Williams NI, Nichols JF, Rauh MJ, Nattiv A. Higher incidence of bone stress injuries with increasing female athlete triad-related risk factors: a prospective multisite study of exercising girls and women. Am J Sports Med. 2014;42:949–58. https://doi.org/10.1177/0363546513520295.

Brown KN, Wengreen HJ, Beals KA. Knowledge of the female athlete triad, and prevalence of triad risk factors among female high school athletes and their coaches. J Pediatr Adolesc Gynecol. 2014;27:278–82. https://doi.org/10.1016/j.jpag.2013.11.014.

Misra M. Neuroendocrine mechanisms in athletes. Handb Clin Neurol. 2014;124:373–86. https://doi.org/10.1016/B978-0-444-59602-4.00025-3.

Weiss K, Whatman C. Biomechanics associated with patellofemoral pain and ACL injuries in sports. Sports Med. 2015;45:1325–37. https://doi.org/10.1007/s40279-015-0353-4.

Diet and Gender 13

Francesca Pasqui, Carolina Poli, and Davide Festi

Key Points

- Women have always played a primary role in this context by preparing meals, ensuring food safety in all historical ages and all cultures.
- Gender differences in behaviours play a part in health disparity.
- Food craving defined as a strong desire to eat shows different character between women and men.
- Several gender differences in health behaviour have reported in many studies.
- Mothers have difficulty in properly perceiving the nutritional status of their children.
- The perception of mothers about the weight of their children is often wrong.
- Gender differences in the prognosis of several pathological conditions and in particular in cardiovascular disease have been described in the literature.

13.1 Introduction

Diet has always been a dominant theme in man's history. Food and ways of finding it has always been one of the determining factors in human survival. Today, moreover, it has been shown that dietary behaviour plays a primary role in maintaining a state of health and well-being. The type, quality and quantity of foods ingested every day are fundamental to the concept of both physical and mental health. It has

F. Pasqui · C. Poli · D. Festi (✉)
Department of Medical and Surgical Sciences, University of Bologna, Bologna, Italy
e-mail: davide.festi@unibo.it

I. Tarricone, A. Riecher-Rössler (eds.), *Health and Gender*,
https://doi.org/10.1007/978-3-030-15038-9_13

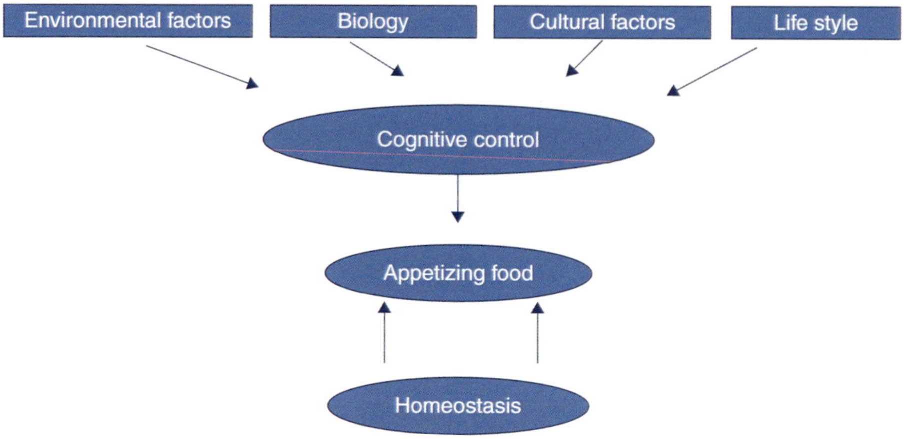

Fig. 13.1 Regulation of food intake is a complex mechanism which leads on homeostasis and it depends on cognitive control. The cognitive control is in relation with environmental, biology, cultural and life style factors

also been shown that a balanced diet is a very important tool both in preventing many illnesses and in managing and treating others.

Regulation of food intake is a complex mechanism, depending by environment and social factors (Fig. 13.1):

Women have always played a primary role in this context by preparing meals, ensuring food safety—with fundamental resulting repercussions in everyday life—and guaranteeing the primary and secondary prevention of health problems depending on the type of food given.

13.2 The Role of Women in History and Culture

The connection between women and food is a seemingly obvious one, since we all eat—men and women—but it is also a relationship with strongly gender-based attributes. If we take a moment to retrace prior stages in history, we can observe that the relationship between women and food has always been very strong, with great attention paid to beauty, health and the family. This can be perceived from numerous sources, such as iconography in which we observe the everyday work of women in preparing bread, pasta and bakery products in addition to making fabrics and tending the vegetable garden.

Going back in time, women were initially involved only in the preparation of domestic meals, while cooking in royal courts and the houses of the aristocracy was done only by men; subsequently, around the sixteenth century, there were female cooks and writers of recipes and nutritional prescriptions who demonstrated abilities that were not only limited to the family kitchen. Discipline and moderation were two behavioural aspects that women were always expected to observe, above all at the table. The rule was to eat small quantities of food and to drink just a drop of wine; only women who had recently given birth were advised to drink more, to help them recover their strength and relieve the strain of childbirth.

Moderation in eating was a very important value since it was seen as necessary to shun the vice of gluttony, regarded as the first pitfall for a young woman aspiring to marriage; drinking copious amounts of wine was only justified if she needed to gain weight. In the sixteenth century, it was particularly recommended for very thin women to take small doses, morning and evening, of a mixture of ground almonds, white poppy seeds, butter and sugar, together with plenty of wine. The tendency in mediaeval times was to project an elegant feminine image with moderation in her gestures, speaking, eating and facial expressions. Moderation was therefore the fundamental rule that had to be observed and followed by every woman to avoid the excesses of vice, gluttony and loquacity.

The transition to the modern age brought with it many changes; feelings began to spread of maternal attachment represented by breastfeeding. Mothers became more sensitive to their responsibilities and to the care and growth of their children, supporting campaigns by doctors and pedagogues that were emerging in that period to stress the importance of maternal breastfeeding and denouncing surrogate wet nurses, seen as bearers of disease.

Women began to occupy roles as cooks in public places outside the home to seek prestige and visibility and to offer their culinary skills not only for financial reward but also for social recognition.

Modernity then also brought with it education on food preparation, childcare, home maintenance, discipline and obedience, as well as the care of clothing. Mothers taught their daughters everything they needed to become good housewives; female education was every woman's duty, and they had to be taught from a young age in order to become wives and mothers and to be loved and respected.

The woman who ate very little and who was obliged to exercise self-discipline—the typical model of the mediaeval and early modern ages—was replaced by a woman restricted to less rigid eating behaviour, as evidenced by the eighteenth and nineteenth centuries.

With the beginning of the eighteenth century, therefore, the norms of beauty and the female shape underwent considerable changes, from thin and slender to plump, with wide hips and a generous bosom. This female model led to a change in eating habits above all in wealthier families; they ate foods rich in fat, butter, sugar, cream and desserts. An excess of weight, however, resulted in a loss of beauty, and overweight or obese women were considered infertile and more prone to illness. A correct diet needed to be combined with adequate exercise.

Between the end of the eighteenth and the beginning of the nineteenth centuries, girls of marriageable age were taught good manners and a correct relationship with food; they were warned not to confuse the appetite of the stomach with that of the palate, and on their first inkling of fullness, the meal had to end; the relationship between women and food was an expression of good taste—they had to know exactly when to eat in public at official receptions or banquets. Within the popular classes, the woman had the central role in the home. She devoted herself to caring for her children, to monitoring the family finances and to seeking out suitable foods for the preparation of meals. The financial role became increasingly important, to the extent of leading women into uprisings in the streets and markets to defend the family purchases. By the beginning of the nineteenth century, the presence of women in "hunger" riots is widely documented. Their protests were motivated by the desire to defend their everyday food supplies, and the social phenomenon that caused them to take to the streets was a rise in prices [1–7].

The different roles of women are therefore gradually highlighted: in the kitchen, in society and at work. Women were probably the first technocrats of food, textiles and communications; as females, mothers and members of society, women were not only responsible for raising their children and distributing food to the members of the family but also for contributing to the social and economic development of society; if they were able to demonstrate their productivity, fertility and respect for social rules, the well-being of the family was assured. Since the time when women were able to assume entrepreneurial, technical and leadership roles, there has been a growth in management of the food production chain and of healthcare systems [8]. Females have therefore always been involved in meal preparation and nutritional choices, both for themselves and their families and also for physiological needs such as pregnancy and breastfeeding—important events in which one individual's health depends strictly on the health of another.

Despite the changes referred to through the various periods of history, women today are unfortunately still victims of hunger, and around half of all pregnant women in developing countries are anaemic; this causes around 110,000 deaths in childbirth every year; the available data confirm that, in the hands of women, an increase in family income improves the health and nutrition of children. Education is naturally fundamental to everything and has been shown to contribute to a 43% reduction in child malnutrition over time (World Food Programme 2015).

13.3 Diet, Health and Beauty: Gender Differences and Possible Mechanisms

We can state today that the binomial of aesthetics and nutrition strongly influences women's dietary choices, since the concept is gaining traction that only a balanced diet makes possible the conservation of real beauty—the supreme desire of all women. In comparing the attitudes of men and women towards health, illness and the relationship with food, many studies have identified gender differences, but the causal mechanisms behind these attitudes have often been overlooked [9].

One study [9]—which assessed four types of behaviour in choosing foods among a large sample of young adults in 23 countries—observed two possible mechanisms that could explain these gender differences in dietary habits, finding that women were more likely to follow a diet and also to be more convinced of the importance of keeping to a healthy diet; the four types of behaviour analysed involved avoiding fats, eating fibre and fruit, and limiting sodium. The women in the study were more likely than men to claim that they avoided high-fat foods, that they ate fruit and fibre and that they limited their intake of foods with a high-sodium content. Beliefs relating to health explained about 40% of the differences in each type of nutritional behaviour; gender differences in the choice of foods therefore seem partly attributable to the fact that women have more control over their weight and partly to the fact that they believe more in the importance of healthy eating [9]. Many differences in behaviour with regard to food were also observed between males and females [10], and differences in choices are not always automatically reflected in differences in energy [11], but this is partly due to alcohol consumption by men which can add a significant amount of energy as liquid calories (drink calories); the diet of women, on the other hand, tends to contain higher amounts of microelements [9].

Many gender differences are also found in attitudes, beliefs and eating choices related to health. Men rate many forms of health-related behaviour as less important compared to women; they are less interested in knowing the value of foods, in acquiring more knowledge about nutrition and health and in worrying about their weight [8].

Recently it has been seen that health-related knowledge and the desire to control weight can explain up to 50% of gender differences in the choice of foods, and men's less healthy food choice profiles can be connected with their poorer nutritional knowledge. However, knowledge about a person's own health, nutritional attitudes and diet seem to be phenomena that vary during that person's lifespan. With increasing age, changes related to the perception of taste also play an important role in the choice of foods [12].

13.4 Food Craving and Food Addiction: Different Choices Between Women and Men

Another point to consider regards food craving, defined as a strong desire to eat—extremely common and experienced by more than 90% of the population [13–16] (Fig. 13.2).

The types of foods preferred vary between men and women, but gender diversity was also assessed in terms of the intensity and frequency of craving and the ability to handle these cravings. A number of studies show that men prefer savoury foods, while women state a greater desire for sweet tastes (chocolate, pastries,

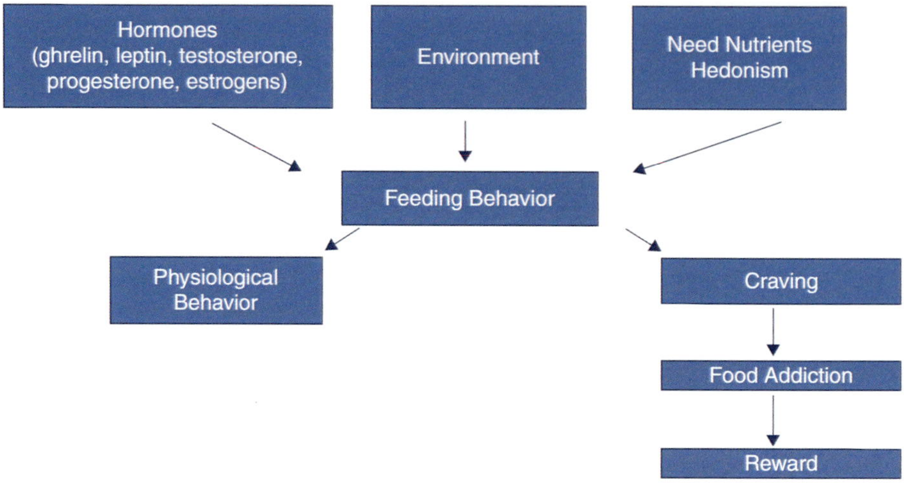

Fig. 13.2 Feeding behavior is often influenced by hormones (grelin, leptin, testosterone...), environment and hedonism. It correlates with physiological and psychological behaviour

ice-cream), and some studies report that over 92% of those with a craving for chocolate are women [13]. Gender differences have been assessed regarding the desire for certain foods among a large sample of university students, discovering that women have a significantly higher desire score than men even when they are under dietary control and have eating disorder symptoms. Desire also appeared higher among women who were already embarked on a weight loss programme than among overweight and obese men; women also frequently reported experiences of craving. In investigations into neural reactivity to food images using magnetic resonance imaging, women showed greater activity related to both taste and desire. In another study, women who were undergoing calorie restriction showed a greater neural reactivity to the mention of high-calorie foods, especially during the luteal phase compared to the follicular phase. A complex combination of biological, sociological and environmental factors probably explains these gender differences in desire and obesity; the sexual hormones (testosterone, progesterone and estrogens) regulate food consumption and can be regarded as important causal factors of gender differences [13].

In the past few decades, research studies on addiction have asserted that the desire for food is similar to using drugs; in the past 15 years, the literature has reported that the neural circuits working for food are the same as those activated by legal drugs like caffeine, alcohol and nicotine and illegal ones like cocaine. Food and cocaine share the same neurobiological pathways, which take the messages driving behaviour to the frontal cerebral cortex. Other important factors such as family, friends, education, language and culture can facilitate or compromise the delicate balance between pleasure and addiction [17]. Women with bulimia and anorexia have a high risk of using substances compared to control groups. Adolescent girls with purging behaviour have an increased risk of beginning to use drugs and to binge drink on alcohol [18, 19].

13.5 Knowledge About Diet, Its Impact on Health and Dissatisfaction with Body Shape

Despite describing better dietary knowledge in relation to health and chronic illnesses, the literature reports gender differences in epidemiology and in the physiopathology of obesity, with a greater incidence of these problems among women than men [20, 21]. In the USA obesity has reached epidemic proportions, and according to the NHANES, about 62% of American women over the age of 20 are overweight, and one in three is obese, with a projected percentage in 2030 of 58% [22]. This in turn carries high risk for various types of cancer (endometrial, breast, ovarian) but also pathologies such as depression, amenorrhoea, PCOS, infertility and obesity; the presence of the latter during pregnancy can be linked to negative outcomes for the foetus. An increased risk of obesity is also found among women with psychiatric disorders and among those who use certain psychotropic drugs [22–24]; during a course of weight loss, it has been observed that women tend to show slower but more sustained weight loss and a reduction in the use of drugs for diabetes. A higher percentage of obesity among women corresponds to a higher likelihood of seeking weight loss therapies [24].

A study carried out in 183 countries also reported that 38% of women are overweight—1% more than among men, with significant geographical differences in obesity [20]; women, in contrast to men, have a higher incidence of excess weight and obesity in developing countries. Genetic, hormonal, environmental and social factors seem to be involved in obesity, as well as the choice of foods and physical activity. Among adolescents there is a strong reduction in physical activity, and this difference continues also into adulthood [20]; and, naturally, a sedentary lifestyle has a role in maintaining this difference compared to males [21, 25].

Differences in dietary choices already appear during adolescence; a study carried out in high-income countries has shown that disorders relating to food quality and quantity are found more frequently among girls, who in turn report greater dissatisfaction with their body shape [21].

13.6 The Role of Mothers in the Dietary Behaviour of Their Children

Mothers are seen to be particularly involved in the dietary behaviour of their children due to the longer time that they spend together, including the time spent preparing meals [26]. Another aspect regards their perception of their children's nutritional condition, and a number of studies report a discrepancy between mothers' perceptions in recognising obesity in their children and reality. As regards the incidence of obesity, this was detected among 6666 children out of a sample of 18,650, but according to the perceptions of their mothers, only 5501 were overweight or obese [27].

If parents—and particularly mothers—do not recognise that their children are obese, it follows that they will not have any thoughts about possible treatment, let alone encourage them to change their lifestyles [27]. In most available studies, the perception of mothers showed an accurate view of the nutritional condition of their children when they were of normal weight but tended to significantly undervalue this nutritional condition if their children were overweight [27–31]. Factors associated with this altered perception among mothers are low education of the mother, the sex (males) and age of the child, the mother's overweight status and ethnicity. Environment also seems to be important; Binkin et al. [29] assessed the perception of mothers in different Italian regions with a low, moderate or high incidence of obesity, and it emerged that the highest rates of undervaluation of nutritional condition were observed in regions with the highest incidence of obesity [27].

Okkio alla Salute, a surveillance system to promote health and healthy growth among primary school children set up in collaboration with all the Italian regions and the Ministry of Education, Universities and Research, stated in its 2014 report that out of 40,000 children examined, 20.9% were overweight and 9.8% were obese; it also observed—in relation to mothers' perceptions of their children's weight—that as many as 48.6% of overweight children were perceived as being of normal weight. Furthermore, 76% of obese children were perceived as slightly overweight, and 13% were even perceived as of normal weight. A lower accuracy of perception is detected in the regions of the South than in the Centre-North, among mothers with lower levels of education and among those who are overweight, confirming the data reported by other studies. As regards their opinions of the quantity of food eaten by their children, 75% of mothers of overweight children and 55% of mothers of obese children think that this quantity is right.

Also as regards physical activity, it emerges that 53% of mothers of physically inactive children believe that their children are doing sufficient physical activity and that 6% even think that they are doing too much.

Emotional responsibility is the binding factor between binge eating of a mother, the nutrition of her child and his/her weight, suggesting that the mother's diet and emotional reactivity are important in understanding the interpersonal context of diet and patterns in the weight of children [32].

Attention should also be paid to social media, since there seems to be a negative relationship between body image and eating disorder symptoms among women who spend time on Facebook [33].

Based on professional practical observations and experiences rather than evidence, treatment approaches also seem to vary by gender, with a higher frequency among women of choosing or using phytotherapeutic, parapharmaceutical, social and other non-accredited products.

13.7 Conclusions

From what is reported above, we can state with certainty that women have had and still have an important role in the management of the home, diet and health and—given their involvement in the motivations for food choices—also in calorie intake, body image dissatisfaction, emotional responses and the well-being of their children and generally in managing the health of the whole family. It is therefore vitally important for health professionals to be increasingly active in providing correct information and in raising awareness of this aspect.

References

1. Appiano A. Bello da mangiare. Il cibo come forma simbolica nell'arte. Booklet Milano; 2000.
2. Dronke P. Donne e cultura nel Medioevo. Scritti medioevali dal II al XIV secolo. Milano: Il Saggiatore; 1986.
3. Woolgar CM. Food and the middle ages. J Mediev Hist. 2010;36:1–19.
4. Muzzarelli MG, Tarozzi F. Il Medioevo e l'età moderna. In: Donne e cibo una relazione nella storia. Milano: Mondadori; 2003.
5. Muzzarelli MG, Re L. Il cibo e le donne nella cultura e nella storia. Bologna: Clueb; 2006.
6. Venel JA. Essai sur la santée et l'education medicinale des jeunes filles destinèes au mariage par Jean-André Venel; 1776.
7. Maretti L, Pieri L, Sagrestani M. I moti della fame nel Mugello. Polistampa; 1998.
8. Pan WH, Hsieh YT, Wahlqvist ML. Gender-specific roles and needs in food-health security. Asia Pac J Clin Nutr. 2009;18:642–6.
9. Wardle J, Haase AM, Steptoe A, Nillapun M, Jonwutiwes K, Bellisle F. Gender differences in food choice: the contribution of health beliefs and dieting. Ann Behav Med. 2004;27: 107–16.
10. World Health Organization. Health and health behaviour among young people: health behaviour in school-age children : a who cross-national study (HBSC): international report. Geneva: World Health Organization; 2000.
11. Troiano RP, Briefel RR, Carroll MD, et al. Energy and fat intakes of children and adolescents in the United States: data from the National Health and Nutrition Examination Surveys. Am J Clin Nutr. 2000;72:1343S–53S.
12. Westenhoefer J. Age and gender dependent profile of food choice. Forum Nutr. 2005;57:44–51.
13. Hallam J, Boswell RG, DeVito EE, Kober H. Gender-related differences in food craving and obesity. Yale J Biol Med. 2016;89:161–73.
14. Osman JL, Sobal J. Chocolate cravings in American and Spanish individuals: biological and culture influences. Appetite. 2006;47:290–301.
15. Withe MA, Williamson DA, Greeway FL, Netemewer RG. Development and validation of the Food craving of the Food Craving Inventory. Obes Res. 2002;10:107–14.
16. Hill AJ. The psychology of food craving. Proc Natl Acad Sci U S A. 2007;66:277–85.
17. Volkov ND, Morales M. The brain on drugs: from reward to addiction. Cell. 2015;162:712–25.
18. Calero EA, Krug I, Davis K, Lopez C, Fernandez AF, Treasure J. Meta analysis on drugs in people with eating disorder. Eur Eat Disord. 2009;17:243–59.
19. Root T, Pisetsky EM, Thorton L, Lichtenstain NL, Pedersen NL, Bulik CM. Patterns of comorbidity of eating disorders and substance in Swedish females. Psychol Med. 2010;40:105–15.
20. Rochlani Y, Pothineni NV, Mehta JL. Metabolic syndrome: does it differ between women and men? Cardiovasc Drugs Ther. 2015;29:329–38.
21. Garawi F, Devries K, Thorogood N, Uauy R. Global differences between women and men in the prevalence of obesity: is there an association with gender inequality? Eur J Clin Nutr. 2014;68:1101–6.
22. Azarbad L, Gonder-Frederick L. Obesity in women. Psychiatr Clin North Am. 2010;33:423–40.
23. Kulie T, Slattengren A, Redmer J, Counts H, Eglash A, Schrager S. Obesity and women's health: an evidence-based review. J Am Board Fam Med. 2011;24:75–85.
24. Ryan DH, Braverman-Panza J. Obesity in women. J Fam Pract. 2014;63:S15–20.
25. Bauman A, Bull F, Chey T, Craig CL, Ainsworth BE, Sallis JF, Bowles HR, Hagstromer M, Sjostrom M, Pratt M. The international prevalence study on physical activity: results from 20 countries. Int J Behav Nutr Phys Act. 2009;31:6–21.
26. Scaglioni S, Salvioni M, Galimberti C. Influence of parental attitudes in the development of children eating behaviour. Br J Nutr. 2008;99(Suppl 1):S22–5.
27. Francescatto C, Santos NS, Coutinho VF, Costa RF. Mothers' perceptions about the nutritional status of their overweight children: a systematic review. J Pediatr. 2014;90:332–43.
28. Baughcum AE, Chamberlin LA, Deeks CM, Powers SW, Whitaker RC. Maternal perceptions of overweight preschool children. Pediatrics. 2000;106:1380–6.

29. Binkin N, Spinelli A, Baglio G, Lamberti A. What is common becomes normal: the effect of obesity prevalence on maternal perception. Nutr Metab Cardiovasc Dis. 2013;23:410–6.
30. Carnell S, Edwards C, Croker H, Boniface D, Wardle J. Parental perceptions of overweight in 3-5 y olds. Int J Obes (Lond). 2005;29:353–5.
31. Boutelle K, Fulkerson JA, Neumark-Sztainer D, Story M. Mothers' perceptions of their adolescents' weight status: are they accurate? Obes Res. 2004;12:1754–7.
32. Saltzman JA, Pineros-Leano M, Liechty JM, Bost KK, Fiese BH. Eating, feeding, and feeling: emotional responsiveness mediates longitudinal associations between maternal binge eating, feeding practices, and child weight. Int J Behav Nutr Phys Act. 2016;13:89.
33. Eckler P, Kalyango Y, Paasch E. Facebook use and negative body image among U.S. college women. Women Health. 2017;57:249–67.

Suggested Reading

Ahmad NN, Butsch WS, Aidarous S. Clinical management of obesity in women: addressing a lifecycle of risk. Obstet Gynecol Clin North Am. 2016;43(2):201–30.

Benton D, Young HA. A meta-analysis of the relationship between brain dopamine receptors and obesity: a matter of changes in behavior rather than food addiction? Int J Obes (Lond). 2016;40:S12–21.

Edwards ES, Sackett SC. Psychosocial variables related to why women are less active than men and related health implications. Clin Med Insights Womens Health. 2016;9(Suppl 1):47–56.

Lundahl A, Kidwell KM, Nelson TD. Parental underestimates of child weight: a meta-analysis. Pediatrics. 2014;133(3):e689–703.

Pickett-Blakely O, Uwakwe L, Rashid F. Obesity in women: the clinical impact on gastrointestinal and reproductive health and disease management. Gastroenterol Clin North Am. 2016;45(2):317–31.

Walker M, Thornton L, De Choudhury M, Teevan J, Bulik CM, Levinson CA, Zerwas S. Facebook use and disordered eating in college-aged women. J Adolesc Health. 2015;57(2):157–63.

Part III

Women's Health at All Stages of Life

14 Motherhood, Childbirth and Perinatal Age

Silvia Savini and Giacomo Faldella

Key Points

- In the last three decades, the western social reality has changed significantly. Mothers are more present on the labour market, while fathers take care of infants and help doing housework.
- The parents play a more and more interchangeable role in infant education, even if strong differences still persist between a role culture model based on a relationship of equality and the practical situation children and infants live every day.
- The chapter refers to an in-depth study of motherhood, childbirth and perinatal ages taking into account different areas such as psychology, sociology and pedagogy.
- In this chapter, increased risks of maternal and perinatal adverse outcomes among mothers due to potential confounding factors have been identified. In particular, two aspects explored of parenting at risk during motherhood and childbirth: preterm birth and migration.
- Specific interventions are significantly essential. These findings underline the importance of the further implementation of pregnancy prevention strategies and healthcare interventions to reduce vulnerability factors for women's health in contemporary society.

S. Savini (✉) · G. Faldella
Department of Medical and Surgical Sciences, Neonatology and Neonatal Intensive Care Unit, S. Orsola-Malpighi Hospital, University of Bologna, Bologna, Italy
e-mail: silvia.savini3@unibo.it

I. Tarricone, A. Riecher-Rössler (eds.), *Health and Gender*,
https://doi.org/10.1007/978-3-030-15038-9_14

14.1 Introduction

From the approach of gender differences, gender study turned into gender psychology. With regard to gender, we can say that it refers not only to individual differences but also to an independent variable that involves thought and behaviour differences. In the same way as culture, gender has marked influence upon any human situation, and it represents an inseparable part of everyday life.

In the last three decades, the western social reality has changed significantly. In fact, mothers are more present on the labour market, while fathers take care of infants and help doing housework. They play a more and more interchangeable role in infant education, even if strong differences still persist between a role culture model based on a relationship of equality and the practical situation children and infants live every day.

The following pages refer to an in-depth study of motherhood, childbirth and perinatal ages taking into account different areas such as psychology, sociology and pedagogy.

14.2 Motherhood and Childbirth

It is now known that with regard to infant mental health, the quality of primary relationships in infant development is fundamental. It is also recognized that, from the first moments of life, biological and behavioural factors interact in the evolutionary process.

The interactive-cognitive perspective highlights the fact that a good reciprocity in the prime relationships and in the early emotional experiences with caregivers involves neurodevelopment [1, 2].

In the twentieth century, ethologists and developmental psychologists, such as Lorenz, Bowlby and Ainsworth, assumed that sensitive responsiveness is the most important aspect of parenting.

This perspective of mother-infant interaction is supported by the concept of emotional availability [3, 4] which consists of the ability to read and to respond adequately to infant signals and to synchronize with their physical and affective needs.

Through the appropriate behavioural care, the mother provides the infant with the necessary stimulation for an adequate social-affective and cognitive development [5]. These aspects can be inadequate in parenting risk situations.

The next two paragraphs intend to explore two aspects of parenting at risk during motherhood and childbirth: preterm birth and migration.

14.2.1 Parenting Risk: Preterm Birth

In the last few decades, progressive improvement in perinatal medicine has led to a significant decrease in infant mortality rates. This improvement has involved a higher incidence of preterm births and a better survival for infants with low birthweight and low gestational age. On the other hand, it has involved increased

Table 14.1 Countries with the highest number of migrants

Country	%
United States	19.1
Germany	4.9
Russian Federation	4.8
Saudi Arabia	4.2
United Kingdom	3.5
United Arab Emirates	3.3
Canada	3.2
France	3.2
Australia	2.8
Spain	2.4
Italy	2.4

Data of Eurostat. The first 11 countries with the highest number of migrants. Year 2015. Absolute values (in millions)

negative sequels for infant development and an emotional burden for the parents.

Preterm birth is considered a risk factor for infant development as long periods of hospitalization in a neonatal intensive care unit (NICU) are needed. In this context, the early separation of the infants from their parents is necessary, but, at a later date, it could be an obstacle to the development of the maternal and paternal relationships.

Preterm birth is a highly stressing event that involves a lot of feelings of concern and loss of control. It is a real moment of emotional crisis for the parents. Kaplan and Mason [6] defined four fundamental processes regarding what parents must face after the birth of a preterm infant.

The first process is immediately after childbirth, when parents must balance their need to have hope on one hand and to face an "early mourning" feeling for the possible loss of the infant on the other. The mothers of preterm infants alternate feelings of hope and optimism and with those of guilt, anxiety and fear [7].

The mothers, at the same time, must recognize and deal with their own sense of failure, since the feeling of guilt adversely affects maternal interactions and their role as mothers [8].

As time goes by, and the parents begin to play a more active role in looking after the infant, they start to rebuild the relationship that had been brutally and traumatically interrupted.

Lastly, it is necessary to face the challenge of understanding what the "special needs" and the development patterns of a preterm infant are compared with a full-term infant.

The preterm birth can be very stressful for the parents who show symptoms not only during the hospitalization period [9] but also in the first years of life of the infants [10–13]. The suffered distress can involve post-traumatic stress disorders [10, 14, 15], and it can deeply influence the furtherance of interactive co-construction and parenting functions.

In conclusion, preterm birth, resulting in a high degree of suffering, involves feelings of anxiety and depression that could compromise the performance of parenting functions and significantly influence the future development of the infant.

In this perspective, the quality of the hospital NICU can play an important role in supporting the difficult experience of families. Giving the mother the opportunity to see and touch her baby with the support of psychologists and medical staff can reduce the feelings of helplessness and increase her commitment [16]. Carrying out the follow-up of preterm infants at an early stage is necessary, not only for the evaluation of medical problems but also for the medium- and long-term neurobehavioural development. Follow-ups are fundamental to support families and build a connection between the doctors who took care of the baby in the hospital and the family paediatrician and, if necessary, public care. As neurosciences show [17, 18], the reciprocal and synchronized communication between the mother and infant produces a better connection of the central nervous system functions [19].

For this reason, it is essential to give psychological support to the parents so that they can use their own resources to observe and better understand the signals, often weak and contradictory, of their preterm infant.

14.2.2 Parenting Risk: Migration

The increasing migration flows in Europe (see Table 14.1 adapted data of Report Caritas 2015) involve not only the need to face the social and cultural dimension of the phenomenon but also the clinical conditions and the needs of the population, represented by migrant parents and their infants.

It is important to bear in mind that migrants are individuals, as we are, and every individual, in all cultures, subjectively processes the cultural heritage that is transmitted in an original and specific way [20]. In this sense, migration is meant not only as a sociological event but also as a potentially traumatic psychological event of great importance.

Migration can imply an interruption of the relationship of continuous exchange and mutual reinforcement between external and internal culture. This interruption can reduce the capacity of the inner cultural system to orient itself in the world and to make use of the experience. For this reason, transcultural clinical psychology speaks about "migratory trauma".

One of the aims of clinical practice is to rebuild the links between the internal representations of the original culture and those of the host society culture, in order to avoid the traumatic experience of a fracture between these two worlds that could create a psychological situation of suffering for the individual. The specific clinical practice also aims to prevent malaise in the new generations. If parents do not process their migratory trauma, this malaise can cause an insecure identity in their infants. The gap between the present world and the original one can easily provoke a disorder in the transmission from generation to generation.

Moro's studies [21] have highlighted the psychological vulnerability of migrant infants. Psychological vulnerability, developed by Anthony [22], is a dynamic concept which affects the developmental process. Every slight internal or external variation can cause serious suffering, a block or an inhibition to the development of the infant's potential.

The nature of this link and the mechanisms concerning the eventual causality between the two factors has still to be established because the existence of a connection does not automatically indicate this causality. Starting from these studies and the clinical practice, migrant infants are vulnerable and belong to a risk group. In conclusion, the first period of vulnerability of these infants is postnatal, during which time the infant and the mother must adapt themselves one to the other.

14.3 Perinatal Age: The Importance of Relationships for Infant Development

Since the second postwar period, René Spitz's studies on the first year of life and the development of institutionalized infants have played a key role [23]. Bowlby's attachment theory is also relevant and has become a common heritage for all professions, which, for various reasons, concern infant development [24–26]. Another important contribution is infant research methodology that has transformed the image of the infant from a passive recipient of maternal care into an active one. This consideration is also due to the development of neuroscience.

Research carried out in recent years on the early stages of infant development has allowed us to understand in greater depth, not only the infant's typical development but also the early atypical development, thus helping to identify the risk factors that most influence his growth. In order to protect the infant's well-being, it is first and foremost important to safeguard his relationships, his affections and, more generally, the family microsystem in which the infant grows and develops [27].

In literature, the expression "risk factors" related to parenthood indicates all those conditions in which the fundamental components of parental function—specifically the care and protection of the infant—are disturbed and adversely affect the quality of the parent-infant relationship, producing potential negative consequences in the developmental process [28, 29].

The risk factors that could influence the parental quality in infant interaction and development are multiple and interact with one other in a complex way: a single factor can increase the risk of different aspects of infant development, while in other circumstances diverse factors could increase the risk of a specific field of infant development [30].

A less sensitive mother-infant interaction, characterized by inconsistent, unstable or poorly responsive cure modes, can have adverse developmental consequences, such as when the caregiver suffers from depression [31, 32] or if the family lives in a state of social poverty [33]. Various motherhood and parenthood risk factors, which increase the likelihood of negative outcomes for the infant, are reported in psychological studies. For example, mothers with a socio-economic or low education level, migrant mothers, mothers with psychological fragility, adolescent mothers or mothers who raise their baby without the help of a partner can have difficulty in the delicate task of being a parent, increasing the likelihood that their infant will develop a degree of discomfort [5, 29, 32, 34–37]. However, the effects on the infant's psychological growth depend on the complex dynamics characterizing the relationship between risk factors and those of protection. The latter comprise those conditions that favour adaptive development and healthy growth of the infant, such as the presence of a supportive social network, which can reduce the negative impact of risk factors [38, 39]. Among the protective factors are also some temperamental peculiarities of the infant (for instance, a positive mood, high consolability), good maternal sensitivity and a secure attachment relationship between mother and infant [28]. The risk and protection factors can be distal or proximal.

Among the distal factors are variables such as the social context in which the infant is born and grows and the family environment. They are an indirect influence, introducing elements of fragility and weakness that make the individual and the family more vulnerable. According to the transactional model [40], the development of the infant depends on the constant and dynamic interaction between the baby and the social-family context. Recent studies confirm that the association of familial discomfort with other risk factors increases the incidence of an insecure attachment in childhood with consequent effects on development [41, 42]. The family stress pattern which states that living conditions interfere with infant development through their direct effects on parenting and parental care [43] shows that the parents who live under unfavourable social conditions are forced to face numerous problems in their daily life that can affect the quality of dyadic interactions with their infant, risking his growth and development [44].

Proximal risk factors, however, relate more closely to neonatal variables, such as temperamental and individual characteristics, the psychological characteristics of the parents and parental care. Unlike distal risk factors, they are a direct influence on relationships and contribute to enhancing the risk, amplifying its effect [38, 39]. Among the variables that influence childhood development, parental responsibility is one of the basic concepts most enriched in recent years by developmental research. Ainsworth [45] defined the concept of responsiveness as the ability to read and respond adequately to the infant's signals, but lately this concept has been expanded considerably. Recent research has emphasized that maternal responsiveness is closely related to some aspects of maternal emotional competence, in particular to the mother's ability to regulate negative emotions and the infant's distress [46–48] and to share positive emotions [28, 49].

Many researchers also understood responsiveness as the ability to attribute to the infant a state of mind, called reflection by Fonagy [50]. Such responsiveness determines a higher quality in relation to the infant [28]. Another key component that influences infant development is the communicative ability in a parent-infant relationship [28].

From the first months of life, communication is bidirectional, on the one hand, to establish secure attachment relationship that can regulate emotions [51] and on the other to establish intersubjective connections to the sharing of emotional states and of information from the surrounding environment, so that the parent performs an adequate scaffolding function [52].

The study of the relationship between maternal responsiveness and communication has shown that these components have medium- and long-term effects on the infant's socio-emotional and relational development [28, 53–55].

14.4 Conclusions

In this chapter, increased risks of maternal and perinatal adverse outcomes among mothers due to potential confounding factors have been identified. Specific interventions are significantly essential. These findings underline the importance of the further implementation of pregnancy prevention strategies and healthcare interventions to reduce vulnerability factors for women's health in contemporary society.

References

1. Schaffer HR. Social development. Oxford: Blackwell; 1996.
2. Bornstein MH, editor. Maternal responsiveness: characteristics and consequences. San Francisco, CA: Jossey-Bass; 1989.
3. Emde RN. Emotional availability: a reciprocal reward system for infants and parents with implications for prevention of psychosocial disorders. In: Taylor PM, editor. Parent-infant relationships. Orlando, FL: Grune & Stratton; 1980. p. 87–115.
4. Biringen Z, Robinson JL, Emde RN. Emotional availability scales: infancy to early childhood version (3rd edition). Unpublished manual, Department of Human Development and Family Studies, Colorado State University, Fort Collins; 1998.
5. Bornstein MH, Bradley RH. Socioeconomic status, parenting, and child development. Mahwah, NJ: Lawrence Erlbaum Associates; 2003. (Monographs in Parenting, Volume 2).
6. Kaplan DM, Mason EA. Maternal reactions to premature birth viewed as an acute emotional disorder. Am J Orthopsychiatry. 1960;30:539–52.
7. Linhares MBM, Carvalho AEV, Bordin MBM, Chimello JT, Martinez FE, Jorge SM. Prematuridade e muito baixo peso ao nascer como fator de risco ao desenvolvimento psicológico da criança. Cadernos de Psicologia e Educação Paidéia. 2000;10:60–9.
8. Shah PE, Clements M, Poehlmann J. Maternal resolution of grief after preterm birth: implications for infant attachment security. Pediatrics. 2011;127(2):284–92.
9. Singer LT, Salvator A, Guo S, Collin M, Lilien L, Baley J. Maternal psychological distress and parenting stress after the birth of a very low-birth-weight infant. JAMA. 1999;281(9):799–805.
10. Kersting A, Dorsch M, Wesselmann U, Lüdorff K, Witthaut J, Ohrmann P, Hörnig-Franz I, Klockenbusch W, Harms E, Arolt V. Maternal posttraumatic stress response after the birth of a very low-birth-weight infant. J Psychosom Res. 2004;57(5):473–6.
11. Jackson K, Ternestedt BM, Magnuson A, Schollin J. Parental stress and toddler behaviour at age 18 months after pre-term birth. Acta Paediatr. 2007;96(2):227–32.
12. Grunau RE, Whitfield MF, Petrie-Thomas J, Synnes AR, Cepeda IL, Keidar A, Rogers M, Mackay M, Hubber-Richard P, Johannesen D. Neonatal pain, parenting stress and interaction, in relation to cognitive and motor development at 8 and 18 months in preterm infants. Pain. 2009;143(1-2):138–46.
13. Huhtala M, Korja R, Lehtonen L, Haataja L, Lapinleimu H, Munck P, Rautava P, The PIPARI Study Group. Parental psychological well-being and cognitive development of very low birth weight infants at 2 years. Acta Paediatr. 2011;100(12):1555–60.

14. DeMier RL, Hynan MT, Hatfield RF, Varner MW, Harris HB, Manniello RL. A measurement model of perinatal stressors: identifying risk for postnatal emotional distress in mothers of high-risk infants. J Clin Psychol. 2000;56(1):89–100.
15. Pierrehumbert B, Nicole A, Muller-Nix C, Forcada-Guex M, Ansermet F. Parental post-traumatic reactions after premature birth: implications for sleeping and eating problems in the infant. Arch Dis Child Fetal Neonatal Ed. 2003;88(5):400–4.
16. Trombini E, Surcinelli P, Piccioni A, Alessandroni R, Faldella G. Environmental factors associated with stress in mothers of preterm newborns. Acta Paediatr. 2008;97(7):894–8.
17. Schore AN. La regolazione degli affetti e la riparazione del sé. Rome: Astrolabio Ubaldini; 2008.
18. Schore AN. I disturbi del sé. La disregolazione degli affetti. Rome: Astrolabio Ubaldini; 2010.
19. Negri R. Il neonato in terapia intensiva. Un modello neuropsicoanalitico di prevenzione. Milano: Raffaello Cortina Press; 2012.
20. Moro MR. Genitori in esilio. Psicopatologia e migrazione. Milano: Raffaello Cortina; 2002.
21. Moro MR. Maternità e amore. Quello di cui hanno bisogno i bambini per crescere bene qui e altrove. Milano: Saggi Frassinelli; 2008.
22. Anthony EJ, Chiland C, Koupernik C. L'Enfant dans sa famille, l'enfant vulnérable. Paris: PUF; 1978.
23. Spitz R. Il primo anno di vita. Roma: Armando; 1965.
24. Bowlby J. Attaccamento e perdita, L'attaccamento alla madre, vol. I. Torino: Boringhieri; 1969.
25. Bowlby J. Attaccamento e perdita, La separazione dalla madre, vol. II. Torino: Boringhieri; 1973.
26. Bowlby J. Attaccamento e perdita, La perdita della madre, vol. III. Torino: Boringhieri; 1980.
27. Malagoli Togliatti M, Lubrano Lavadera A. I figli che affrontano la separazione dei genitori. Psicologia Clinica Dello Sviluppo. 2009;XIII(1):3–39.
28. Riva Crugnola C. La relazione genitore-bambino. Tra adeguatezza e rischio. Milano: Il Mulino; 2012.
29. Candelori C, Mancone A. Manuale di psicopatologia dell'infanzia. Milano: Raffaello Cortina; 2001.
30. Ammaniti M, et al. La prevenzione del maltrattamento: il sostegno ai genitori. In: La prevenzione del disagio nell'infanzia e nell'adolescenza. di Firenze: Istituto degli Innocenti; 2002.
31. Field T. Psychologically depressed parents. In: Bornstein MH, editor. Handbook of parenting, vol. 4. Mahwah, NJ: Erlbaum; 1995.
32. Tronick EZ, Field T. Maternal depression and infant disturbance. In: New directions for child development, vol. 34. London: Jossey-Bass; 1986.
33. Halpern R. Poverty and infant development. In: Zeanah CH, editor. Handbook of infant mental health. New York, NY: Guilford; 1993.
34. Cederna G, Inverno A, Rebesani M. Dossier: Il Paese di Pollicino. L'Italia ha dimenticato i bambini. Roma: Save the Children Italia onlus; 2012.
35. Mayes L, Fonagy P, Target M. Developmental science and psychoanalysis. Integration and innovation. London: Karnac; 2007.
36. Oyserman D, Mowbray CT, Meares PA, Firminger KB. Parenting among mothers with a serious mental illness. Am J Orthopsychiatry. 2000;70(3):296–315.
37. Kelly JF, Barnard KE. Assessment of parent-child interaction: implications for early intervention. In: Handbook of early childhood intervention, vol. 2. New York, NY: Cambridge University Press; 2000. p. 258–89.
38. Di Blasio P. Tra rischio e Prevenzione. Milano: Unicopli; 2005.
39. Schaffer HR. Introducing child psychology. Oxford: Blackwell; 2004.
40. Sameroff AJ. Ecological perspectives on developmental risk. In: Osofsky JD, Fitzgerald HE, editors. WAIMH handbook of infant mental health: infant mental health in groups at high risk, vol. IV. New York, NY: Wiley; 2000.

41. Costantino E, Cassibba R, Liso G, Gatto S, Godelli S. Sviluppo socio-emotivo e rischio psicosociale in età scolare: il ruolo dell'attaccamento. Maltrattamento e Abuso all'Infanzia. 2007;9:5–26.
42. Weinfield NS, Whaley GJL, Egeland B. Continuity, discontinuity, and coherence in attachment from infancy to late adolescence: sequelae of organization and disorganization. Attach Hum Dev. 2004;6:73–97.
43. Belsky J, Pasco Fearon RM. Infant-mother attachment security, contextual risk, and early development: a moderational analysis. Dev Psychopathol. 2002;14:293–310.
44. Crnic KA, Gaze C, Hoffman C. Cumulative parenting stress across the preschool period: relations to maternal parenting and child behavior at age 5. Infant Child Dev. 2005;14:117–32.
45. Ainsworth MDS, Blear MC, Waters E, Wall S. Patterns of attachment. A psychological study of strange situation. Hillsdale, NJ: Erlbaum; 1978.
46. McElwain NL, Booth-LForce C. Maternal sensitivity to infant distress and nondistress as predictors of infant-mother attachment security. J Fam Psychol. 2006;20(2):247–55.
47. Tronick EZ, Weinberg MK. Le madri depresse e i loro bambini: l'insuccesso nella formazione di stati di coscienza diadici. In Depressione post-partum e sviluppo del bambino. CIC: Roma; 1997.
48. Tronick EZ. Emotions and emotional communication in infant. Am Psychol. 1989;44(2):112–9.
49. Hennighausen KH, Lyons-Ruth K. Disorganization of behavioral and attentional strategies toward primary attachment figures: from biologic to dialogic processes. The 92 Dahlem workshop report: attachment and bonding: a new sintesy. Cambridge, MA: MIT Press; 2005.
50. Fonagy P, Target M. Attachment and reflective function: their role in self-organization. Dev Psychopathol. 1997;9:679–700.
51. Trevarthen C. Communication and cooperation in early infancy. A description of primary intersubjectivity. In Before speech: the beginnings of human communication. Cambridge, MA: Cambridge University Press; 1979.
52. Tomasello M. Origins of human communication. Cambridge, MA: Harvard University Press; 2008.
53. Cohn MA, Fredrickson BL, Brown SL, Mikels JA, Conway AM. Happiness unpacked: positive emotions increase life satisfaction by building resilience. Emotion. 2009;9:361–8.
54. Feng X, Shaw DS, Skuban EM, Lane T. Emotional exchange in mother-child dyads: stability, mutual influence, and the association with maternal depression and child problem behaviours. J Fam Psychol. 2007;21:714–25.
55. Mantymaa M, Puura K, Luoma I, Salmelin RK, Tamminem T. Early mother-infant interaction, parental mental health and symptoms of behavioral and emotional problems in toddlers. Infant Behav Dev. 2004;27:134–49.

Childhood

15

Antonia Parmeggiani and Evamaria Lanzarini

Key Points

- Infancy and early childhood are key periods in an individual's neural and behavioural development, because the brain undergoes important changes at a faster rate than in other life periods. For this reason, significant events occurring in these age periods can leave a neurobiological footprint on the child's developing nervous system.
- There is strong evidence that traumatic events occurring during infancy and childhood are associated with poor health outcomes, which persist into adulthood. As a result, adults who have experienced early traumas live shorter and challenging lives while suffering from higher rates of chronic and mental illnesses than others who grew up under the care of warm and sensitive parents and in a stable and supportive community.
- The diversity of clinical pictures and health outcomes resulting from genetic predisposition and environmental exposure has prompted recent investigations into the differences between males and females in the way the brain develops during the early years of life. By considering these differences, gender-specific therapeutic approaches could be designed to help children fully develop their resilience.
- "Resilience" is a dynamic concept that results from an interplay among protective factors that facilitates a better-than-expected outcome in children who have been exposed to early traumas. Since the environment plays an important role in mediating genetic expression, protective factors can be enhanced and improved with focused intervention, to help the child build his/her resilience.

A. Parmeggiani (✉) · E. Lanzarini
Department of Medical and Surgical Sciences, University of Bologna, Bologna, Italy
e-mail: antonia.parmeggiani@unibo.it

I. Tarricone, A. Riecher-Rössler (eds.), *Health and Gender*,
https://doi.org/10.1007/978-3-030-15038-9_15

- Increasing evidence exists that the foundations of a healthy and happy life are established even before birth, if not earlier. Therefore, women's health must be safeguarded at all ages in order to protect the well-being of subsequent generations.

15.1 Introduction

Health, as defined by the World Health Organization in 1946 [1], is "a state of complete physical, mental and social well-being and not merely the absence of disease or infirmity". The interaction between each individual and his/her natural, cultural and socioeconomic environment plays a critical role in maintaining a healthy state throughout his/her entire lifespan. With regard to the early stages of human development, research has shown that an interplay exists between genetic and environmental factors, which can have long-term effects on the health status of the individual as an adult.

In particular, early childhood represents a period in human development of great vulnerability to stressful events because the brain undergoes important changes.

In this chapter, we focus our attention on women's health during childhood (3–11 years old). However, since infancy and childhood constitute a continuum when referring to human development, we will also briefly consider the first 2 years of an individual's life.

The term "infant" will refer to both male and female gender.

15.2 Infancy

During infancy, the child almost completes his/her psychomotor development and acquires language and relational skills; this gives the infant increasing autonomy until he/she is able to begin exploring the world independently. For these reasons, genetic and acquired conditions that emerge in this life period can have a long-term impact on an individual's development.

15.2.1 Attachment

Since birth, the infant relies completely on the help of his/her caregivers on which his/her survival depends. The infant establishes a bond with the caregiver—whether a parent or a parent's substitute—to receive protection, comfort and assistance. John Bowlby proposed the so-called attachment theory, in which he described the strong bond that exists between the infant and his/her caregiver. The caregiver's proximity to the infant is key to giving him/her protection under threatening conditions. When the infant cries or smiles, he/she is using his/her social competences, albeit still immature, to maintain or restore proximity to the caregiver [2]. When the infant learns to crawl or to walk, the caregiver becomes a "secure base" from which he/she can venture out to explore the world and to which he/she can return safely.

The literature shows some evidence that the quality of the infant's attachment to the caregiver is predictive of a number of important developmental outcomes, including the degree of independence in preschool, the ability to forge peer relations in middle childhood and the development of internalizing and externalizing behaviour problems [3].

Mary Ainsworth designed a test to assess the quality of infants' attachment, which she called the "Strange Situation" test. The attachment quality was categorized in three groups: "secure", "avoidant" and "resistant" [4]. About a decade later, Mary Main and Judith Solomon noted that some children showed odd and unexpected reactions during the test, which did not fit in any of the three categories described by Ainsworth. It was then that "disorganized attachment" was introduced as a new and distinct category that was associated with a negative outcome [5]. In fact, an insecure (avoidant/resistant) or disorganized attachment is associated with the development of internalizing (e.g. depressive symptoms, anxiety) and externalizing (e.g. conduct disorders, oppositional defiant disorder) behaviours [6, 7].

Parental behaviours (e.g. parental availability during distress in contrast to maltreatment) and challenges (e.g. mental illness in a parent, domestic violence and challenging living conditions such as low income, substance abuse in the household, belonging to a minority group, single parenting, adolescent parenting and low parental education level) are the most important factors wielding influence over the quality of attachment.

Conversely, the child's own temperament affects the quality of the parent-infant interaction and their attachment relationships.

15.2.2 Risk and Protective Factors for Mental Health During Infancy

Urie Bronfenbrenner postulated that every person interacts with five systems that are more or less close to the individual itself (ecological system theory). He identified "proximal" influences wielded by such systems as family, school and peer groups, which are closer to the child, and "distal" influences exercised by such systems as mass media, industry, social services, neighbours and local policies. In the same way, he divided stressors into proximal and distal [8].

Depression and anxiety are among the most common mental health issues affecting parents, which can have a long-term impact on the child's mental health at this sensitive time of his/her development. Both genetic and environmental factors could explain this association. A mother suffering from depression is less reactive to the child's signals. This, in turn, affects negatively the mother-child interactions [9]. Maternal depression may also be linked to a lower family income and the related difficulty for parents to achieve financial stability and social recognition and to access healthcare services. These challenges further increase the risk of subsequent impaired development in the child [10]. A recent study shows that mothers who reported elevated levels of adversity and prenatal depression were more likely to live in disadvantaged socioeconomic conditions and that low prenatal family income was associated with children's behavioural problems at 5 years after birth [11].

Daniel Bagner and his research team examined the specific effect of maternal depression during the first year of a child's life and found that infants of mothers suffering from major depressive disorders during this period showed behavioural problems regardless of the child's age or gender at the time of evaluation [12]. While he found no difference between boys and girls, Carter and colleagues observed that both prenatal and postnatal maternal depressive symptoms were associated with externalizing behaviour problems in boys only and that the quality of the mother-infant interactions at 4 months was associated with externalizing and internalizing behaviour problems in girls only [13].

Cook et al. [14] demonstrated that a positive parenting style in a child's first years of life can predict academic skills up to fifth grade (approximately 10 years old).

Another proximal risk factor for mental health in infancy is adolescent parenting. Being a parent at an age when the individual is still developing presents challenges that are linked to higher rates of negative outcomes of the offspring. Adolescent parenting has been associated with poorer adaptation to the parental role, poorer social support and increased risk for depression [15]. Distal risk factors in infancy as poverty or sudden catastrophes like natural disasters, accidents and armed conflicts are conditions and events in which the caregivers are unable to protect the infant from negative experiences or care for his/her basic needs. If the caregiver is able to restore the infant's sense of safety by helping him/her cope with the traumatic experience and achieve a successful emotion regulation, the effects of the infant's exposure to trauma can be mitigated [16].

Parental warmth, availability and sensitivity and a positive family atmosphere are essential indicators of a good relationship [17]. Distal protective factors include the caregiver's social network and easy access to social services and the healthcare system.

15.2.3 Gender Differences in Infancy

Gender differences in health issues during early childhood are less evident than in other stages of human development. However, increasing attention has been given to finding differences between the sexes in the early years of life at both biological (e.g. differences in the structure of certain brain areas) and behavioural levels, with the aim of developing gender-specific therapeutic approaches.

Connelan et al. [18] reported that female newborns tend to look at human faces longer than male newborns, who, instead, pay more attention to object manipulation.

In the kindergarten years, boys tend to isolate themselves and be unruly, while girls show cooperation and sociability. This seems to suggest higher levels of empathy in female children during their first years of life. Male children, on the other hand, show greater difficulty in attributing mental states to others [19].

Between 18 months and 2 years of age, the child engages in symbolic play. Relevant behavioural differences between the sexes are evident also during other play activities in children's early years of life. Girls tend to play together and collaborate, while boys tend to isolate themselves. These differences appear to originate, at least in part, from the parents' behaviours towards their children. In fact, parents tend to behave differently with their female and male children from the very first years of their lives.

15.2.4 Neuropsychiatric Conditions in Infancy

Neurologic and psychiatric conditions and diseases occurring during infancy can negatively influence a child's cognitive and psychological development. Some of these conditions tend to have a different prevalence in the two sexes. Autism spectrum disorders, for instance, occur more in males (male:female ratio of 4:1). Language disorders also show a higher prevalence in males. X-linked diseases, like Duchenne dystrophy or fragile-X syndrome, are commonly exhibited only by males, while females are asymptomatic or paucisymptomatic carriers.

Rett syndrome, linked to mutations of the MECP2 gene, located on the X-chromosome, affects almost only females due to the higher prenatal lethality levels of this genetic mutation in males.

15.3 Childhood

Childhood is a critical period for the development of an individual's social skills. The child learns to distinguish between right and wrong on the basis of what is socially acceptable, following existing moral and ethical values. Both boys and girls undergo physical changes. During this time of personal profound changes, the occurrence of traumatic events can radically disrupt the normal developmental process and have long-lasting consequences on the individual's physical and mental health.

15.3.1 Adverse Childhood Experiences

Individuals who were subjected to maltreatment in childhood are at increased risk for psychological and global functioning deficits [20].

Maltreatment refers to both physical or sexual and psychological abuse. Psychological abuse and neglect are more difficult to quantify but can be as traumatic as physical maltreatment.

Institutional deprivation is the most extreme form of psychological mistreatment because it involves neglect both in human interaction and conversation. Studies show that profound institutional deprivation and child abuse have similar biological consequences [21].

Prevalence of maltreatment in childhood does not differ between males and females, with the exception of sexual abuse which is more frequently experienced by females and disabled children.

The Adverse Childhood Experiences (ACEs) Study was the first study that described the long-term connection between childhood abuse and household dysfunction with adult health status and mortality. Almost two-thirds of the study participants reported at least one ACE, and approximately one-fifth reported three or more ACEs, which meant that ACEs are common and tend to occur together. ACE exposure increased the risk for chronic health conditions (e.g. heart disease and cancer), the presence of health behaviour risk factors (e.g. smoking, promiscuity, alcoholism and substance abuse), mental illnesses (e.g. depressed affect), fewer life opportunities (e.g. education) and decreased life expectancy.

A possible explanation for the lifelong influence of ACEs on an individual's health and well-being could be that the exposure to acute or chronic stressors during childhood, when the brain is rapidly developing and cognition is still consolidating, leads to a disruption of the individual's neurodevelopment with lasting effects on the brain's structures and functions. This leads, in turn, to social, emotional and cognitive impairment, which facilitates an individual's adoption of health-risk behaviours [22] (Table 15.1, Fig. 15.1).

Early sexual debut (before 15 years old) has been linked to exposure to ACEs. Some authors suggest that young individuals seek protection outside of the family when the family has been unable to protect them from early traumas. This need and search for protection may be responsible for their reduced ability to estimate the

Table 15.1 Health and well-being outcomes associated with exposure to multiple ACEs

Outcomes associated with exposure to multiple ACEs	
Prevalent diseases	Ischemic heart disease, cancer, chronic lung disease, skeletal fractures, sexually transmitted diseases, liver disease
Adoption of health-risk behaviours	Smoking, alcohol abuse, promiscuity, obesity, illicit drug use, injection drug use, multiple somatic symptoms
Mental health	Depressive disorders, anxiety, hallucinations, panic reactions, sleep disturbances, memory disturbances, poor anger control
Sexual and reproductive health	Early sexual debut, teen pregnancy, unintended pregnancy, teen paternity, foetal death
General health and social problems	High perceived stress, impaired job performance, relationship problems, alcoholic marriage, bullying, domestic abuse, premature mortality

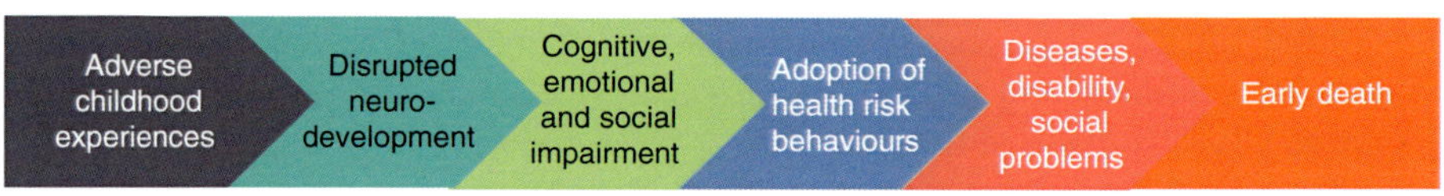

Fig. 15.1 Mechanism by which adverse childhood experiences influence health and well-being throughout the lifespan (*Adapted from CDC—Centers for Disease Control and Prevention*)

consequences connected with sexual risky behaviours while attempting to achieve close interpersonal relations [23]. Early sexual debut is also associated with inconsistent use of contraceptive, multiple unintended pregnancies, drugs/alcohol use, experience of physical intimate partner violence and contact with multiple sexual partners [24].

Taken together, these circumstances can explain the decrease in life expectancy that has been observed in people who had ACEs. Brown et al. [25] found that individuals with six or more ACEs died on average nearly 20 years earlier than those without ACEs. Studies also report that exposure to ACEs increases the risk of suicide attempts not only among children and adolescents but also in adults with a history of ACEs, which confirms ACEs' long-term impact on individuals' lives [26].

Bullying is a common childhood traumatic experience and has been therefore included between the ACEs.

Victims of bullying during childhood or adolescence are at greater risk of developing psychiatric disorders during adulthood. The Great Smoky Mountains Study revealed that victims of bullying are at higher risk of anxiety disorders in adulthood, while people who are at the same time victims and bullies are more prone to adult depression and panic disorder. These findings remained significant even when preexisting psychiatric disorders were taken into account. When considering the gender, the risk for adult psychopathology is similar between male and female victims and bully-victims. However, male bully-victims show higher rates of suicidality, while females suffer more often from agoraphobia during adulthood. Interestingly, bullies are at risk only of developing an antisocial personality disorder regardless of their gender [27].

The environment can influence the risk of being bullied; physical maltreatment by parents, maternal depression and low socioeconomic status facilitate peer victimization [28]. However, even personal characteristics such as emotional and behavioural problems may increase, in a child, the risk of being victimized by his/her peers [29]. Furthermore, being a victim of violence places the child at increased risk of further violence (revictimization) and exposure to multiple forms of abuse and Internet harassment (polyvictimization). Being bullied is not a casual occurrence; traumatic environmental factors and predisposing personal traits play a role in the risk of experiencing peer violence, which in turn leads to a higher risk of adverse outcomes.

Other stressful events, which have been recently taken into account as regards ACEs, include forced marriage, exposure to crime and collective violence in a community and early conscription.

Gender-based differences in the development of negative outcomes associated with ACEs exposure have been recently investigated. For example, Brown et al. [24] report stronger associations between ACEs and sexual debut at a younger age for women rather than men. However, other factors probably play a role in this association. In fact, it is well-known that adverse childhood experiences tend to occur together [22] and that families of children who experience ACEs tend to be less stable and show higher rates of divorce. The absence of the father in a home has been linked to earlier sexual debut and increased risky sexual behaviours in girls, but not in boys [30].

Comprising verbal aggression, criticism and hostility towards the child, a harsh parenting style has been mostly related to a diagnosis of conduct disorder or oppositional defiant disorder in the offspring [31]. With regard to this issue, a longitudinal study was conducted on a large sample of monozygotic twin pairs [32]. The authors found that only for the couples who showed marked different levels of parent-twin conflict or externalizing symptom's score a direct correlation existed between the high levels of parent-child conflict and a higher prevalence of externalizing behaviours at age 14. However, this association was not replicated between age 14 and 17 [33]. These findings demonstrate that since monozygotic twins share 100% of the genetic and environmental factors, the environment (in this case, the parenting style) can predict a change in child behaviour in early adolescence, but not in late adolescence, probably on account of a weaker influence of the parent-child relationship as the child grows into adulthood.

On the contrary, parental warmth, which includes affection, admiration and a positive attitude towards the child, appears to play a protective role against childhood disorders [34].

The levels of parental monitoring have been found to predict norm-breaking behaviours during adolescence [35]. Adverse childhood events like the incarceration or mental illness of a parent causing a lack of parental supervision could partly explain the adverse outcomes experienced by their offspring [24].

Parents' divorce is associated with a range of negative outcomes, including academic failures, behavioural problems and difficulties in peer relations [36]. The negative influence of divorce on children's well-being is mediated by the marital conflicts preceding the parents' separation, the economic difficulties following it and the reduced parental monitoring [37].

Environmental risk factors outside of the family and the peer group (e.g. neighbourhood and socioeconomic status) play a significant role in a child's health. A study conducted in the United States involved families from high-poverty neighbourhoods, who were given vouchers to move to a low-poverty area, showed, initially, a beneficial effect on school achievements for both boys and girls. At a later follow-up, only girls maintained a significative benefit from the intervention. The authors also observed lasting effects on reduced levels of psychological distress and obesity only in girls [38].

Another negative environmental factor is represented by war. Children experiencing a war are exposed to a wide range of traumatic experiences such as losing one or both parents, being raped or taken prisoner, suffering famine and thirst and seeing people being killed. This obviously leads to high rates of psychiatric disorders, especially post-traumatic stress disorder [39].

The socioeconomic status of a child's family also affects his/her health with regard to executive function and language skills, for parents in low-income families tend to expose their children to lower levels of cognitive stimulation and higher degree of stress and family conflicts [40].

15.4 Resilience

"Resilience" should not be seen as a personal trait but rather as the result of an interplay among protective factors that facilitates a better-than-expected outcome in children who have been exposed to early traumas [17, 41].

Protective factors include the individual's psychological, social and biological features and the characteristics of the family or the community where he/she lives. In this regard, social abilities can be particularly important in adulthood, when an individual may reach a critical personal milestone like marriage, which can help him/her depart from previous maladaptive trajectories [42].

Because resilience is a sum of individual and environmental protective factors, it tends to vary in response to different social circumstances [43]. A recent study examined the protective factors associated with physical health in a sample of adolescents and adults exposed to high levels of distress including child abuse. The authors found that those individuals who were able to modulate their emotions, engaged in purposeful activities for themselves or had stronger interpersonal skills to cope with various occurrences in their lives perceived their lives as healthier. The strongest association observed was between emotion regulation and perceived quality of life [44]. This conclusion is particularly important as it suggests that protective factors connected with the self-regulation of emotion can be enhanced and improved with focused intervention.

Resilience is closely related also to the quality of parenting. In particular, living with nurturing parents who organize consistent family routines for their offspring and teach them good self-care skills helps children cope with traumas by fostering a positive appraisal style and effective executive functions [45].

Last but not least, exposure to mild forms of stress during childhood has a positive effect on the child's mental and physical health because it gives him/her an opportunity to learn how to deal with challenges—a knowledge from which he/she will benefit later in life.

15.5 The Biology of Environmental Effects

Evidence of biological differences between children who experience traumatic events and others who do not is emerging in the literature on the topic. If traumas occurring in particularly sensitive periods of a child's life can leave a neurobiological footprint on the child's developing nervous system, this may help explain why there seems to be a transgenerational transmission of vulnerability to mental illnesses.

The hypothalamic-pituitary-adrenal axis (HPA axis) is involved in the neuroendocrine response to stressful events. In nature, stress triggers the activation of the HPA axis, which results in the production of glucocorticoids by the adrenal glands. Steroid hormone receptors are present in many parts of the brain and function as transcription factors for the regulation of gene expression.

Thus, the presence of very high levels of cortisol, as can happen after a severe acute stress, or a stable increase in its production, as in response to chronic stress, can influence the brain's structural development. However, the effects of this response may be different and largely depend on the areas of the brain that are either developing or declining when a person is experiencing stress [46].

Infants born from mothers who experienced stress during pregnancy have higher cortisol levels compared to control subjects [47], probably on account of their exposure to high maternal cortisol levels during the last months of the pregnancy. High maternal cortisol levels have a programming effect on the HPA axis of the newborn, and this is believed to give the child an incremented sensitivity to stressful events occurring during his/her life. This hypersensitivity to stress could partially mediate the negative health outcomes described in individuals exposed to ACEs.

During early childhood, exposure to stress can have variable effects on the production of glucocorticoids. In fact, some children show higher level of cortisol than controls, while others exhibit hypocortisolism. This could be mediated by a downregulation of the HPA axis at the level of the pituitary gland in response to the chronic corticotropin-releasing hormone drive from the hypothalamus. Thus, some children show hypersensitivity to stress, while others do not.

Stressful events occurring during infancy, childhood or adolescence tend to alter the amygdala microstructure and its connections with other parts of the brain. It has been suggested that these alterations may increase the risk of psychiatric illnesses, particularly mood disorders.

A recent study found that higher maternal cortisol levels in early pregnancy were associated with a larger right amygdala volume in girls but not in boys. Furthermore, larger amygdalas were associated with more affective symptoms in girls [48].

Several studies have also demonstrated that prenatal depressive symptoms in the mother are associated with greater functional connections between the child's amygdala and other regions of the limbic systems. These alterations would be responsible for the child's hyperactivity to novelty or threatening events and for increasing the risk of mood disorders [49, 50].

Valentino et al. [51] have demonstrated that differences exist between boys and girls in the way in which the corticotropin-releasing factor—the major orchestrator of stress response—interacts with the major arousal system, the locus coeruleus (LC)-norepinephrine system. These differences would give girls a greater magnitude of arousal in response to emotion-related stimuli, which translates into an enhanced sensitivity to acute stress and a decreased ability to adapt to chronic or repeated stress. This could explain why depression and post-traumatic stress disorder have a higher prevalence in women than in men.

Recent research suggests a robust association between early-life stress exposure and telomere length [52]. Telomeres are the terminal parts of chromosomes and serve as protection against damages. With each cell division, telomeres become shorter, until cells lose their ability to divide further. Exposure to severe stress could accelerate the shortening of their length, thus conferring a higher risk of chronic diseases and early death.

A recent study has shown an altered expression of the kappa opioid receptor gene in a region of the insula that influences glucocorticoid receptor binding. In this study, this alteration was present in individuals who had died by suicide and had a history of child abuse. It was not found in others who had died by suicide but had no history of child abuse, or in the control group, which included individuals who had died in a car accident [53]. The authors concluded that the different expressions of genes that mediate the glucocorticoid's activity of transcription regulation could be the result of the individual's exposure to abuse in the early years of life.

15.5.1 Psychiatric Disorders in Childhood

Unlike children affected by externalizing disorders, children affected by internalizing disorders (mood and anxiety disorders) most often show quiet and inner distress rather than overt socially negative or disruptive behaviour. For this reason, it is more difficult to detect this type of disorders in young children, since their verbal skills are less developed and their ability to describe feelings is limited [54].

Externalizing disorders consist in disruptive, hyperactive and aggressive behaviours and are a strong predictor of adult violence and crime [55].

Several studies report an equal prevalence of internalizing disorders in prepubertal girls and boys. After puberty, the prevalence of these disorders is higher in girls, while in boys externalizing disorders are most dominant.

A higher prevalence of conduct and tic disorders has been described in boys than in girls in childhood. Eating disorders, depression and anxiety disorders affect predominantly females.

Reyes-Rodriguez et al. [56] have described a prevalence of post-traumatic stress disorder (13%) in women suffering from anorexia nervosa. Among them, 40.8% reported a sex-related trauma during childhood.

15.6 Conclusion

Infancy and early childhood are key periods in an individual's neural and behavioural development.

There is strong evidence that traumatic events occurring at this age are associated with poor health outcomes, which persist into adulthood. Furthermore, increasing evidence exists that the foundations of a healthy and happy life are established even before birth, if not earlier. Therefore, women's health must be safeguarded at all ages in order to protect the well-being of subsequent generations.

In recent years a greater effort has been made to investigate the mechanisms of resilience rather than to study the negative effects of chronic stress. Since the environment plays an important role in mediating genetic expression, all health professionals who work with children must keep in mind the importance of addressing both primary and secondary preventions of trauma, identifying treatable trauma sequelae and building resilience.

The diversity of clinical pictures and health outcomes resulting from genetic predisposition and environmental exposure has prompted recent investigations into the differences between males and females in the way the brain develops during the early years of life. By considering these differences, gender-specific therapeutic approaches could be designed to help children fully develop their resilience.

References

1. WHO. Constitution of the World Health Organization. New York. Geneva: WHO; 1946. http://apps.who.int/gb/bd/PDF/bd47/EN/constitution-en.pdf?ua=1. Accessed 11 Oct 2017.
2. Bowlby J. Developmental psychiatry comes of age. Am J Psychiatry. 1988;145(1):1–10.
3. Maccoby E. Parenting and its effects on children: on reading and misreading behavior genetics. Annu Rev Psychol. 2002;51(1):1–27. https://doi.org/10.1146/annurev.psych.51.1.1.
4. Ainsworth M. The Bowlby-Ainsworth attachment theory. Behav Brain Sci. 1978;1(03):436.
5. Main M, Solomon J. Procedures for identifying infants as disorganized/disoriented during the Ainsworth Strange Situation. In: Greenberg MT, Cicchetti D, Cummings EM, editors. The John D. and Catherine T. MacArthur Foundation series on mental health and development. Attachment in the preschool years: theory, research, and intervention. Chicago, IL, US: University of Chicago Press; 1990. p. 121–60.
6. Groh AM, et al. The significance of insecure and disorganized attachment for children's internalizing symptoms: a meta-analytic study. Child Dev. 2012;83:591–610.
7. Madigan S, Atkinson L, Laurin K, Benoit D. Attachment and internalizing behavior in early childhood: A meta-analysis. Dev Psychol. 2013;49(4):672–89. https://doi.org/10.1037/a0028793.
8. Bronfenbrenner U. Toward an experimental ecology of human development. Am Psychol. 1977;32:513–31.
9. Stein A, Craske M, Lehtonen A, Harvey A, Savage-McGlynn E, et al. Maternal cognitions and mother-infant interaction in postnatal depression and generalized anxiety disorder. J Abnorm Psychol. 2012;121(4):795–809. https://doi.org/10.1037/a0026847.
10. Brooks-Gunn J, Duncan GJ. The effects of poverty on children and youth. Future Child. 1997;7:55–71.
11. Bouvette-Turcot A, Unternaehrer E, Gaudreau H, et al. The joint contribution of maternal history of early adversity and adulthood depression to socioeconomic status and potential relevance for offspring development. J Affect Disord. 2017;207:26–31.
12. Bagner D, Pettit J, Lewinsohn P, et al. Effect of maternal depression on child behavior: a sensitive period? Am Acad Child Adolesc Psychiatry. 2010;49(7):699–707.
13. Carter A, Garrity-Rokous F, Chazan-Cohen R, et al. Maternal depression and comorbidity: predicting early parenting, attachment security, and toddler social-emotional problems and competencies. Am Acad Child Adolesc Psychiatry. 2001;40(1):18–26.
14. Cook GA, et al. Fathers' and mothers' cognitive stimulation in early play with toddlers: predictors of 5th grade reading and math. Fam Sci. 2011;2:131–45.
15. Reid V, Meadows-Oliver M. Postpartum depression in adolescent mothers: an integrative review of the literature. J Pediatr Health Care. 2007;21(5):289–98. https://doi.org/10.1016/J.PEDHC.2006.05.010.
16. Scheeringa M, Peebles C, Cook C, Zeanah C. Toward establishing procedural, criterion, and discriminant validity for PTSD in early childhood. J Am Acad Child Adolesc Psychiatry. 2001;40(1):52–60. https://doi.org/10.1097/00004583-200101000-00016.

17. Rutter M. Resilience as a dynamic concept. Dev Psychopathol. 2012;24:335–44.
18. Connellan J, Baron-Cohen S, Wheelwright S, Batki A, Ahluwalia J. Sex differences in human neonatal social perception. Infant Behav Dev. 2000;23(1):113–8.
19. Baron-Cohen S. The extreme male brain theory of autism. Trends Cogn Sci. 2002;6(6):248–54.
20. Jonas S, Bebbington P, McManus S, et al. Sexual abuse and psychiatric disorder in England: results from the 2007 Adult Psychiatric Morbidity Survey. Psychol Med. 2011;41(04):709–19.
21. Rutter M, Sonuga-Barke EJX. Conclusions: overview of fidings from the E.R.A. study, inferences, and research implications. In: Deprivation-specifi psychological patterns: effects of institutional deprivation, vol. 75. Oxford: Monographs of the Society for Research in Child Development; 2010. p. 212–29. https://doi.org/10.1111/j.1540-5834.2010.00557.x.
22. Felitti V, Anda R, Nordenberg D, et al. Relationship of childhood abuse and household dysfunction to many of the leading causes of death in adults. The adverse childhood experiences (ACE) study. Am J Prev Med. 1998;14(4):245–58.
23. Hillis S, Anda R, Felitti V, Marchbanks P. Adverse childhood experiences and sexual risk behaviors in women: a retrospective cohort study. Fam Plann Perspect. 2001;33(5):206.
24. Brown M, Masho S, Perera R, et al. Sex and sexual orientation disparities in adverse childhood experiences and early age at sexual debut in the United States: results from a nationally representative sample. Child Abuse Negl. 2015;46:89–102.
25. Brown D, Anda R, Tiemeier H, et al. Adverse childhood experiences and the risk of premature mortality. Am J Prev Med. 2009;37(5):389–96.
26. Dube S, Anda R, Felitti V, Chapman D, Williamson D, Giles W. Childhood abuse, household dysfunction, and the risk of attempted suicide throughout the life span. JAMA. 2001;286(24):3089.
27. Copeland W, Wolke D, Angold A, Costello E. Adult psychiatric outcomes of bullying and being bullied by peers in childhood and adolescence. JAMA Psychiat. 2013;70(4):419.
28. Bowes L, Arseneault L, Maughan B, et al. School, neighborhood, and family factors are associated with children's bullying involvement: a nationally representative longitudinal study. Am Acad Child Adolesc Psychiatry. 2009;48(5):545–53.
29. Barker E, Boivin M, Brendgen M, et al. Predictive validity and early predictors of peer-victimization trajectories in preschool. Arch Gen Psychiatry. 2008;65(10):1185.
30. James J, Ellis B, Schlomer G, et al. Sex-specific pathways to early puberty, sexual debut, and sexual risk taking: tests of an integrated evolutionary–developmental model. Dev Psychopathol. 2012;48(3):687–702.
31. Hoeve M, Dubas J, Eichelsheim V, et al. The relationship between parenting and delinquency: a meta-analysis. J Abnorm Child Psychol. 2009;37(6):749–75.
32. Iacono W, Carlson S, Taylor J, et al. Behavioral disinhibition and the development of substance-use disorders: findings from the Minnesota Twin Family Study. Dev Psychopathol. 1999;11(4):869–900.
33. Burt S, McGue M, Iacono W, et al. Differential parent-child relationships and adolescent externalizing symptoms: cross-lagged analyses within a monozygotic twin differences design. Dev Psychol. 2006;42(6):1289–98.
34. Davidov M, Grusec J. Untangling the links of parental responsiveness to distress and warmth to child outcomes. Child Dev. 2006;77(1):44–58.
35. Kerr M, Stattin H. What parents know, how they know it, and several forms of adolescent adjustment: further support for a reinterpretation of monitoring. Dev Psychol. 2000;36(3):366–80.
36. Amato P. Children of divorce in the 1990s: an update of the Amato and Keith (1991) meta-analysis. J Fam Psychol. 2001;15(3):355–70.
37. Amato PR. Research on divorce: continuing trends and new developments. J Marriage Fam. 2010;72:650–66.
38. Ludwig J, Duncan G, Gennetian L, et al. Neighborhood effects on the long-term well-being of low-income adults. Science. 2012;337(6101):1505–10.
39. Attanayake V, McKay R, Joffres M, Singh S, Burkle F, Mills E. Prevalence of mental disorders among children exposed to war: a systematic review of 7,920 children. Med Confl Surviv. 2009;25(1):4–19.

40. Hackman D, Farah M. Socioeconomic status and the developing brain. Trends Cogn Sci. 2009;13(2):65–73.
41. Rutter M. Resilience: clinical implications. J Child Psychol Psychiatry. 2013;54:474–87.
42. Jaffee S, Lombardi C, Coley R. Using complementary methods to test whether marriage limits men's antisocial behavior. Dev Psychopathol. 2013;25(01):65–77.
43. Luthar SS, Zelazo LB. Research on resilience: an integrative review. In: Resilience and vulnerability: adaptation in the context of childhood adversities. Cambridge: Cambridge University Press; 2003. p. 510–49.
44. Banyard V, Hamby S, Grych J. Health effects of adverse childhood events: identifying promising protective factors at the intersection of mental and physical well-being. Child Abuse Negl. 2017;65:88–98.
45. Traub F, Boynton-Jarrett R. Modifiable resilience factors to childhood adversity for clinical pediatric practice. Pediatrics. 2017;139(5):e20162569. https://doi.org/10.1542/peds.2016-2569.
46. Lupien S, McEwen B, Gunnar M, et al. Effects of stress throughout the lifespan on the brain, behaviour and cognition. Nat Rev Neurosci. 2009;10(6):434–45.
47. Davis EP, Glynn LM, Waffarn F, et al. Prenatal maternal stress programs infant stress regulation. J Child Psychol Psychiatry. 2011;52(2):119–29.
48. Buss C, Davis E, Shahbaba B, et al. Maternal cortisol over the course of pregnancy and subsequent child amygdala and hippocampus volumes and affective problems. Proc Natl Acad Sci U S A. 2012;109(20):E1312–9.
49. Rifkin-Graboi A, Bai J, Chen H, Hameed W, Sim L, Tint M, Leutscher-Broekman B, Chong Y, Gluckman P, Fortier M, Meaney M, Qiu A. Prenatal maternal depression associates with microstructure of right amygdala in neonates at birth. Biol Psychiatry. 2013;74(11):837–44.
50. Qiu A, Anh T, Li Y, Chen H, Rifkin-Graboi A, Broekman B, Kwek K, Saw S, Chong Y, Gluckman P, Fortier M, Meaney M. Prenatal maternal depression alters amygdala functional connectivity in 6-month-old infants. Transl Psychiatry. 2015;5(2):e508.
51. Valentino R, Reyes B, Van Bockstaele E, Bangasser D. Molecular and cellular sex differences at the intersection of stress and arousal. Neuropharmacology. 2012;62(1):13–20.
52. Price LH, et al. Telomeres and early-life stress: an overview. Biol Psychiatry. 2013;73:15–23.
53. Lutz P, Gross J, Dhir S, Maussion G, Yang J, et al. Epigenetic regulation of the kappa opioid receptor by child abuse. Biol Psychiatry. 2018;84(10):751–61.
54. Tandon M, Cardeli E, Luby J. Internalizing disorders in early childhood: a review of depressive and anxiety disorders. Child Adolesc Psychiatr Clin N Am. 2009;18(3):593–610.
55. Liu J. Childhood externalizing behavior: theory and implications. J Child Adolesc Psychiatr Nurs. 2004;17(3):93–103.
56. Reyes-Rodríguez M, Holle A, Ulman T, Thornton L, Klump K, et al. Post traumatic stress disorder in anorexia nervosa. Psychosom Med. 2011;73(6):491.

Young Women in the "Digital Generation"—New Risks and New Opportunities

16

Anna Rita Atti, Lucia Rossi, and Diana De Ronchi

Key Points
- Adolescents' brains are particularly sensitive to surrounding influences.
- The most of mental disorders start by the mid-teens and the mid-20s.
- Less than half of adolescents with mental health problems receive an appropriate care.
- Digital natives are in between new risks (hyper-connection and Internet addiction, Web-based unhealthy lifestyle promotion, cyberbullying, grooming) and new opportunities (Web-based professional help)
- There's a strong need for developing a proper digital education encompassing families, institutions, media, and therapists.

A person between 10 and 19 years of age is conventionally framed as an adolescent. Apart from age, biological changes and social transitions occurring in those years have a deep influence in adolescence advent. Such changes are largely socioculturally mediated, and therefore adolescence occurs at different moments in different areas of the globe and across different societies. In addition, two other variables need to be taken into account to define adolescence: (1) sex, as adolescent girls reach biological maturity up to 2 years ahead of adolescent boys, and (2) gender, as expectations and societal norms differ significantly between boys and girls in most societies.

Adolescence, "the conjugator of childhood and adulthood" as suggested by the psychologist Louise J Kaplan, represents one of the more complex phases of human development as during the "teen years" childhood experiences sediment to become the foundation of the adult identity. Adolescence is probably the most important transitional period in life as adolescents' brains are particularly sensitive to surrounding influences [1] (Fig. 16.1).

A. R. Atti (✉) · L. Rossi · D. De Ronchi
Department of Biomedical and NeuroMotor Sciences, University of Bologna, Bologna, Italy
e-mail: annarita.atti@unibo.it

I. Tarricone, A. Riecher-Rössler (eds.), *Health and Gender*,
https://doi.org/10.1007/978-3-030-15038-9_16

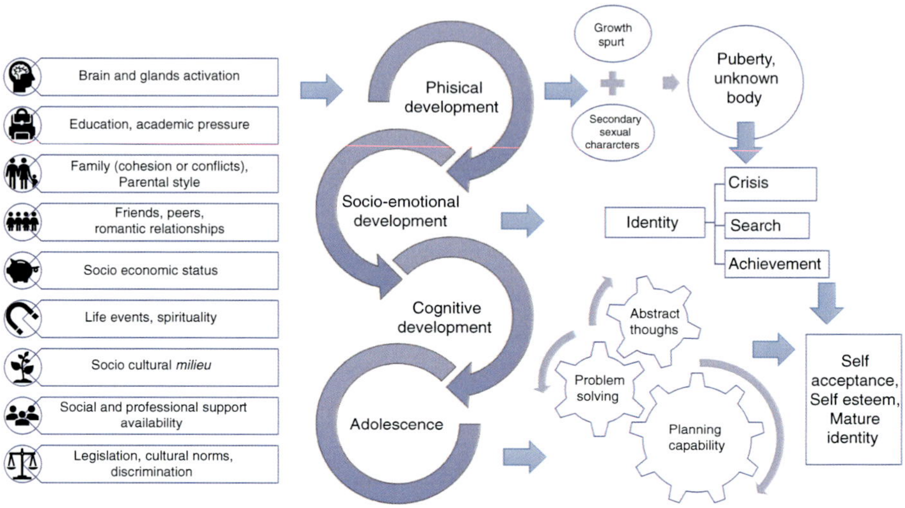

Fig. 16.1 Adolescence at a glance

Adolescents experience, at different levels, many interplaying factors influencing both current and future physical and mental health. The adolescent is a subject in between the past and the future, he/she is in a process of personal transformation, childhood seems really far, and sudden changes, both physical and psychological, must be faced. Adolescent boys and girls have to learn to recognize themselves in new bodies. According to the "Report of the *American Psychological Association* (APA) Task Force on the Sexualisation of Girls" [2], this is especially relevant for young women who face the objectivation and sexualisation of female icons in contemporary Western media. The report highlights the sexualized content of mainstream teen magazines, music videos, and music lyrics and the trend towards sexy clothing sponsored for young girls. "The world has not paid enough attention to the health of adolescents", warns the *Family, Women's and Children's Health*, of the WHO, as psychological health appears to be more fragile in this age group with respect to the other age groups.

The first cause of illness and disability in this age group is depression, whereas suicide ranks number three among causes of death. The probability of depressive symptoms affecting adolescents' daily living rises from around 5% in early adolescence to 15% by late adolescence [3]. The female preponderance in adolescent depression is impressive (about 2:1) with even larger gender difference in middle to late adolescence [3]. Unfortunately, even in high-income countries, less than half of adolescents with mental health problems receive an appropriate care, whereas in low- and middle-income countries, the access to treatment is scarce.

Promoting healthy behaviours during adolescence is critical for the prevention of health problems in adulthood: roughly, half of all lifetime mental disorders in most studies start by the mid-teens and three-fourths by the mid-20s [4]. Several factors influence adolescent vulnerability to physical and mental problems. Besides individual factors (gender, education) and family and peer influences, at an institutional level (school, health system, religious affiliation), the availability of facilities, education, and preventive programmes has a strong impact on young mental health. In addition, cultural practices and unwritten norms spread by mass media and digital interactive media have an additional power especially on adolescents. Table 16.1 reported a list of both risk and protective factors in early and late adolescence (see Table 16.1).

16.1 The Digital Generation

The constant exposition to new technologies is a critical factor for an adolescent's mental health. Individuals born between the end of the 1990s and the early 2000s are known as "digital natives". Having grown up surrounded by technologies, the "digital" generation has developed different thinking and learning patterns from the previous "paper" generations [5]. "Digital natives" are synthetic and fast, and they have a different concept of space, time, and an altered idea of confidentiality and identity and, in everyday life, exhibit constantly "multitasking" behaviours. They are hyper-connected and constantly engaged in exchanging virtual information, activities for which they use a new figurative language [6]. New technologies have therefore changed the bond with their own identity, the relationship with inner psychic life, and the processes of consolidation of self-sense. Today's relationships are multifaceted, simultaneous, and short-lived [7]. The ways of communicating between friends, boyfriends, and family members have changed together with new ways of controlling and monitoring interactions. The network provides adolescents with opportunities never experienced, such as the access to a wide array of resources and information and the possibility to communicate in real time with peers from all over the planet. This is a unique chance for facilitating learning and intercultural knowledge but at risk of unclear or even dangerous information. Indeed, information found on social network home pages are generally quick and superficial and thus are at risk of being exploited and misused. The major risk is related to the amplification: even a single aberrant content can have a wide media coverage because thousands of users share it. Exposure to this kind of information could have repercussions on those who are still incapable of critical evaluation, such as adolescents.

The use of the Internet can be dangerous but can also provide useful information such as health promotion and sexual education. Furthermore, some benefits in adolescents lacking of daily off-line relationships need to be recognized. However, despite the large potential and abundant usage by young people, limited research is available on apps and health promotion for adolescents. Apps can enable users to set targets, enhance self-monitoring, and increase awareness [8]. A literature review, for example, identified 193 articles on Apps use as health promotion tools and a need for culturally appropriate and tailored health messages to increase knowledge and awareness of health behaviours such as healthy eating. Participants prefer

Table 16.1 Risk and protective factors in early and late adolescence

	Risk factors			Protective factors		
	Individual	Family	School, peers, community	Individual	Family	School, peers, community
Early adolescence	Poor impulse control Low harm avoidance Sensation seeking Lack of behavioural self-control/ regulation Aggressiveness Antisocial behaviour Early substance use	Permissive parenting or harsh discipline Parent–child conflict Inadequate supervision and monitoring Low parental warmth or hostility Low parental aspirations for child Child abuse/ maltreatment Substance use among parents or siblings or favourable attitudes towards alcohol and/ or drugs	School failure Low commitment to school Peer rejection Deviant peer group Peer attitudes towards drugs Interpersonal alienation Extreme poverty for those children antisocial in childhood	Mastery of academic skills (math, reading, writing) Following rules for behaviour at home, at school, and in public places Ability to make friends Good peer relationships	Consistent discipline Language-based, rather than physical, discipline Extended family support	Healthy peer groups School engagement Positive teacher expectations Effective classroom management Positive partnering between school and family School policies and practices to reduce bullying High academic standards

Late adolescence	Behavioural disengagement coping Negative emotionality Conduct disorder Favourable attitudes towards drugs Rebelliousness Early substance use Antisocial behaviour Lack of commitment to conventional adult roles	Substance use among parents Lack of adult supervision Poor attachment with parents Balance of autonomy and relatedness to family Progressive development of behavioural and emotional autonomy	School failure Low commitment to school Not college bound Aggression towards peers Norms (e.g. advertising) favourable towards alcohol use Accessibility/ availability Substance-using peers	Positive physical development Emotional self-regulation High self-esteem Good coping skills and problem-solving skills Engagement and connections in two or more of the following contexts: at school, with peers, in athletics, employment, religion, culture Future orientation	Family provides structure, limits, rules, monitoring, and predictability Supportive relationships with family members Clear expectations for behaviour and values	Presence of mentors and support for development of skills and interests Opportunities for engagement within school and community Positive norms Clear expectations for behaviour Physical and psychological safety Opportunities for exploration

applications that are quick and easy to administer and those that increase awareness of food intake and weight management [9]. Overweight is a risk factor for cardiovascular diseases and diabetes during adolescence and adulthood and a key condition to monitor, prevent, and treat. It has been shown that healthy lifestyle is not only associated with physical benefits but also psychological health. Indeed, the importance of the role of exercise in the treatment of adolescent depression [10] is well demonstrated, and Web-based stimuli could provide regular and cost-effective positive reinforcement.

16.2 Risky Situations

In the following paragraphs, we describe a number of possible Web-related at-risk situations, and we suggest potentially protective factors for an adolescent's mental health exploring the most well-known gender differences.

16.2.1 Hyper-connection and Internet Addiction

According to the data of the main reason why adolescents use the Internet is for communicative or social motivations (94% of the young). Other frequent incentives to Internet use are recreational (music, movies, games) and education (material research, learning sites). Noticeably, the age of first contact with smartphones and the Web has considerably lowered over the years. This has many advantages including the increased ability of younger subjects to use technologies, but this can also lead to a continuous use of smartphones both in solitude and in social situations [11] which can lead up to technology addiction. According to a study made in 2006 about cell phone addiction, 22.1% of adolescents and 27.9% of young people can be considered cell phone addicts.

16.2.2 Web-Based Unhealthy Lifestyle Promotion (Pro-ana, Pro-drinking, Pro-suicide)

The shift of social life online has opened the doors to the "online trends" phenomenon. Among the most dangerous social modes, there are those related to eating disorders (pro-ana or pro-mia websites), addiction, self-harm, and even suicide. Such website promotes diet restriction, vomiting, and other disruptive behaviours including self-harm and alcohol or drug use as a way to achieve perfection and to increase the sense of mastery. In some "drinking games", the largest amount of alcohol should be consumed as quickly as possible as power demonstration. Harmless websites teach the smartest way of self-harming or committing suicide. The only powerful strategy against this phenomenon is spreading information and knowledge on healthy lifestyles, alcohol, and drug-related diseases. Second step is to provide health and psychological facilities together with tailored preventive programmes targeting adolescents.

16.2.3 Cyberbullying

Cyberbullying, a term coined in 2005, is characterized by the use of technological information and communications to support intentionally repetitive and hostile behaviour of an individual or group of individuals who intend to harm someone. Different categories of cyberbullying have been identified so far: flaming (sending vulgar or aggressive messages), online harassment (sending offensive messages by repetitive email), cyberstalking (sending repetitive threats), masquerade (sending another person by damaging the reputation of the victim), and outing (disclosing confidential information about another person). The phenomenon of cyberbullying is particularly dangerous because the victim can be reached at any time and in any place and ignores the identity of cyberbully. Furthermore, differently from real life, the victim is unable to respond to violent actions so that the aggression of the perpetrator can be mitigated. Various studies identify cyberbullying as a gender-related phenomenon: the female sex would seem to be predominant in the role of victim of cyberbullying acts, while the genders seem to be equally represented among attackers [12, 13]. The ways in which victims are bullied often involve the social dimension rather than the physical dimension, for example, through exclusion: girls, who are also favoured in this sense by a more early verbal development than boys are, mainly act this kind of behaviour on. Cyberbullying has very often a psychopathological outcome for the victim, with both psychological and physical damages. Victims may tend to isolate themselves from their family and friends and not reveal what they are being tormented by shame: the psychophysical repercussions may reach the so-called bullycide. This term refers both to the suicide which the victim may be instigated because of unsustainable acts of prevarication and to the murder which has been carried out by the victim against the victimiser. As bullying usually originates in the school, analysing classroom social dynamics, fostering a group spirit, and speaking openly about the phenomenon are tools that should be used by teachers in this direction.

16.2.4 Grooming

Grooming is an increasingly widespread problem involving children and adolescents who are contacted by paedophiles via social networks, chat rooms, and online games. This phenomenon involves mainly girls. According to the *National Adolescence Observatory*, about two out of ten adolescents have been contacted online by unknown adults at least once. This phenomenon is increasing over time: from 6% to 11% from 2000 to 2011. The identity of attenders of forums/blogs can be kept anonymous. Online you can hide your real identity and show yourself under other appearances and profiles that do not correspond to the truth and have interactions avoiding direct contact. The approval research also pushes a significant number of attenders to publish intimate photos: this behaviour can occur both in the messaging between two (the so-called sexting) and on social networks, making those who carry out this type of practice easy prey to blackmail. Especially girls are often blackmailed in exchange for sexual practices. According to data from the National Adolescence Observatory, 4.5% of children would have published hard material from friends online without their consent.

16.3 Conclusions

In our opinion, adolescents do have choices to reduce the risk of possible detrimental mental health consequences in adulthood. A set of resources is necessary to protect the "digital natives". Besides personal resources, a deep knowledge and proper education on new technologies is required. Beside school, a proper "digital education" has to comprise families, institutions, media and therapists.

Education has to build a strong critical sense and has to help the young in improving their "resilience". Resilience is defined as "the protective factors and processes that, despite experiences with situations shown to carry significant risks for developing psychopathology, contribute to good outcome" [14]. Being resilient is a personal resource that develops throughout life, reflecting the ability to cope with different life condition using protective resources [15, 16]. Empirical evidence indicates three resilience characteristics in a person's life, serving as a principle for the construction of resilience: personal characteristics and resources of the individual, a stable and supportive family environment, and social resources outside the family [14, 17]. Although findings are not consistent, females seem to report higher scores on social and interpersonal resources, whereas males rate themselves higher on personal dispositions [14].

Considering both physical and mental health, the "digital generation" faces new risks but also has new opportunities. For example, young people are often reluctant to seek professional help for their problems. Indeed, adolescents often underestimate the need for outside help and attempt to deal with their problems on their own. Programmes targeted at adolescents can also operate through new technology, for example, using the Internet. Some children and young people may prefer the Internet to "face to face" contact when having mental health or everyday problems. Web coaches in Sweden provide their help for young people on the Internet. Other programmes aim to provide adolescents with information and to help them solve their problems by getting online advices from counsellors and peers.

References

1. Knudsen EI. Sensitive Periods in the development of the brain and behavior. Cogn Neurosci. 2004;16(8):1412–25.
2. APA. Report of the task force on the sexualization of girls. Washington, DC: APA; 2007. https://www.apa.org/pi/women/programs/girls/report.aspx.
3. Thapar A, Collishaw S, Pine DS, Thapar AK. Depression in adolescence. Lancet. 2012;379(9820):1056–67. https://doi.org/10.1016/S0140-6736(11)60871-4.

4. Kessler RC, Amminger GP, Aguilar-Gaxiola S, Alonso J, Lee S, Ustün TB. Age of onset of mental disorders: a review of recent literature. Curr Opin Psychiatry. 2007;20(4):359–64.
5. Helsper EJ, Eynon R. Digital natives: where is the evidence? Br Educ Res J. 2010;36(3):503–20. https://doi.org/10.1080/01411920902989227.
6. Kennedy G, Judd T, Dalgarno B, Waycott J. Beyond natives and immigrants: exploring types of net generation students. J Comput Assist Learn. 2010;26(5):332–43.
7. Cain MS, Leonard JA, Gabrieli JDE, Finn AS. Media multitasking in adolescence. Psychon Bull Rev. 2016;23:1932–41.
8. Dute DJ, Bemelmans WJE, Breda J. Using mobile apps to promote a healthy lifestyle among adolescents and students: a review of the theoretical basis and lessons learned. JMIR Mhealth Uhealth. 2016;4(2):e39. https://doi.org/10.2196/mhealth.3559. PMID: 27150850.
9. Coughlin SS, Whitehead M, Sheats JQ, Mastromonico J, Hardy D, Smith SA. Smartphone applications for promoting healthy diet and nutrition: a literature review. Jacobs J Food Nutr. 2015;2(3):021. PubMed PMID: 26819969; PubMed Central PMCID: PMC4725321.
10. Avenevoli S, Swendsen J, He JP, Burstein M, Merikangas KR. Major depression in the national comorbidity survey-adolescent supplement: prevalence, correlates, and treatment. J Am Acad Child Adolesc Psychiatry. 2015;54(1):37–44.e2. https://doi.org/10.1016/j.jaac.2014.10.010. PMID: 25524788.
11. Aljomaa SS, Al Qudah MF, Albursan IS, Bakhiet SF, Abduljabbar AS. Smartphone addiction among university students in the light of some variables. Comput Hum Behav. 2016;61:155–64. https://doi.org/10.1016/j.chb.2016.03.041.
12. Hinduja S, Patchin JW. Bullying, cyberbullying, and suicide. Arch Suicide Res. 2010;14(3):206–21. https://doi.org/10.1080/13811118.2010.494133.
13. Robin M, Kowalski RM, Limber SP, Agatston PW. Cyberbullying: bullying in the digital age. 2nd ed. London: Wiley-Blackwell; 2012. isbn:978-1-444-33481-4.
14. Friborg O, Hjemdal O, Rosenvinge JH, Martinussen M, Aslaksen PM, Flaten MA. Resilience as a moderator of pain and stress. J Psychosom Res. 2006;61(2):213–9.
15. Davydov D, Stewart R, Karen R, Isabelle C. Resilience and mental health. Clin Psychol Rev. 2010;30:479–95. https://doi.org/10.1016/j.cpr.2010.03.003.
16. Zolkoski SM, Bullock LM. Resilience in children and youth: a review. Child Youth Serv Rev. 2012;34(12):2295–303.
17. Luthar SS, Sawyer JA, Brown PJ. Conceptual issues in studies of resilience: past, present, and future research (Conference Paper). Ann N Y Acad Sci. 2006;1094:105–15.

Suggested Reading

Bor W, Dean AJ, Najman J, Hayatbakhsh R. Are child and adolescent mental health problems increasing in the 21st century? A systematic review. Aust N Z J Psychiatry. 2014;48(7):606–16. https://doi.org/10.1177/0004867414533834.

Chadi N, Bagley SM, Hadland SE. Addressing adolescents' and young adults' substance use disorders. Med Clin North Am. 2018;102(4):603–20. https://doi.org/10.1016/j.mcna.2018.02.015. Review. PubMed PMID: 29933818.

Crockett LJ, Silbereisen RK, editors. Negotiating adolescence in times of social change. Cambridge: Cambridge University Press; 2000.

Lerner RM, Steinberg L, editors. Handbook of adolescent psychology: Individual bases of adolescent development. 3rd ed. Hoboken, NJ: John Wiley & Sons Inc.; 2009. https://doi.org/10.1002/9780470479193.

Madigan S, Villani V, Azzopardi C, Laut D, Smith T, Temple JR, Browne D, Dimitropoulos G. The prevalence of unwanted online sexual exposure and solicitation among youth: a meta-analysis. J Adolesc Health. 2018; https://doi.org/10.1016/j.jadohealth.2018.03.012. pii:S1054-139X(18)30134-4. Review. PubMed PMID: 29921546.

Santrock W. Adolescence. New York, NY: McGraw-Hill Higher Education; 2005.

Sowar K, Thurber D, Vanderploeg JJ, Haldane EC. Psychiatric community crisis services for youth. Child Adolesc Psychiatr Clin N Am. 2018;27(3):479–90. https://doi.org/10.1016/j.chc.2018.03.002. Review. PubMed PMID: 29933796.

Tay JL, Tay YF, Klainin-Yobas P. Effectiveness of information and communication technologies interventions to increase mental health literacy: a systematic review. Early Interv Psychiatry. 2018; https://doi.org/10.1111/eip.12695. Review. PubMed PMID: 29897166.

Vahedi Z, Sibalis A, Sutherland JE. Are media literacy interventions effective at changing attitudes and intentions towards risky health behaviors in adolescents? A meta-analytic review. J Adolesc. 2018;67:140–52. https://doi.org/10.1016/j.adolescence.2018.06.007. Review. PubMed PMID:29957493.

Wozney L, McGrath PJ, Gehring ND, Bennett K, Huguet A, Hartling L, Dyson MP, Soleimani A, Newton AS. eMental Healthcare technologies for anxiety and depression in childhood and adolescence: systematic review of studies reporting implementation outcomes. JMIR Ment Health. 2018;5(2):e48. https://doi.org/10.2196/mental.9655. Review. PubMed PMID: 29945858; PubMed Central PMCID:PMC6039769.

List of Web Resources for Mental Health Promotion and Prevention

http://ec.europa.eu/health/ph_determinants/life_style/mental/mental_health_compass_en.htm.
http://www.mentalhealthpromotion.net/?i=promenpol.en.
http://www.friendsinfo.net/.
http://www.coolness-training.de/.
http://info.stakes.fi/aikalisa/EN.

Sexual Health, LGBT, and Human Rights 17

Manlio Converti and Antonio Ventriglio

Key Points

- **Lesbians** represent the bigger group among LGBT: women attracted by the same sex or both. Their healthcare and needs of support may differ.
- **Intersex** individuals may present a combination of many different possible chromosomal or phenotypic genetic variations and may suffer mutilation at birth.
- **Transsexual (transgender)** people face tremendous amount of stigma in the society, where sexual orientation or identity is often confused with gender, thereby creating further problems and contributing to discrimination and stigma. Gender refers to the body you feel or you fit in. Cisgender people accept their body at birth. Transgender do not accept their body and ask for surgical and/or hormonal changes.
- **Tomboy** or **sissies** are people with opposite sex behavior, with manneristic or unenforceable ways to be.
- **Gender role** can be very strongly socially influenced, and gender variation may be better accepted in some cultures compared with others.
- Women are often subjected to **misogyny,** but being LGBT may further experience **homophobia** or **transphobia**. In this chapter term **lesbophobia** is used to highlight various issues that lesbians may face.

M. Converti (✉)
AMIGAY, Italian LGBT Medical Association, and Asl Napoli 2 Nord, UOSM Giugliano, Territorial Mental Health Service, Giugliano, Italy

A. Ventriglio
Department of Clinical and Experimental Medicine, University of Foggia, Foggia, Italy
e-mail: a.ventriglio@libero.it

I. Tarricone, A. Riecher-Rössler (eds.), *Health and Gender*,
https://doi.org/10.1007/978-3-030-15038-9_17

17.1 Introduction to Sex Orienteering

Sex orienteering has been coined to describe LGBT sub-minorities in all their main nuances (Table 17.1). This is a useful instrument especially for adolescents who may be **questioning** about their own sexual orientation. They may be still confused about their own differences, especially between gender identity and sexual orientation. There may be another gap between self-well-being and illness, especially in a familiar or social perspective. Eventually the sex orienteering psychoeducational tool is somewhat helping for them to understand themselves better.

Gender role (or sex role) is a sociocultural role encompassing a range of behaviors and attitudes based on an individual actual or perceived sex or sexuality. Moreover, it influences the social representation of any LGBT sub-minority, modeling and naming the roles of their own feminine, male, or mixed behaviors. Within this framework, it is of interest to differentiate the identity gender, the sexual orientation, the gender behavior, and intersexual condition, since they refer to different life experiences and unmet needs.

Intersexual condition may occur as a result of bodily or hormonal differences. These people are often infertile. The surgery may be carried out at a very early stage in life and sometimes without their consent to a feminine status. Thus, their womanhood may prove to be problematic, because a vagina does not assign gender or sexual orientation. When they become adults, they might disagree with their condition and commit suicide [1, 2].

Transgender people are born XX or XY with normal sex organs and hormones. During the childhood, we call **gender variant** those boys telling they are girls and vice versa. These children are usually desisting during the adolescence because they understand they were confusing their homosexual orientation with a transgender

Table 17.1 The sex orienteering

LGBT minority	Cause	Binary majority
Innovation Out of schemes New roles	Gender roles	Ordinary people Preconstituted roles
Intersexuals	Chromosomes Phenotypes	XX-XY Penis or vagina
Tomboy Sissy Queer	Gender behavior	Male or female
Gender variant Transexuals Transgender MtF FtM	Gender identity	Cisgender Man or woman
Lesbian Homosexual Bisexual Pansexual Asexual	Sexual orientation	Heterosexual Straights

MtF male to female, *FtM* female to male

identity [3, 4]. Actually, some legislation is permitting the use of triptorelin to stop adolescent changes in persistent gender variants. Only when become adults, they can usually conform their bodies to the opposite sex. Only 10% is really asking to change their sex: the appearance and the social consideration usually are their main goal [4].

The few sociological studies about **tomboys** and **sissies** poorly explain about the **gender behavior**. Therefore, their status is not necessarily indicating any specific gender identity neither any sexual orientation. Being a tomboy may be used as well to gain male privileges where masculinity is a requirement [5–7].

Lesbian or **bisexual women** are often rarely considered in gender studies even if they are the biggest feminine LGBT group. International studies report some consistent differences between heterosexual, bisexual, homosexual woman, and gay and lesbians, so we presume we need to **focus on more specialized studies** [8–11].

17.2 Definition of Gender

It is important here to acknowledge the WHO (World Health Organization) definition of gender [12]:

> Gender refers to the socially constructed characteristics of women and men – such as norms, roles and relationships of and between groups of women and men … When individuals or groups do not "fit" established gender norms they often face stigma, discriminatory practices or social exclusion – all of which adversely affect health (…) …
>
> Gender requires us to ensure that health policy, programs, services and delivery models are responsive to the needs of women, men, girls and boys in all their diversity.
>
> Gender norms, roles and relations influence people's susceptibility to different health conditions and diseases and affect their enjoyment of good mental, physical health and well-being. They also have a bearing on people's access to and uptake of health services and on the health outcomes they experience throughout the life-course (…) …

17.3 The Feminine and the Feminist Perspective of Gender

The attribution of feminine role to lesbians is relatively easily acceptable in many countries. The main lesbian associations are sometimes uncomfortable with the transgender people, denying the womanhood of MtF (male to female) transsexual people [13, 14]. In the same way, women medical association or feminist groups are denying lesbian representative rights, usually simply avoiding speaking about them.

17.4 Lesbian, Transgender, and Intersexual Differences: The Coming Out

LGBT individuals have always been a minority, historically and consistently, even though social acceptance may well have varied. This may have contributed to **minority stress** and consequent high levels of discrimination and stigma. Not surprisingly, this affects their own self-esteem and increases stress, which in turn has contributed to higher than expected levels of various psychiatric disorders and changes in their lifestyle [15], including physical complaints.

Coming out is the phenomenon by which the individuals firstly acknowledge to themselves their own sexual orientation or uneven gender identity and then gradually start to tell others about it. Usually they firstly tell their friends before their own family. Employers and other peers are usually involved much later. This process is largely voluntary, but in some circumstances (e.g., to hinder someone career or for political reasons) people may be outed without their own consent (**outing**). Thus, perceived or real threat of **outing** may contribute further to stress and distress.

People may need some **help to disclose** and special support [16–20], since they may feel unsafe and may think there is no going back after the outing. There have been arguments that staying in the "closet" may be better for some individuals (e.g., people living in developing countries, very religious family of origin, other ethnicity in a western country, very poor family of origin, very poor sociocultural context) [21]. Nevertheless, here we consider the coming out and its related **social and sanitary support** really changing worldwide and affecting the LGBT life.

The coming out not just represents LGBT political acting to contrast homophobia worldwide but a specific resilient and safe way of living a healthy life. In fact, it is demonstrated to be psychologically, socially, and physically healthy to come out [22].

The social support to the coming out should firstly involve the family of LGBT people. Relatives and parents should be helped to accept the chance to deal an intersexual child and its consequences. Specific courses and scholar interventions could also reduce familiar and social homophobia against LGBT child and their coming out in the adolescence.

Specific undergraduate healthcare education and professional training programs are needed to ameliorate and change the health trajectory for lesbian women and transgender men or women, supporting and educating the key stakeholders [23]. It is a difficult target to reduce lesbophobia and misogyny also for the missing research and tools on women and their role in the society. Social support to their coming out remains the only known good instrument to help them in the life course [24].

17.5 Lesbian, Transgender, and Intersexual: A Medical History

Lesbianism is not a recent phenomenon and has existed throughout history and across all cultures. Since Saffo, the ancient Greek poet from Lesbo Island, few others were famous, also in the medical field.

However, we can recall Madeleine Pelletier, first French psychiatrist, cross-dresser; Marie Equi, USA's first social doctor, openly lesbian, who adopted with her beloved partner a child; or Dr. Alan L. Hart, radiologist and tuberculosis researcher, born woman, lived disguised as a man, twice really married with women and beloved adoptive father, too [25–27]. We cannot forget Evelyn Hooker, the first psychologist researcher to dismantle the myth that homosexual men and women are inherently unhealthy [28].

Especially in western countries, we actually see also transsexual people graduating in medicine; facing this big problem, they usually change sex during the university courses. It is very important to improve the bureaucracy, permitting a third gender to be included in the administration of public trails.

17.6 The Lesbian Violence Risk

Violence against women is common, but violence against lesbians is much higher, as they are not seen as conforming to the standard model of women's roles in the society [29, 30].

Many countries still consider only combined marriages, also in the early age. In many others men believe it may be therapeutic to rape a lesbian woman in order to covert her [31, 32]. Also, it is of note the high risk of a lesbian partner violence [33]. Peer education and services against sexual violence in colleges and universities need to be developed further [34]. Interestingly, the Olympic Committees are also considering the sexual violence against LGBT people as a sport-related problem to deal with [35].

17.7 Vulnerable Factors for Lesbians Health

Health issues among lesbians and transgender women considered to be important are (Table 17.2) substance abuse, sexual health and sexually transmitted diseases, early and later pregnancy difference, obesity and other eating disorders, cardiovascular prevention, cancer prevention and screening, depression and other

Table 17.2 The gender medicine gap

LGBT minority	Cause	Solution
Intersexuals	Newborn Mutilation	Consider their will, psychological, hormonal or surgeons help
Gender Variant	Transphobia Rape Bullying	Consider their will, psychological, hormonal, or surgeons help
Tomboy Sissy Queer	Bullying	Psychological and social support
Transexuals Transgender MtF FtM	Transition rights	Rights with or without sexual transition Hormones and surgeon free familial and social support
Lesbian Bisexual FtM transsexuals FtM transgender	Eating disorders, obesity, pregnancy, breast cancer, HPV-related cancers, candida, substance abuse (tobacco or alcohol) rape, cardiovascular risk, child abuse, partner abuse, loneliness depression, suicide risk	Specific anamnestic Gayfriendly approach Active support to coming out Specific spot and material for prevention, diagnostic and healthcare

MtF male to female, *FtM* female to male

psychological disorders, social isolation, suicide, and personal and intimate partner violence [15, 36].

After decades of debating, actually the scientific community considers those differences mostly caused by neglecting oneself health or direct hit of lesbophobia.

These differences in lesbian health care needs may be partly due to lesbophobia. When health professionals avoid LGBT patients, it may be due to sanitary or health lesbophobia. Contrarily, lesbian "heterosexism introverted" would reduce compliance to preventive or medical programs [37, 38].

17.8 Protective Health Factors for Lesbians

The main protective factor is an open and positive speaking by nurses and doctors around sexual orientation and gender identities since the first sanitary interview. It helps them to reduce their fear of any lesbophobic reaction [39, 40].

Fight against stigma is another big deal. Many American scientific associations (American Academy of Family Physicians, American Academy of Nursing, American Academy of Pediatrics, American College of Emergency Physicians, American College of Nurse-Midwives, American College of Obstetrics and Gynecology, American College of Physicians, American Medical Association, American Psychiatric Association, American Psychological Association, and American Public Health Association) have already included this aim in their statements [41].

Adolescence and childhood are very problematic moments of human life when **questioning** people are much more represented than LGBT well-confirmed one. As stated above, sex orienteering tool (Table 17.1) can help those people someway.

17.9 Genomic Differences

The only important genomic differences to be considered may be the **intersexual** condition at birth. Their genital mutilation is now considered a crime in some western legislations [42, 43].

17.10 Differences in Work Places

The gender role and expectations for women are still an issue in the workplaces especially if lesbian or transgender individuals [44]. Apart from unequal salaries, issues reported are often related to motherhood, artificial insemination, surrogacy, and adoption, all them need to be accepted in a job contract.

Anti-discriminatory legislation and enlightenment targeting negative attitudes and prejudice against lesbians and gay men could decrease the negative bias that they face in accessing a new job [44].

Transgender workers report a double rate of unemployment if compared to the general population [45]. Most of MtF transgender people are still involved in prostitution, as the only possible source of income; they may experience homelessness or poverty since their relatives reject sometimes them during the childhood or adolescence [15]. The lack of documents corresponding to their sex change is possible reason of unemployment [44].

Support their recognition in the society and families is a big deal for the modern society.

17.11 Educational Factors

Especially for young women who are "struggling" with their sexual orientation or are coming out, schools and universities may also be stressful places. Teaching about sexual orientation and around lesbian and transgender historical contribution will also help [45–47]. This can create safe spaces against bullying in the real and cyber world, through lesbian and straight alliances [48].

17.12 Problems Related to *Migration*

Lesbians may seek refuge or asylum in countries, which are probably supportive. Migration experience is not simple and leads to problems in the pre-migration phase as well as post-migration adjustment. During the migration process, the risk of being raped or being trafficked is high [31].

These problematic issues suggest sometime a need for a series of differentiated relocation places for regular and irregular LGBT migrants [49].

17.13 Role of Media, Cinema, Music, or Dance

Worldwide LGBT expressions into the media are sometimes censored or hidden or falsified [50, 51]. The slow rising of LGBT-positive representations or spontaneous coming outs began when media, cinema, music, and sport stars came out. Kissing or dancing between women is still a lesbophobic issue.

Bessie Jackson and her "bull dagger" woman, Rae Bourbon, singing around "her change of sex" to female, are some of LGBT well-known singers.

Marlene Dietrich kissed in man dresses a woman on screen in Morocco.

Greta Garbo kissed also a woman in Queen Christina, and both movie stars have a thrilling love and spying affair during the Second World War.

Maud Allen was depicted as an extraordinary dancer, spy, and lesbian too [50, 51].

17.14 Sports and LGBT

Lesbian or tomboy runners existed also during the historical Olympic Games as representative of Sparta. Actually, there is a ban in lesbophobic countries, although international games are officially open to their participation. Coming out is still rare: Nicole Bonamino in Italy is the only sport-lesbian known. In general, few lesbians and very few transsexual people are really playing sports [52].

Some transsexual people are also considered for doping in any competitive sport because of their status [53].

An international self-organized group born in 1970 called LGBT Open Games aims to change legislation and improve sport participation.

Halbrook group investigated also the role of sport as a distraction from sexuality, the problem of invisibility and isolation within sports, and the importance for self-well-being to come out within a team [54].

17.15 Dietary Problems

Many studies exemplify the role of lesbophobia in the **eating disorders** among LGBT people. Sexual variations may be the background on any eating disorder and should be assessed. In addition, obesity may be predictable in some "closeted" lesbian. Many studies suggested it might be due to "internalized heterosexism" [55–57].

The prediction of **obesity** is also important for closed lesbians, especially during the adolescence. It has been reported it may be a self-contempt caused by internalized heterosexism or as a prize for male disdain [58].

17.16 Motherhood

A major challenge in the society is the issue of motherhood for lesbian individuals as this raises political issues and further stigma.

The motherhood for LGBT people can be seen as both a ghost and a mourning [59]. There is no evidence to suggest that LGBT individuals would be bad parents. After decades of debating, quite all the reviews on this subject confirmed there is any difference in growing with straight or LGBT parents. Lesbian or transgender relatives assure their children also an adequate social environment and education [60].

Motherhood in lesbian women can be a result of natural sex or semen donation by a friend. Motherhood should be also a protective special factor against the mourning risk in their fantasies.

17.17 Sexual Health and Human Rights

Transgender women (MtF (Male to Female)) are at higher risk for HIV (human immunodeficiency virus) and other STI (sexual transmitted illnesses), especially if forced to prostitution. Little is known around lesbian sexual health [8–10].

Mammography, Pap test, and vaccines against HPV (human papillomavirus) and HAV (hepatitis A virus) must be considered for lesbians too, supporting them specifically [8–10, 15, 36, 37]. It has been shown that the life expectancy is highly reduced for lesbians because they neglect their health or healthcare system do not support them enough [17].

Still quite never Women's Health Spots identify lesbian or transgender women as subject of interest in their claim to prevention, neither to ameliorate life styles [36, 37]. The lesbophobia or indifference against lesbians may affect negatively prevention, diagnostic, and caring programs for this population.

Candida is the first STI to be detected [61], and **breast cancer** [62] is the most common cancer for lesbian and bisexual women. Is a big aim to help them fighting obesity, smoking, alcohol or drug abuse, as well as to help them specifically to prevent Candida or other STI and breast cancer through health advertisments directed to LGBT women [36, 37].

Transsexual condition is more problematic and less studied, because of the adverse legislations too [63].

17.18 Elder Age

The Stonewall generation is today reaching the elder age, forcing to rethink the movement itself, not only around the adolescent and youth rights.

The main problem of each elderly is the stress of mourning, the isolation, and loneliness, but LGBT people used to experience it since adolescence. The main usual problem for an elder lesbian or transgender woman remains to fight against lesbophobia, when they are more fragile and needing help [64, 65].

17.19 Other Specifics

New technologies are once again increasing the likelihood of people remaining in the closet. It is easier to date privately and sometimes also working and buying online. On the opposite, cyberbullying can arise depressive mood and suicidal risk [66, 67].

The coming out is the only consistent tool for real and welcoming relationships.

Adversities from family and societies stop aspirations and needs for lesbians. Media, celebrities, and Lesbian-Transgender Pride events are helpful to support coming out and LGBT rights in the real life [68, 69].

References

1. Schweizer K, et al. Coping with diverse sex development: treatment experiences and psychosocial support during childhood and adolescence and adult well-being. J Pediatr Psychol. 2017;42(5):504–19.
2. Falhammar H, et al. Health status in 1040 adults with disorders of sex development (DSD): a European multicenter study. Endoc Conn. 2018;7(3):466–78.
3. Drescher J, Cohen-Kettenis PT, Reed GM. Gender incongruence of childhood in the ICD-11: controversies, proposal, and rationale. Lancet Psychiatry. 2016;3(3):297–304.

4. Judge C, et al. Gender dysphoria – prevalence and co-morbidities in an Irish adult population. Front Endocrinol (Lausanne). 2014;5:87.
5. Hilgenkamp HD, Livingsston MM. Tomboys, masculine characteristics, and self-ratings of confidence in career success. Psychol Rep. 2002;90(3 Pt 1):743–9.
6. Craig T. Lacroix. Tomboy as protective identity. J Lesbian Stud. 2011;15(4):450–65.
7. Hall JM. Tomboys: meanings, marginalization, and misunderstandings. J Issues Ment Health Nurs. 2008;29(6):555–65.
8. Diamant AL, et al. Health behaviors, health status and access to and use of health care: a population-based study of lesbian, bisexual and heterosexual women. Arch Fam Med. 2000;9:1043–51.
9. Valanis BG, et al. Sexual orientation and health: comparisons in the Women's Health Initiative sample. Arch Fam Med. 2000;9:843–53.
10. White J, et al. Health risk factors and health seeking behaviour in lesbians. J Womens Health. 1997;6:103–12.
11. Cochran SD, et al. Cancer-related risk indicators and preventive screening behaviors among lesbians and bisexual women. Am J Public Health. 2001;91:591–7.
12. http://www.who.int/gender-equity-rights/understanding/gender-definition/en/.
13. https://www.gay.it/donne/news/arcilesbica-le-donne-trans-la-biologia-conta.
14. https://www.independent.co.uk/voices/anti-trans-protests-london-pride-transgender-transphobia-terf-lgbt-feminist-a8448521.html.
15. Hatzenbuehler ML, Pachankis JE. Stigma and minority stress as social determinants of health among lesbian, gay, bisexual, and transgender youth: research evidence and clinical implications. Pediatr Clin North Am. 2016;63(6):985–97.
16. Giammattei SV. Beyond the binary: trans-negotiations in couple and family therapy. Fam Process. 2015;54(3):418–34.
17. St. Pierre M. Under what conditions do lesbians disclose their sexual orientation to primary healthcare providers? A review of the literature. J Lesbian Stud. 2012;16(2):199–219.
18. Heatherington L, Lavner JA. Coming to terms with coming out: review and recommendations for family systems-focused research. J Fam Psychol. 2008;22(3):329–43.
19. Goldfried MR, Goldfried AP. The importance of parental support in the lives of gay, lesbian, and bisexual individuals. J Clin Psychol. 2001;57(5):681–93.
20. Benton J. Making schools safer and healthier for lesbian, gay, bisexual, and questioning students. J Sch Nurs. 2003;19(5):251–9.
21. Green RJ. "Lesbians, gay men, and their parents": a critique of LaSala and the prevailing clinical "wisdom". Fam Process. 2000;39(2):257–66.
22. Bry LJ, et al. Management of a concealable stigmatized identity: a qualitative study of concealment, disclosure and role flexing among young, resilient sexual and gender minority individuals. J Homosex. 2017;64(6):745.
23. Rodgers SM. Transitional age lesbian, gay, bisexual, transgender, and questioning youth: issues of diversity, integrated identities, and mental health. Child Adolesc Psychiatr Clin N Am. 2017;26(2):297.
24. McCann E, Brown M. The inclusion of LGBT+ health issues within undergraduate healthcare education and professional training programmes: a systematic review. Nurse Educ Today. 2018;64:204.
25. http://www.encyclopedia.com/women/encyclopedias-almanacs-transcripts-and-maps/pelletier-madeleine-1874-1939.
26. https://en.wikipedia.org/wiki/Marie_Equi.
27. http://ftmitalia.blogspot.it/2015/03/ftm-story.html?m=1.
28. American Psychology Association history about Evelyn Hooker. http://www.apa.org/research/action/gay.aspx.
29. Rothman EF, Exner D, Baughman AL. The prevalence of sexual assault against people who identify as gay, lesbian, or bisexual in the United States: a systematic review. Trauma Violence Abuse. 2011;12(2):55–66.

30. Blondeel K, de Vasconcelos S, García-Moreno C, Stephenson R, Temmerman M, Toskin I. Violence motivated by perception of sexual orientation and gender identity: a systematic review. Bull World Health Organ. 2018;96(1):29–41L.
31. https://en.wikipedia.org/wiki/LGBTQ_migration.
32. Calton JM, Cattaneo LB, Gebhard KT. Barriers to help seeking for lesbian, gay, bisexual, transgender, and queer survivors of intimate partner violence. Trauma Violence Abuse. 2016;17(5):585–600.
33. Edwards KM, Littleton HL, Sylaska KM, Crossman AL, Craig M. College campus community readiness to address intimate partner violence among LGBTQ+ young adults: a conceptual and empirical examination. Am J Community Psychol. 2016;58(1-2):16–26.
34. Mountjoy M, Brackenridge C, Arrington M, Blauwet C, Carska-Sheppard A, Fasting K, Kirby S, Leahy T, Marks S, Martin K, Starr K, Tiivas A, Budgett R. International Olympic Committee consensus statement: harassment and abuse (non-accidental violence) in sport. Br J Sports Med. 2016;50(17):1019–29.
35. Schulman JK, Erickson-Schroth L. Mental health in sexual minority and transgender women. Psychiatr Clin North Am. 2017;40(2):309–19.
36. Turčan P. [Specifics of medical care for lesbians]. [Article in Czech]. Ceska Gynekol 2015;80(2):104-114
37. Floyd SR, Pierce DM, Geraci SA. Preventive and primary care for lesbian, gay and bisexual patients. Am J Med Sci. 2016;352(6):637–43.
38. Bjarnadottir RI, Bockting W, Dowding DW. Patient perspectives on answering questions about sexual orientation and gender identity: an integrative review. J Clin Nurs. 2017;26(13-14):1814–33.
39. U.S. Transgender Survey Report. 2015. http://www.ustranssurvey.org/reports.
40. USA Medical and Nurse position statements about LGBT Health Rights. https://www.google.com/url?sa=t&rct=j&q=&esrc=s&source=web&cd=1&cad=rja&uact=8&ved=2ahUKEwjp15rNpM7cAhVJG5oKHRL8AngQFjAAegQICRAB&url=http%3A%2F%2Fwww.glma.org%2F_data%2Fn_0001%2Fresources%2Flive%2FGLMA%2520Compendium%2520of%2520Health%2520Profession%2520Association%2520LGBT%2520Policy%2520and%2520Position%2520Statements.pdf&usg=AOvVaw1Td8CKdQwE7eCsGx6J4gSY.
41. https://www.intersexequality.com/tag/glma-statement-intersex/.
42. https://www.linkiesta.it/it/article/2018/05/19/intersessuali-e-invisibili-anche-in-italia-subiscono-pregiudizi-e-muti/38151/.
43. Fric K. Access to the labour market for gays and lesbians: research review. J Gay Lesb Soc Serv. 2017;29:319.
44. https://www.hrc.org/blog/transgender-workers-at-greater-risk-for-unemployment-and-poverty.
45. http://www.stonewall.org.uk/get-involved/education/secondary-schools.
46. Erhard RL, Ben-Ami E. The schooling experience of lesbian, gay, and bisexual youth in Israel: falling below and rising above as a matter of social ecology. J Homosex. 2016;63(2):193–227.
47. Lim FA, Hsu R. Nursing students' attitudes toward lesbian, gay, bisexual, and transgender persons: an integrative review. Nurs Educ Perspect. 2016;37(3):144–52.
48. Marx RA, Kettrey HH. Gay-straight alliances are associated with lower levels of school-based victimization of LGBTQ+ youth: a systematic review and meta-analysis. J Youth Adolesc. 2016;45(7):1269–82.
49. Walsh CF. "It really is not just gay, but African American gay": the impact of community and church on the experiences of black lesbians living in North Central Florida. J Homosex. 2016;63(9):1236–52.
50. https://en.wikipedia.org/wiki/Media_portrayal_of_LGBT_people.
51. https://it.wikipedia.org/wiki/Storia_del_lesbismo#Il_XX_secolo_2.
52. https://en.wikipedia.org/wiki/Homosexuality_in_modern_sports.
53. Jones BA. Sport and transgender people: a systematic review of the literature relating to sport participation and competitive sport policies. Sports Med. 2017;47(4):701–16.

54. Halbrook MK, et al. High school coaches' experiences with openly lesbian, gay, and bisexual athletes. J Homosex. 2018;17:1–19.
55. Calzo JP, et al. Eating disorders and disordered weight and shape control behaviors in sexual minority populations. Curr Psychiatry Rep. 2017;19(8):49.
56. McClain Z, Peebles R. Body image and eating disorders among lesbian, gay, bisexual, and transgender youth. Pediatr Clin North Am. 2016;63(6):1079–90.
57. Jones BA, et al. Body dissatisfaction and disordered eating in trans people: a systematic review of the literature. Int Rev Psychiatry. 2016;28(1):81–94.
58. Eliason MJ, Fogel SC. An ecological framework for sexual minority women's health: factors associated with greater body mass. J Homosex. 2015;62(7):845–82.
59. Hodson K, Meads C, Bewley S. Lesbian and bisexual women's likelihood of becoming pregnant: a systematic review and meta-analysis. BJOG. 2017;124(3):393–402.
60. Rubio B, et al. Transition to parenthood and quality of parenting among gay, lesbian and heterosexual couples who conceived through assisted reproduction. J Fam Stud. 2017; https://doi.org/10.1080/13229400.2017.1413005.
61. Bailey JV, Benato R, Owen C, Kavanagh J. Vulvovaginal candidiasis in women who have sex with women. Sex Transm Dis. 2008;35(6):533–6.
62. Lisy K, et al. Experiences and unmet needs of lesbian, gay and bisexual people with cancer care: a systematic review and meta-synthesis. Psychooncology. 2018;27:1480.
63. Nikolić D. Breast cancer and its impact in male transsexuals. Breast Cancer Res Treat. 2018;171:565.
64. Caceres BA, Frank MO. Successful ageing in lesbian, gay and bisexual older people: a concept analysis. Int J Older People Nurs. 2016;11(3):184–93.
65. Waite H. Old lesbians: gendered histories and persistent challenges. Australas J Ageing. 2015;34(Suppl 2):8–13.
66. Huang ET, Williams H, Hocking JS, Lim MS. Safe sex messages within dating and entertainment smartphone apps: a review. JMIR Mhealth Uhealth. 2016;4(4):e124.
67. Escobar-Viera CG, et al. For better or for worse? A systematic review of the evidence on social media use and depression among lesbian, gay, and bisexual minorities. JMIR Ment Health. 2018;5:e10496.
68. Berg RC, Munthe-Kaas HM, Ross MW. Internalized homonegativity: a systematic mapping review of empirical research. J Homosex. 2016;63(4):541–58.
69. Doyle DM, Molix L. Author manuscript; Social stigma and sexual minorities' romantic relationship functioning: a meta-analytic review. Pers Soc Psychol Bull. 2015;41:1363.

Senility

18

Marco Domenicali and Annagiulia Gramenzi

Key Points

- The male-female health-survival paradox: females live longer than males but with poorer health.
- Sarcopenia and osteoarthritis are frequent during senility and present several gender-related differences.

Senility is a term used to describe a decline in an older adult's physical and cognitive health. Like dementia, senility can cause changes in mental health, such as memory loss or a decline in judgment. But senility symptoms can also include physical changes such as:

- Stiff joints
- Change in posture
- Decreased strength
- Wrinkling of the skin
- Loss of vision or hearing
- Brittle bones or bone loss

Women live longer than men, and this difference in life expectancy is a worldwide phenomenon indicating that the difference in mortality seems strongly influenced by gender defined as the combination between biological and social factors [1–3]. However, the survival advantage of women is counterbalanced by a poorer

M. Domenicali (✉) · A. Gramenzi
Dipartimento di Scienze Mediche e Chirurgiche, Alma Mater Studiorum - Università di Bologna, Bologna, Italy
e-mail: m.domenicali@unibo.it

I. Tarricone, A. Riecher-Rössler (eds.), *Health and Gender*,
https://doi.org/10.1007/978-3-030-15038-9_18

quality of life in advanced age due to an increased prevalence of a variety of disabling nonlethal pathological conditions [4, 5]. This so-called mortality-morbidity paradox has several plausible hypotheses [6]. The first is that simply by virtue of reaching advanced old age, women are more likely to develop every age-related disease. A second possible explanation may be found in a higher female attention to physical discomfort and illness that led the women to seek medical attention more frequently than men. In general, women are more medicalized in terms of frequency of medical visits, days of hospitalization, and number of drugs routinely administrated [7, 8]. In addition, the higher susceptibility and severity of arthritis and musculoskeletal disease among older women [1, 6] widely contributes to their worse health and functional status. In any case, humans are currently the only species in which the mortality-morbidity paradox has been observed.

18.1 Disability

The overall prevalence and severity of disability among older women will continue to increase in line with the growing aging population and the higher proportion of elderly women in the oldest age groups. It has been consistently shown that women have higher prevalence rates of disability in activities of daily living (ADL), instrumental activities of daily living (IADL), and physical tasks compared to men [9]. Furthermore, among adults with disabilities, women experience higher rates of limitations in both basic and complex activity limitations than men [10].

Several health, disease, behavioral, and sociodemographic factors as well as gender-based discrimination contribute to the higher prevalence of disability in women compared to men. Women have a longer duration of life lived with disability, in part due to higher prevalence of nonfatal chronic conditions, constitutional factors such as body composition, lower muscle strength and lower bone density, and higher rates of modifiable lifestyle factors such as sedentary behavior and obesity [11]. Several of these factors are modifiable and provide important targets for researchers, clinicians, and public health practitioners in their efforts to reduce the burden of disability in the older population and improve older women's quality of life even though gender differences in comorbidity and disability appear to be still poorly considered and investigated despite their biomedical and social relevance. The burden of disability in older women has wide-ranging and profound effects on older women themselves, their families, and the health-care system. Therefore, clinical studies aimed at understanding the gender-related factors in the physical, social, and economic environments that are associated with women's disabilities in later life are urgently needed.

18.2 Sarcopenia

Age-related loss in skeletal muscle mass and function, a condition commonly referred to as sarcopenia, could explain at least in part the high physical disability rate in older men and women. Reduced muscle mass in older age can have significant consequences for day-to-day living. For example, the Framingham study showed that 40% of women aged 55–64 and 65% of women aged 75–84 were unable to lift 4.5 kg [12]. Prevalence estimates for sarcopenia vary widely in different clinical settings, depending on the population studied, the measurement techniques, and the operational definition used [13]. Although considerable variation in the rate of skeletal muscle mass loss does exist, progressive loss of muscle mass appears inevitable, with annual rate of decline of 1–2% from as early as age 50 reaching more than 50% in individuals above the age of 80 [14, 15], and muscle strength decline of 1.5% per year between ages 50 and 60 increasing to 3% annually [14]. To prevent or treat sarcopenia, predictors of skeletal muscle mass loss should be identified, even though the multifactorial etiology makes them difficult to discern, especially in elderly patients exhibiting several of these extrinsic and intrinsic morbidities at the same time [16]. Epidemiological data for older sex-specific sarcopenia have been conflicting [13]. Since gender greatly influences muscle mass, several studies had suggested that men experience a greater decline in muscle mass than women [13, 17]. However, it has been recently shown that in older women sarcopenia confers a higher mortality risk despite its lower prevalence compared to their male counterparts [18].

18.3 Osteoarthritis and Osteoporosis

Osteoarthritis and osteoporosis are major causes of chronic disability in older adults and are associated with chronic pain and limited quality of life and disability. Gender differences exist in the presentation of these musculoskeletal diseases, and recognition of the differences between men and women's burden of disease and response to treatment is key in optimizing care. Between the ages of 60 and 90 years, women are more likely than men to suffer from osteoarthritis, and women experience more severe arthritis in the knee [19, 20]. Although the presentation of osteoarthritis does not differ between men and women, symptom severity does. Additionally, women are three times less likely than men to undergo hip or knee arthroplasty [20]. Osteoporosis is three times more common in women than in men, partly because women have a lower peak bone mass and partly because of the hormonal changes that occur at menopause and the effect of pregnancy which can alter calcium composition in a woman's body in the absence of appropriate diet and/or administration of calcium supplements [21]. The gender gap in diagnosis and treatment of osteoporosis after a fragility fracture is wide. In particular it has been consistently shown that only few male patients with hip fractures undergoes bone mineral density testing and most of them does not receive any osteoporosis treatment [19]. On the other side while both osteoarthritis and osteoporosis and consequent fractures, spontaneous or caused by falls, place an enormous burden on the health-care system and society, often they do not get the attention they deserve because they are incorrectly seen as an inevitable part of aging especially in women or less serious than such conditions as heart disease or cancer.

References

1. Ostan R, Monti D, Gueresi P, Bussolotto M, Franceschi C, Baggio G. Gender, aging and longevity in humans: an update of an intriguing/neglected scenario paving the way to a gender-specific medicine. Clin Sci (Lond). 2016;130:1711–25.
2. Regitz-Zagrosek V. Sex and gender differences in health. EMBO Rep. 2012;13:596–603.
3. Barford A, Dorling D. Life expectancy: women now on top everywhere. BMJ. 2006;332:808.
4. Van Oyen H, Nusselder W, Jagger C, Kolip P, Cambois E, Robine JM. Gender differences in healthy life years within the EU: an exploration of the "health-survival" paradox. Int J Public Health. 2013;58:143–55.
5. Jagger C, Gillies C, Moscone F, Cambois E, Van Oyen H, Nusselder W, Robine J-M. Inequalities in healthy life years in the 25 countries of the European Union in 2005: a cross-national meta-regression analysis. Lancet. 2008;372:2124–31.
6. Austad SN, Fischer KE. Sex differences in lifespan. Cell Metab. 2016;23:1022–33.
7. Christensen K, Doblhammer G, Rau R, Vaupel JW. Ageing populations: the challenges ahead. Lancet. 2009;374:1196–208.
8. Austad SN, Bartke A. Sex differences in longevity and in responses to anti-aging interventions: a mini-review. Gerontology. 2015;62:40–6.
9. Leveille SG, Resnick HE, Balfour J. Gender differences in disability: evidence and underlying reasons. Aging Clin Exp Res. 2000;12:106–12.
10. Murtagh KN, Hubert HB. Gender differences in physical disability among an elderly cohort. Am J Public Health. 2004;94:1406–11.
11. Clegg A, Young J, Iliffe S, Rikkert MO, Rockwood K. Frailty in elderly people. Lancet. 2013;381:752–62.
12. Jetté A, Branch L. The Framingham disability study. II. Physical disability among the aging. Am J Public Health. 1981;71:1211–6.
13. Cruz-Jentoft AJ, Landi F, Schneider SM, Zúñiga C, Arai H, Boirie Y, Chen LK, Fielding RA, Martin FC, Michel JP, Sieber C, Stout JR, Studenski SA, Vellas B, Woo J, Zamboni M, Cederholm T. Prevalence of and interventions for sarcopenia in ageing adults: a systematic review. Report of the International Sarcopenia Initiative (EWGSOP and IWGS). Age Ageing. 2014;43:748–59.
14. von Haehling S, Morley JE, Anker SD. An overview of sarcopenia: facts and numbers on prevalence and clinical impact. J Cachexia Sarcopenia Muscle. 2010;1:129–33.
15. Baumgartner RN, Koehler KM, Gallagher D, et al. Epidemiology of sarcopenia among the elderly in New Mexico. Am J Epidemiol. 1998;147:755–63.
16. Biolo G, Cederholm T, Muscaritoli M. Muscle contractile and metabolic dysfunction is a common feature of sarcopenia of aging and chronic diseases: from sarcopenic obesity to cachexia. Clin Nutr. 2014;33:737–48.
17. Gallagher D, Visser M, DeMeersman RE, et al. Appendicular skeletal muscle mass: effects of age, gender, and ethnicity. J Appl Physiol. 1997;83:229–39.
18. Batsis JA, Mackenzie TA, Barre LK, et al. Sarcopenia, sarcopenic obesity and mortality in older adults: results from the National Health and Nutrition Examination Survey III. Eur J Clin Nutr. 2014;68:1001–7.
19. Wolf JM, Cannada L, Van Heest AE, O'Connor MI, Ladd AL. Male and female differences in musculoskeletal disease. J Am Acad Orthop Surg. 2015;23:339–47.
20. O'Connor MI. Sex differences in osteoarthritis of the hip and knee. J Am Acad Orthop Surg. 2007;15(Suppl 1):S22–5.
21. Cawthon PM. Gender differences in osteoporosis and fractures. Clin Orthop Relat Res. 2011;469:1900–5.

Part IV

Gender Aspects in Medical Disorders and Care

Heart and Vascular Disorders: Gender Differences in Acute Coronary Syndrome

19

Olivia Manfrini and Edina Cenko

Abbreviations

ACS	Acute coronary syndrome
AMI	Acute myocardial infarction
CVD	Cardiovascular diseases
DAPT	Dual antiplatelet therapy
ECG	Electrocardiogram
NSTE-ACS	Non-ST-segment elevation acute coronary syndrome
PCI	Percutaneous coronary intervention
ST	ST segment at ECG
STEMI	ST-segment elevation myocardial infarction

Key Points

- Cardiovascular disease is the first single cause of mortality, both in men and women.
- Sex differences in clinical presentation have detrimental consequences for timely diagnosis and treatment, resulting in high risk of death for women.
- In both women and men, the most common symptom is typical chest pain/discomfort; however, women often present with atypical chest pain and angina equivalent symptoms such as fatigue, dyspnea, diaphoresis, weakness, and nausea/vomiting.

O. Manfrini (✉) · E. Cenko
Dipartimento di Medicina Specialistica, Diagnostica e Sperimentale, Università di Bologna, Bologna, Italy
e-mail: Olivia.manfrini@unibo.it; edina.cenko2@unibo.it

I. Tarricone, A. Riecher-Rössler (eds.), *Health and Gender*,
https://doi.org/10.1007/978-3-030-15038-9_19

- In case of suspicion of a heart attack it necessary to call immediately the emergency service: "time is heart muscle", more time passes without restoring blood flow, the greater the damage to the heart muscle and the risk of death.
- In the setting of AMI, women have more complications such as shock, heart failure, reinfarction, recurrent ischemia/reinfarction, bleeding, and stroke than men.

19.1 Introduction

Diseases of the heart and circulatory system, also called cardiovascular diseases (CVD), are the leading cause of mortality globally, both in men and in women [1–3]. The "Europe Cardiovascular Disease Statistics 2017" reported that CVD is currently responsible for over 3.9 million deaths in 1 year, that is, 45% of all deaths. Specifically, CVD accounts for 1.8 million deaths (40% of all deaths) in men, and 2.1 million deaths (49% of all deaths) in women. By comparison, cancer—the next most common cause of death—accounts for just under 1.1 million deaths (24%) in men and just under 900,000 deaths (20%) in women [1].

The main forms of CVD are ischemic heart disease and stroke. Stroke is the second most common single cause of death, accounting for 9% of deaths in men and 13% of deaths in women each year in Europe [1]. Ischemic heart disease is the first single cause of mortality [2, 3], responsible for 19% and 20% of all deaths in Europe each year among men and women, respectively [1].

In most patients, either men or women, ischemic heart disease shows up the first time acutely with the so-called acute coronary syndrome (generally speaking "heart attack") that can be unstable angina or acute myocardial infarction (AMI), and it occurs when a part of the heart muscle suddenly does not receive enough blood flow [4–7]. Emerging data highlight several gender differences in pathophysiology, clinical presentation, and outcome [8–10].

Since early statistics performed in 1984, it was evident that more women die of AMI than men [11]. However, only in 1990, two studies published in the *New England Journal of Medicine* provided evidence that there was sex bias in the management of ischemic heart disease [12, 13]. Women were significantly less likely to undergo coronary angiography and coronary revascularization when admitted to the hospital with a diagnosis of AMI, unstable or stable angina, or chest pain. The reason for the aforementioned disparity was attributed to the fact that early research studies were exclusively conducted in male populations, so that neither women nor their doctors could fully have recognized that AMI was the leading cause of death even in women, who often do not exhibit those typical male signs and symptoms [12–14]. Actually, when a woman presented herself clinically as a man, she had the same propensity to be treated like a man. As a result of this observation, Bernadine Healy, at that time chief of National Institutes of Health (Bethesda, MD, USA), had provocatively named "Ischemic Heart Disease in Women" as Yentl syndrome (inspired by Yentl, the nineteenth-century heroine of Isaac Bashevis Singer's short story, who had to disguise herself as a man to attend school and study the Talmud) [14]. Despite that alarming evidence, just because the first step toward surviving a heart attack is learning to recognize symptoms, and women frequently don't have the typical (of the male gender) clinical presentation, for many years, women had dramatically high mortality rates for ischemic heart disease, mainly due to be underdiagnosed and undertreated [11, 15–17]. Indeed, with the great advances in medical and percutaneous treatments of the following next 10 years, the mortality rate for acute coronary syndrome (ACS) decreased rapidly in male, but not in female [1–3, 11]. Only, over the first decade of the twenty-first century (at least in the USA and Western European countries), there have been marked reductions in CVD also in women [15–18]. Nevertheless, sex differences in clinical presentation still have detrimental consequences for timely diagnosis and timely treatment, resulting in high risk of death for women in many countries [19, 20]. Especially young women who have a higher short-term mortality than men in the same age group [21].

19.2 Pathophysiology and Coronary Anatomy

ACSs are due to a sudden interruption of the coronary blood flow [4, 5, 22]. The most common causes are:

1. Coronary thrombosis due to rupture of a lipid-rich plaque (over 75% of men and 55% of women with fatal myocardial infarction)
2. Coronary thrombosis due to erosion of a fibrous plaque (more frequent in women, especially premenopausal women, than men, as well as in non ST-segment elevation ACS than ST-segment elevation myocardial infarction)
3. Coronary spasm (frequently superimposed to plaque rupture or erosion, but rare without it, except in cocaine users)
4. Microvascular dysfunction (uncommon; more frequent in women than men)
5. Spontaneous coronary dissection (uncommon; more frequent in women than men)
6. Percutaneous coronary intervention or coronary bypass graft surgery

Some ex vivo studies associated plaque rupture to male pattern and plaque erosion to female pattern of lesion's morphology [22]. However, in vivo studies with high-resolution imaging technique (such as intravascular optical coherence tomography) reported contrasting results [23].

Anyhow, regarding the coronary tree, women usually have smaller coronary arteries and less severe obstructive lesions than men. In addition, women more frequently than man suffer of microvascular dysfunction and have myocardial ischemia and infarction with normal coronary arteries [24–26]. The prevalence of ACS with normal or nonobstructive coronary arteries ranges from 7% to 32% of patients based on relevant studies [11].

19.3 Clinical Presentation

Most of the time, ACS occurs out of the blue, in people apparently healthy [4]. These persons, especially women, often have more than one major cardiovascular risk factor, including current smoking, hypertension, type 2 diabetes mellitus, and hypercholesterolemia [4]. Also, obesity, anxiety, depression, and acute stress are risk factors for ACS; Mediterranean diet (diet rich of vegetable, fruit, fish, and olive oil) and regular exercise (e.g., 30 min of walking five times a week) seem to prevent it [4].

Regarding psychosocial risk factors, women, especially young women with early-onset AMI, have a disproportional burden of it. The prevalence of depression is about 20% in post-myocardial infarction patients (several times higher than in the general population) and is about twice as high in women with AMI than in men with AMI [27].

The maximum incidence of ACS is around 65 years old in male versus 72 years old in women. Below the age of 60, it occurs 3–4 times more in men, but after the age of 75, women represent the majority of patients [4]. The older age of women with ACS compared with men is thought to be due to the protective role of circulating estrogens. However, studies evaluating hormone replacement therapy in postmenopausal women have been convincingly negative [4].

In both women and men, the most common symptom is "typical chest pain/discomfort" [4]. However, women often present with atypical chest pain and angina equivalent symptoms such as fatigue, dyspnea, diaphoresis, weakness, and indigestion [4, 11].

Typical chest pain/discomfort. It is the feeling of pressure, tightness around the chest, or squeezing in the central chest. Patients show the location of the pain with a clenched first or the entire palm, but not with a finger, since the pain is not located at a specific point on the chest, but seems to be widespread [4]. The pain may radiate to the jaw, neck, one or both shoulders and arm, epigastrium, and back. Moreover, the pain does not change with any thorax movement or deep breathing [4].

Typical additional symptoms are dyspnea, nausea, vomiting, and diaphoresis [4].

Atypical chest pain. The pain is defined atypical when it is sharp, pleuritic, burning, aching soreness, or reproducible. Other characteristics could be heartburn or indigestion and pain just in the upper back, neck, jaw, arm, shoulder, or epigastrium [4].

Atypical additional symptoms are unusual fatigue, flu-like symptoms, generalized scared/anxiety feeling, dizziness, or palpitations.

The rate of patients with ACS without typical chest pain/discomfort ranges from 7.8% to 58.8%, accordingly to the study population and the type of ACS [28]. Atypical complaints are more often observed in the elderly, in women, and in patients with diabetes, chronic renal disease, congestive heart failure, chronic obstructive pulmonary disease, or stroke [29, 31]. Those patients would benefit from aggressive treatment, but often receive few drugs [29].

Women are more likely to present with more symptoms but less chest pain compared with men. Unusual or unexplained fatigue (tiredness) is one of the most common symptoms of heart attack in women.

Symptoms due to myocardial ischemia last for several minutes. When chest pain/discomfort and/or other symptoms last for more than 20 min, the damage deriving from myocardial ischemia turns to myocardial necrosis [4].

Of note, about one of five heart attacks is silent [4].

19.4 Diagnosis and Management

Management of patients with ACS is based on the results of randomized clinical trials, registries, and expert opinions [4–7]. Women and men receive equal benefit from reperfusion and anti-ischemic therapy.

Diagnosis of ACS is usually based on symptoms and ECG signs. In patients with a suspicion of "heart attack," 12-lead ECG should be obtained and interpreted as early as practicable, including in the ambulance. The ambulance service has a critical role in the management of ACS because it is not only a mode of transport but also a place for initial diagnosis, triage, and treatment.

Typical ECG signs of acute heart damage are ST-segment elevation/depression $\geq$0.2 mV in men and 0.15 mV in women (in $\geq$2 contiguous leads), T-wave inversions, and new left bundle branch block.

On the basis of ECG manifestation, ACSs are classified in ST-segment elevation myocardial infarction (30%), non ST-segment elevation myocardial infarction (25%), or unstable angina (35%). The last two are also grouped as non ST-segment elevation ACS.

ST-segment elevation (or new left bundle branch block) is usually caused by a sudden complete occlusion of a coronary artery. Fundamentally, all these patients have an extensive ischemia and will develop myocardial necrosis which is usually from the endocardium to the epicardium (transmural myocardial infarction).

ST-segment depression and/or T-wave inversions are usually caused by sudden severe reduction of the coronary blood flow. Some patients will develop myocardial necrosis (subendocardial myocardial infarction); others will not (unstable angina).

Compared with men, women more commonly present with non-ST-segment elevation ACS.

In vivo, the final diagnosis of AMI is made through serial measurements of circulating biomarkers of myocardial necrosis. Today the most used are high-sensitive cardiac troponin T and I, which have a typical rise and fall over the time. Treatment strategies are not based nor delayed by the results of blood samples.

19.4.1 Treatment of Non-ST-segment Elevation Acute Coronary Syndrome (NSTE-ACS) [6]

The goals of pharmacological therapy are to inhibit platelet aggregation and thrombus formation, to decrease myocardial oxygen demand (secondary to a decrease in heart rate, blood pressure, preload, or myocardial contractility), and to increase myocardial oxygen supply (by administration of oxygen or through coronary vasodilation). Invasive coronary angiography allows to confirm the diagnosis, identify the culprit lesion, and establish the indication for coronary revascularization. Diagnostic angiography (with the intent to perform revascularization if appropriate accordingly to coronary anatomy) is recommended (1) immediately, in patients whose ischemic symptoms are not relieved by nitrates and beta-blockers and those with hemodynamic or electrical instability; (2) within 24 h of hospital admission, in patients with high-risk features (diabetes mellitus, congestive heart failure, post-infarction angina, recent percutaneous coronary intervention, and prior coronary artery bypass graft); and (3) according to physician's choice of conservative strategy versus an early invasive strategy.

Dual antiplatelet therapy (*DAPT*). Aspirin should be administered in all patients without contraindications as soon as possible and continued indefinitely. Moreover, in addition to ASA, a $P2Y_{12}$ inhibitor (clopidogrel, prasugrel, or ticagrelor) should be recommended for up to 12 months.

Anticoagulation. Anticoagulants are used to inhibit thrombin generation and/or activity, thereby reducing thrombus-related events, in the acute phase. Parenteral anticoagulation is recommended at the time of diagnosis according to both ischemic and bleeding risks.

Nitrates. Patients should be titrated upward until symptoms are relieved and in hypertensive patients until blood pressure is normalized, unless side effects (notably headache or hypotension) occur.

Beta-blockers. The administration of beta-blockers should begin in the hospital and be continued after de-hospitalization in all patients without contraindications. Beta-blockers inhibit the myocardial effects of circulating catecholamines and reduce myocardial oxygen consumption by lowering heart rate, blood pressure, and myocardial contractility.

ACE-inhibitor. ACE-inhibitors should be considered in all patients, especially in those with evidence of heart failure, left ventricular systolic dysfunction, diabetes, or an anterior infarct.

19.4.2 Treatment of ST-Segment Elevation Myocardial Infarction (STEMI) [7]

Reperfusion. Reperfusion therapy is the primary therapeutic goal. Dissolution of the intracoronary thrombus (by fibrinolysis) or removal of the intracoronary thrombus (by primary percutaneous coronary intervention), provides the best chance for mortality reduction. Women have a more favorable outcome with percutaneous coronary intervention compared with thrombolytic therapy.

Primary percutaneous coronary intervention (PCI) is the recommended reperfusion therapy over fibrinolysis if performed by an experienced team within 120 min from the first medical contact. Primary PCI should be done within 12 h from symptom onset, but even later if symptoms and ST-segment elevation are still there or have been stuttering. When primary PCI cannot be performed within 120 min from first medical contact, fibrinolysis should be considered.

The use of stent over balloon angioplasty alone should be preferred because it reduces the incidence of restenosis and the rate of re-intervention. For the same reason, stents coated with medication (drug-eluting stents) should be preferred to bare-metal stents. However, since drug-eluting stents carry a high risk of intracoronary acute thrombosis, prolonged dual antiplatelet therapy is mandatory in all patients receiving drug-eluting stents. Thus, drug-eluting stents should be preferred over bare-metal stents if the patient has no contraindications to prolonged dual antiplatelet therapy (indication for oral anticoagulation or estimated high long-term bleeding risk) and is likely to be compliant.

Adjunctive medical therapy. All patients (including those who do not reach the hospital within 12 h from symptoms onset or who have contraindications to pharmacological and mechanical reperfusion strategies) should be treated as soon as possible with an optimal medical therapy, including oxygen, antiplatelet agents and anticoagulant, beta-blocker, ACE-I, and statins, unless otherwise contraindicated.

19.5 Prognosis

In national registries, inhospital mortality of ACS varies between 4% and 15% [6, 7, 20]. The rate of major adverse cardiac events (death, reinfarction, revascularization, heart failure, and stroke) is significantly higher for STEMI than NSTE-ACS and for patients with severe coronary artery stenosis than normal angiograms [6, 7] (the rate of inhospital death in the population with normal angiograms is about 2%, not nil) [30].

In the setting of AMI, "time is heart muscle"; more time passes without restoring blood flow, the greater is the damage to the heart muscle and the risk of death [4]. Lack of awareness of risk, interpretation of symptoms as nonurgent and temporary, inaccurate symptom attribution, low education and socioeconomic levels, living alone, and barriers to self-care are the most frequent factors for delay in seeking medical attention, as well as in the case of elderly and/or women and having comorbidity (stroke, chronic obstructive pulmonary disease, chronic kidney disease, and heart failure) [6, 7, 29]. Women with AMI do not have different all-cause mortality but have higher excess mortality compared with men. Women have more complications, like shock, heart failure, reinfarction, recurrent ischemia/MI, bleeding and stroke than men, whereas ventricular arrhythmias occur at similar rates [6, 7] (Table 19.1).

Table 19.1 Hypertension

Normal	<120 mmHg	and	<80 mmHg
Elevated	120–129 mmHg	and	<80 mmHg
Hypertension			
Stage 1	130–139 mmHg	or	80–89 mmHg
Stage 2	≥140 mmHg	or	≥90 mmHg

References

1. Wilkins E, Wilson L, Wickramasinghe K, Bhatnagar P, Leal J, Luengo-Fernandez R, et al. European Cardiovascular Disease Statistics 2017. European Heart Network, Brussels. http://www.ehnheart.org/images/CVD-statistics-report-August-2017.pdf. Accessed 12 Jan 2018.
2. Go AS, Mozaffarian D, Roger VL, Benjamin EJ, Berry JD, Blaha MJ, et al., American Heart Association Statistics Committee and Stroke Statistics Subcommittee. Executive summary: heart disease and stroke statistics--2014 update: a report from the American Heart Association. Circulation. 2014;129:399–410. https://doi.org/10.1161/01.cir.0000442015.53336.12.
3. Benjamin EJ, Blaha MJ, Chiuve SE, Cushman M, Das SR, Deo R, et al. Heart disease and stroke statistics—2017 update: a report from the American Heart Association. Circulation. 2017;135(10):e146–603. https://doi.org/10.1161/CIR.0000000000000485.
4. Mann D, Zipes D, Libby P, Bonow R. Braunwald's heart disease: a textbook of cardiovascular medicine. 10th ed. Philadelphia, PA: Saunders; 2014.
5. Thygesen K, Alpert JS, Jaffe AS, Simoons ML, Chaitman BR, White HD, et al. Third universal definition of myocardial infarction. J Am Coll Cardiol. 2012;60:1581–98. https://doi.org/10.1016/j.jacc.2012.08.001.
6. Roffi M, Patrono C, Collet JP, Mueller C, Valgimigli M, Andreotti F, et al. 2015 ESC Guidelines for the management of acute coronary syndromes in patients presenting without persistent ST-segment elevation: Task Force for the Management of Acute Coronary Syndromes in patients presenting without persistent ST-segment elevation of the European Society of Cardiology (ESC). Eur Heart J. 2016;37:267–315. https://doi.org/10.1093/eurheartj/ehv320.
7. Windecker S, Kolh P, Alfonso F, Collet JP, Cremer J, Falk V, et al. 2014 ESC/EACTS Guidelines on myocardial revascularization: the Task Force on Myocardial Revascularization of the European Society of Cardiology (ESC) and the European Association for Cardio-Thoracic Surgery (EACTS) developed with the special contribution of the European Association of Percutaneous Cardiovascular Interventions (EAPCI). Eur Heart J. 2014;35:2541–619. https://doi.org/10.1093/eurheartj/ehu278.
8. Shaw LJ, Bugiardini R, Merz CN. Women and ischemic heart disease: evolving knowledge. J Am Coll Cardiol. 2009;54:1561–75. https://doi.org/10.1016/j.jacc.2009.04.098.
9. Vaccarino V, Badimon L, Corti R, de Wit C, Dorobantu M, Manfrini O, et al. Presentation, management, and outcomes of ischaemic heart disease in women. Nat Rev Cardiol. 2013;10:508–18. https://doi.org/10.1038/nrcardio.2013.93.
10. Vaccarino V, Badimon L, Corti R, de Wit C, Dorobantu M, Hall A, et al., Working Group on Coronary Pathophysiology and Microcirculation. Ischaemic heart disease in women: are there sex differences in pathophysiology and risk factors? Position paper from the working group on coronary pathophysiology and microcirculation of the European Society of Cardiology. Cardiovasc Res. 2011;90:9–17. https://doi.org/10.1093/cvr/cvq394.
11. Mehta LS, Beckie TM, DeVon HA, Grines CL, Krumholz HM, Johnson MN, et al. Acute myocardial infarction in women. A scientific statement from the American Heart Association. Circulation. 2016;133:916–47. https://doi.org/10.1161/CIR.0000000000000351.
12. Ayanian JZ, Epstein AM. Differences in the use of procedures between women and men hospitalized for coronary heart disease. N Engl J Med. 1991;325:221–5.
13. Steingart RM, Packer M, Hamm P, Coglianese ME, Gersh B, Geltman EM, et al. Sex differences in the management of coronary artery disease. Survival and Ventricular Enlargement Investigators. N Engl J Med. 1991;325:226–30.
14. Healy B. The Yentl syndrome. N Engl J Med. 1991;325:274–6.
15. Bugiardini R, Yan AT, Yan RT, Fitchett D, Langer A, Manfrini O, Goodman SG, Canadian Acute Coronary Syndrome Registry I and II Investigators. Factors influencing underutilization of evidence-based therapies in women. Eur Heart J. 2011;32:1337–44. https://doi.org/10.1093/eurheartj/ehr027.
16. Bugiardini R, Estrada JL, Nikus K, Hall AS, Manfrini O. Gender bias in acute coronary syndromes. Curr Vasc Pharmacol. 2010;8:276–84.

17. Poon S, Goodman SG, Yan RT, Bugiardini R, Bierman AS, Eagle KA, et al. Bridging the gender gap: insights from a contemporary analysis of sex-related differences in the treatment and outcomes of patients with acute coronary syndromes. Am Heart J. 2012;163:66–73. https://doi.org/10.1016/j.ahj.2011.09.025.
18. Vaccarino V, Parsons L, Peterson ED, Rogers WJ, Kiefe CI, Canto J. Sex differences in mortality after acute myocardial infarction changes from 1994 to 2006. Arch Intern Med. 2009;169:1767–74.
19. Bugiardini R, Ricci B, Cenko E, Vasiljevic Z, Kedev S, Davidovic G, et al. Delayed care and mortality among women and men with myocardial infarction. J Am Heart Assoc. 2017;6. pii:e005968. https://doi.org/10.1161/JAHA.117.005968.
20. Bugiardini R, Manfrini O, Majstorović Stakić M, Cenko E, Boytsov S, Merkely B, et al. Exploring in-hospital death from myocardial infarction in Eastern Europe: from the International Registry of Acute Coronary Syndromes in Transitional Countries (ISACS-TC); on the Behalf of the Working Group on Coronary Pathophysiology & Microcirculation of the European Society of Cardiology. Curr Vasc Pharmacol. 2014;12:903–9.
21. Ricci B, Cenko E, Vasiljevic Z, Stankovic G, Kedev S, Kalpak O, et al. Acute coronary syndrome: the risk to young women. J Am Heart Assoc. 2017;6. pii:e007519. https://doi.org/10.1161/JAHA.117.007519.
22. Falk E, Nakano M, Bentzon JF, Finn AV, Virmani R. Update on acute coronary syndromes: the pathologists' view. Eur Heart J. 2013;34:719–28. https://doi.org/10.1093/eurheartj/ehs411.
23. Guagliumi G, Capodanno D, Saia F, Musumeci G, Tarantini G, Garbo R, et al. Mechanisms of atherothrombosis and vascular response to primary percutaneous coronary intervention in women versus men with acute myocardial infarction: results of the OCTAVIA study. JACC Cardiovasc Interv. 2014;7:958–68. https://doi.org/10.1016/j.jcin.2014.05.011.
24. Bugiardini R, Bairey Merz CN. Angina with "normal" coronary arteries: a changing philosophy. JAMA. 2005;293:477–84.
25. Cenko E, Bugiardini R. Barriers to risk stratification accuracy in ischemic heart disease in women: the role of non-obstructive coronary artery disease. Curr Pharm Des. 2016;22:3928–34.
26. Cenko E, Bugiardini R. Vasotonic Angina as a cause of myocardial ischemia in women. Cardiovasc Drugs Ther. 2015;29:339–45. https://doi.org/10.1007/s10557-015-6595-4.
27. Lichtman JH, Froelicher ES, Blumenthal JA, Carney RM, Doering LV, Frasure-Smith N, et al., on behalf of the American Heart Association Statistics Committee of the Council on Epidemiology and Prevention and the Council on Cardiovascular and Stroke Nursing. Depression as a risk factor for poor prognosis among patients with acute coronary syndrome: systematic review and recommendations: a scientific statement from the American Heart Association. Circulation. 2014;129:1350–69. https://doi.org/10.1161/CIR.0000000000000019.
28. Ricci B, Cenko E, Varotti E, Puddu PE, Manfrini O. Atypical chest pain in ACS: a trap especially for women. Curr Pharm Des. 2016;22:3877–84.
29. Manfrini O, Ricci B, Cenko E, Dorobantu M, Kalpak O, Kedev S, et al., ISACS-TC Investigators. Association between comorbidities and absence of chest pain in acute coronary syndrome with in-hospital outcome. Int J Cardiol. 2016;Suppl:S37–43. https://doi.org/10.1016/j.ijcard.2016.06.221.
30. Bugiardini R. Women, 'non-specific' chest pain, and normal or near-normal coronary angiograms are not synonymous with favourable outcome. Eur Heart J. 2006;27:1387–9.
31. Bugiardini R, Manfrini O, De Ferrari GM. Unanswered questions for management of acute coronary syndrome: risk stratification of patients with minimal disease or normal findings on coronary angiography. Arch Intern Med. 2006;166:1391–5.

Endocrine Disorders

20

Alessandra Gambineri, Paola Altieri,
and Daniela Ibarra-Gasparini

Key Points

- The imbalance in sex hormones has an important impact in metabolic diseases, with androgens playing an interesting sexually dimorphic role.
- In women but not in men, androgens, at supraphysiological levels, decrease insulin sensitivity and promote adipose tissue accumulation.
- In both sexes estrogens promote energy homeostasis, improve body fat distribution, enhance insulin sensitivity, and improve β-cell function.
- Both hyperandrogenic and hypoestrogenic conditions in women have been linked with obesity, insulin resistance, and type 2 diabetes mellitus.
- Treatments aimed at correcting hyperandrogenism and hypoestrogenism may prevent the development of metabolic disorders in women.

20.1 Introduction

The different balance in the sex hormones, androgens and estrogens, is a cardinal aspect of the biology of gender difference and plays a fundamental role in maintaining the physiological state at each age of life [1]. However, the imbalance in sex hormones is involved in some metabolic diseases, with androgens playing an interesting sexually dimorphic role. The sexual dimorphism of androgens in the pathophysiology of metabolic disorders leads to inequalities in both preventive strategies and treatment between women and men.

A. Gambineri (✉) · P. Altieri · D. Ibarra-Gasparini
Endocrinology Unit, Department of Medical and Surgical Science, S. Orsola-Malpighi Hospital, Alma Mater University of Bologna, Bologna, Italy
e-mail: alessandra.gambiner3@unibo.it

I. Tarricone, A. Riecher-Rössler (eds.), *Health and Gender*,
https://doi.org/10.1007/978-3-030-15038-9_20

This review focuses on the relationship between sex hormones and metabolic disorders in women.

20.2 Role of Androgens in Metabolic Target Tissues

Androgens exert key effects on metabolic target tissues, particularly in adipose tissue and skeletal muscle (Table 20.1).

Adipose tissue expansion is a consequence of both hyperplasia (adipogenesis), which is driven by the proliferation of preadipocytes and their differentiation into adipocytes, and hypertrophy, which is driven by the accumulation of lipids in differentiated adipocytes. In females, androgens impair adipogenesis by inhibiting the proliferation and differentiation of mesenchymal stem cells and preadipocytes [2] with a compensatory adipocyte hypertrophy which could induce adipocyte dysfunction which manifests itself in insulin resistance (IR), intracellular stress, and inflammation [3]. In fact, hypertrophic adipose tissue is insulin resistant, produces high amount of free fatty acids, secretes high levels of proinflammatory cytokines, particularly tumor necrosis factor-alpha (TNF-alpha) and interleukin-6 (IL-6), and low levels of adiponectin [3].

Androgens also exert a direct effect on adipose insulin sensitivity. In particular, testosterone (T) directly induces IR in female subcutaneous adipocytes in vitro and inhibits insulin-stimulated glucose uptake by impairing the phosphorylation of protein kinase C via an androgen receptor-mediated mechanism [4]. In vivo human studies have demonstrated that T and its precursor dehydroepiandrosterone sulfate (DHEAS) at physiological levels stimulate lipolysis in a sex- and depot-specific manner. In particular, DHEAS seems to be able to stimulate lipolysis preferably in subcutaneous fat in women and in visceral fat in men [5]. Conversely, by comparing the expression profile of omental adipocytes in obese women with an androgen excess with the profile of obese controls with normal androgens, an enhanced lipogenesis has been found in hyperandrogenic females [6, 7]. This thus highlights the possible role of androgens in promoting adipose lipid accumulation in women if at supraphysiological concentrations.

At the level of skeletal muscle, androgens enhance the differentiation of stem cells to myotubes, as well as skeletal muscle protein synthesis, lipid oxidation,

Table 20.1 Effects of androgens in metabolic target tissues

Target tissue	Effects
Adipose tissue	• Impair adipogenesis • Stimulate adipocyte hypertrophy • Decrease insulin sensitivity • Increase inflammation • Decrease lipid storage • Increase lipolysis
Skeletal muscle	• Stimulate differentiation of stem cells to myotubes • Stimulate protein synthesis • Increase insulin sensitivity • Stimulate lipid oxidation • Stimulate glucose uptake

insulin sensitivity and glucose usage, and mitochondrial function in both men and women but with sex-specific gradual differences [8]. However, in oophorectomized female rats, T administration impairs insulin sensitivity at the level of skeletal muscle by interfering with insulin signalling and by inducing some changes in the myocyte morphology, such as a decrement in insulin-sensitive type I fibers, an increment in less sensitive type IIb fibers, a decrement in capillarization, and the inhibition of glycogen synthase expression and activity [9].

20.3 Role of Estrogens in Metabolic Target Tissues

Estrogens also exert key effects on metabolic target tissues (Fig. 20.1).

Estrogens have historically been viewed as major regulators of adipose tissue in adult females; however recent works have indicated that estrogens are significantly involved in the regulation of adipose tissue also in men. Estrogens have, in fact, a direct effect on adipocytes through the inhibition of lipogenesis in both sexes. In addition, estrogens have an important metabolic effect on other target organs, particularly on the skeletal muscle, liver, pancreatic β cells, and the brain. In terms of the skeletal muscle and the liver, estrogens improve peripheral insulin sensitivity, and they increase fatty acid oxidation in the skeletal muscle, thus protecting other tissues such as the liver and adipose tissue from the accumulation of fat [10]. Regarding pancreatic β cells, estrogens stimulate glucose-stimulated insulin biosynthesis and protect these cells against various injuries such as oxidative stress, amyloid polypeptide toxicity, lipotoxicity, and apoptosis [10].

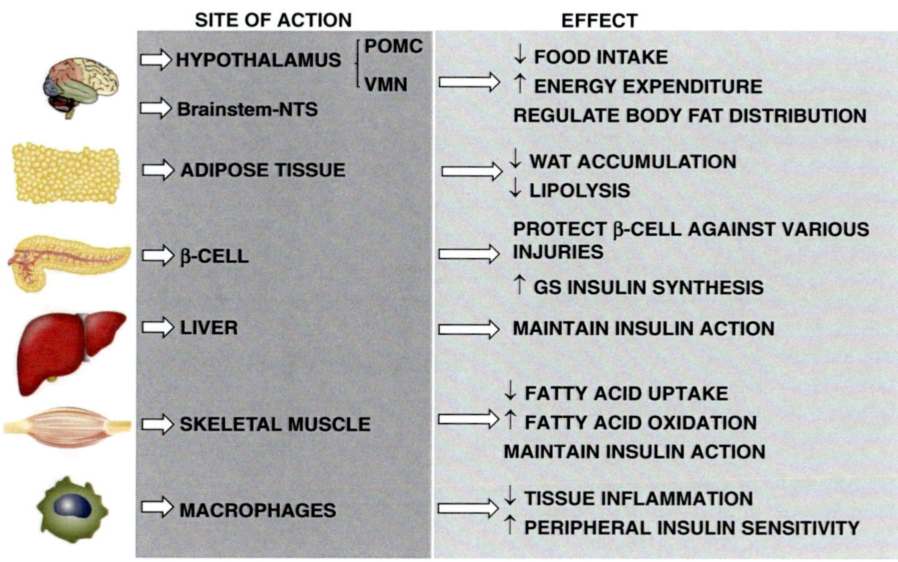

Fig. 20.1 Effects of estrogens in metabolic target tissues. *POMC* proopiomelanocortin, *VMN* ventromedial neurons, *NTS* nucleus tractus solitarius, *WAT* white adipose tissue, *GS* glucose-stimulated

Estrogens also have an important direct central effect with a subsequent regulation in the energy balance. In the hypothalamus, estrogens suppress food intake by acting directly on the proopiomelanocortin neurons in the arcuate nucleus and, at the same time, stimulating physical activity and energy expenditure and regulating body fat distribution by reducing visceral fat deposition. This occurs through direct action on the ventromedial nuclei [10] with an overall inhibitory effect on adipose deposition in both sexes.

20.4 Hyperandrogenism, Obesity, Insulin Resistance, and Type 2 Diabetes Mellitus in Women

Considering the in vivo effects of androgens in metabolic target tissues, it is possible that with circulating androgen levels in the range of female androgen excess, the net effect of androgens on the adipose tissue drives the systemic phenotype and gives rise to metabolic diseases.

Thus, hyperandrogenic conditions in women, such as polycystic ovary syndrome (PCOS), congenital adrenal hyperplasia, and androgen secreting tumors, have been linked with obesity, IR, and type 2 diabetes mellitus (T2DM).

PCOS is the most common hyperandrogenic disorder in women with a prevalence in fertile European women of around 6–8% [11]. In these women, hyperandrogenism is associated with chronic anovulation and infertility. The definition of PCOS is based on the presence of hyperandrogenism, chronic oligo-anovulation, and polycystic ovarian morphology by ultrasound, after the exclusion of other causes of hyperandrogenism [11].

Although the Androgen Excess (AE)-PCOS Society emphasized the primary role of hyperandrogenism in the diagnostic workup of PCOS, the definition of this disorder is still under debate, and associated metabolic alterations, chiefly IR and obesity, are commonly present but not included in the diagnostic criteria [11]. Studies using the euglycemic-hyperinsulinemic clamp technique or the intravenous insulin test have clearly demonstrated that obese PCOS women have significantly lower insulin sensitivity than their non-obese PCOS counterparts and, therefore, a more severe IR state [12].

Insulin sensitivity has been estimated to be reduced by 50% even in lean PCOS subjects. However in obese PCOS women a twofold decrease occurs with respect to obese non-PCOS women, thus suggesting that IR is of common occurrence in PCOS but also that obesity further decreases IR [12]. The prevalence of the metabolic syndrome is also commonly higher in women with PCOS than in the general female population [13].

Interestingly, recent studies have demonstrated a high incidence of T2DM in PCOS. In particular, in a large cohort of UK women with PCOS (mean age of 29.6 years), the incidence of T2DM was 3.6 per 1000 person-years, with increasing rates according to age [14]. In addition, in a prospective study in Italy, the incidence of T2DM was found to be 1.05 per 100 person-years, which was 5.8 times higher than the general age-matched national female population [15]. Finally, in a recent study from the UK, the relative risk of T2DM in a large cohort of women extracted from the General Practice Research Database (a longitudinal, anonymized research database derived from nearly 600 primary care practices in the UK), the crude rates of T2DM were 5.7 and 1.7 per 1000 patient-years for cases and controls, respectively [16].

The prevalence of T2DM may vary from country to country as demonstrated by different epidemiological surveys and can be attributed to environmental and dietary factors and/or specific genetic or epigenetic background. In any case, PCOS is now considered by all the scientific societies as a disorder at risk for T2DM. Alarmingly, impaired glucose tolerance (IGT) state and T2DM have also been found to be highly prevalent among PCOS adolescents [17]. This condition increases the need for an early diagnosis and preventive strategies.

Overall, the literature supports the notion that PCOS is associated with an increased susceptibility to develop T2DM at any age and that androgens are the main link between PCOS and T2DM. To support this assumption, there are only few data that demonstrate that antiandrogenic therapy in women affected by PCOS is able to improve IR, decrease abdominal adiposity [18], and probably prevent metabolic complications such as T2DM (personal data). More studies are warranted to confirm these data.

20.5 Hypoestrogenism, Obesity, Insulin Resistance, and Diabetes in Women

The role of hypoestrogenism in the development of dysmetabolic conditions in women is emphasized by clinical models of estrogen deficiency.

After menopause a precipitous decline in insulin sensitivity parallels an increase in fat mass, with a prevalent visceral accumulation, and elevations in circulating inflammatory markers, low-density lipoprotein (LDL), triglycerides, and fatty acids and an increased prevalence of T2DM, which is indirectly correlated with circulating levels of estradiol [19].

Accordingly, extreme forms of hypoestrogenism induced by the exogenous administration of aromatase inhibitors, such as anastrozole, exemestane, and letrozole, in females as adjuvant therapy of breast cancer are associated with metabolic syndrome and diabetes [20].

In addition, our group recently demonstrated for the first time an important association between Turner syndrome (TS), a genetic form of hypoestrogenism, with diabetes [21]. We found diabetes in 12.5% of adults with TS against a 2.8% prevalence of T2DM in the general female Italian population of a similar age. Interestingly, the insulin response to the glucose load observed in our cases of diabetes at diagnosis suggests that early insufficient insulin secretion characterizes diabetes in TS. These data support the role of hypoestrogenism in the pathogenesis of diabetes in TS, although the role of other still unknown factors intrinsic to the syndrome cannot be ruled out.

Overall, these data demonstrate that estrogen deficiency, whatever the origin and the severity, makes women more prone to metabolic complications. However, treating estrogen deficiency is not straightforward, since estrogens and estrogen receptor (ER) agonists have been linked with carcinogenesis and/or progression of aggressive cancers [22]. Furthermore, the randomized controlled trials on the clinical events associated with hormonal replacement therapy (HRT) have clearly demonstrated that the risk of stroke and other cardiovascular events is higher for women over 60 years that use conjugated estrogens [23, 24]. Therefore, HRT is now recommended for women under 60 years of age, or less than 10 years postmenopause [25], when metabolic complications are less frequent and estrogens could be used mostly as a preventive strategy. *Clinician should consider HRT particularly for postmenopausal women more vulnerable to psychotic episodes, since it has been demonstrated the aggravation of mental disorders after menopause and the beneficial effect of HRT on psychotic disorders* [26, 27].

However, the therapeutic index is narrow since supraphysiological levels of estrogens may be as detrimental as estrogen deficiency, and thus a targeted treatment strategy would be necessary. Unresolved questions regarding treatments with estradiol or its conjugated versions include which patient population can safely benefit from this therapy, what new agents of HRT can be used to optimize the benefits and eliminate the risks of estrogen therapy, and whether it is preferable to use estrogen therapy to prevent or to treat metabolic complications.

20.6 Conclusions

In summary, the bulk of evidence suggests that hyperandrogenism or hypoestrogenism in women facilitates the appearance of metabolic complications, such as diabetes, mainly via the promotion of metabolically unfavorable changes in body composition. Treatments aimed at correcting hyperandrogenism or hypoestrogenism may prevent the development of metabolic disorders, but more studies are warranted.

References

1. Federman DD. The biology of human sex differences. N Engl J Med. 2006;354:1507–14.
2. O'Reilly MW, House PJ, Tomlinson JW. Understanding androgen action in adipose tissue. J Steroid Biochem Mol Biol. 2014;143:277–84.
3. Kloting N, Bluher M. Adipocyte dysfunction, inflammation and metabolic syndrome. Rev Endocr Metab Disord. 2014;15:277–87.
4. Corbould A. Chronic testosterone treatment induces selective insulin resistance in subcutaneous adipocytes of women. J Endocrinol. 2007;192:585–94.
5. Hernandez-Morante JJ, Perez-de-Heredia F, Lujan JA, Zamora S, Garaulet M. Role of DHEA-S on body fat distribution: gender- and depot-specific stimulation of adipose tissue lipolysis. Steroids. 2008;73:209–15.
6. Corton M, Botella-Carretero JI, Benguria A, Villuendas G, Zaballos A, San Millan JL, Escobar-Morreale HF, Peral B. Differential gene expression profile in omental adipose tissue in women with polycystic ovary syndrome. J Clin Endocrinol Metab. 2007;92:328–37.

7. Corton M, Botella-Carretero JI, Lopez JA, Camafeita E, San Millan JL, Escobar-Morreale HF, Peral B. Proteomic analysis of human omental adipose tissue in the polycystic ovary syndrome using two-dimensional difference gel electrophoresis and mass spectrometry. Hum Reprod. 2008;23:651–61.
8. Schiffer L, Kempegowda P, Arlt W, O'Reilly MW. The sexually dimorphic role of androgens in human metabolic disease. Eur J Endocrinol. 2017;177:R125–43.
9. Rincon J, Holmäng A, Wahlström EO, Lönnroth P, Björntorp P, Zierath JR, Wallberg-Henriksson H. Mechanisms behind insulin resistance in rat skeletal muscle after oophorectomy and additional testosterone treatment. Diabetes. 1996;45:615–21.
10. Mauvais-Jarvis F, Clegg DJ, Hevener AL. The role of estrogens in control of energy balance and glucose homeostasis. Endocr Rev. 2013;34:309–38.
11. Conway G, Dewailly D, Diamanti-Kandarakis E, Escobar-Morreale HF, Franks S, Gambineri A, Kelestimur F, Macut D, Micic D, Pasquali R, et al. The polycystic ovary syndrome: a position statement from the European Society of Endocrinology. Eur J Endocrinol. 2014;171:P1–P29.
12. Tosi F, Bonora E, Moghetti P. Insulin resistance in a large cohort of women with polycystic ovary syndrome: a comparison between euglycaemic-hyperinsulinaemic clamp and surrogate indexes. Hum Reprod. 2017;32:2515–21.
13. Gambineri A, Repaci A, Patton L, Grassi I, Pocognoli P, Cognigni GE, Pasqui F, Pagotto U, Pasquali R. Prominent role of low HDL-cholesterol in explaining the high prevalence of the metabolic syndrome in polycystic ovary syndrome. Nutr Metab Cardiovasc Dis. 2009;19:797–804.
14. Wang ET, Calderon-Margalit R, Cedars MI, Daviglus ML, Merkin SS, Schreiner PJ, Sternfeld B, Wellons M, Schwartz SM, Lewis CE, Williams OD, Siscovick DS, Bibbins-Domingo K. Polycystic ovary syndrome and risk for long-term diabetes and dyslipidemia. Obstet Gynecol. 2011;117:6–13.
15. Gambineri A, Patton L, Altieri P, Pagotto U, Pizzi C, Manzoli L, Pasquali R. Polycystic ovary syndrome is a risk factor for type 2 diabetes: results from a long-term prospective study. Diabetes. 2012;61:2369–74.
16. Morgan CL, Jenkins-Jones S, Currie CJ, Rees DA. Evaluation of adverse outcome in young women with polycystic ovary syndrome versus matched, reference controls: a retrospective, observational study. J Clin Endocrinol Metab. 2012;97:3251–60.
17. Palmert MR, Gordon CM, Kartashov AI, Legro RS, Emans SJ, Dunaif A. Screening for abnormal glucose tolerance in adolescents with polycystic ovary syndrome. J Clin Endocrinol Metab. 2002;87:1017–23.
18. Gambineri A, Patton L, Vaccina A, Cacciari M, Morselli-Labate AM, Cavazza C, Pagotto U, Pasquali R. Treatment with flutamide, metformin, and their combination added to a hypocaloric diet in overweight-obese women with polycystic ovary syndrome: a randomized, 12-month, placebo-controlled study. J Clin Endocrinol Metab. 2006;91:3970–80.
19. Muka T, Nano J, Jaspers L, Meun C, Bramer WM, Hofman A, Dehghan A, Kavousi M, Laven JS, Franco OH. Associations of steroid sex hormones and sex hormone-binding globulin with the risk of Type 2 diabetes in women: a population-based cohort study and meta-analysis. Diabetes. 2017;66:577–86.
20. Smith IE, Dowsett M. Aromatase inhibitors in breast cancer. N Engl J Med. 2003;348:2431–42.
21. Ibarra-Gasparini D, Altieri P, Scarano E, Perri A, Morselli-Labate AM, Pagotto U, Mazzanti L, Pasquali R, Gambineri A. New insights on diabetes in Turner syndrome: results from an observational study in adulthood. Endocrine. 2018;59(3):651–60.
22. Gupte AA, Pownall HJ, Hamilton DJ. Estrogen: an emerging regulator of insulin action and mitochondrial function. J Diabetes Res. 2015;2015:916585.
23. Rossouw JE, Anderson GL, Prentice RL, LaCroix AZ, Kooperberg C, Stefanick ML, Jackson RD, Beresford SA, Howard BV, Johnson KC, Kotchen JM, Ockene J, Writing Group for the Women's Health Initiative Investigators. Risks and benefits of estrogen plus progestin in healthy postmenopausal women: principal results From the Women's Health Initiative randomized controlled trial. J Am Med Assoc. 2002;288:321–33.

24. Hulley S, Grady D, Bush T, Furberg C, Herrington D, Riggs B, Vittinghoff E. Randomized trial of estrogen plus progestin for secondary prevention of coronary heart disease in postmenopausal women. Heart and Estrogen/progestin Replacement Study (HERS) Research Group. J Am Med Assoc. 1998;280:605–13.
25. de Villiers TJ, Hall JE, Pinkerton JV, Pérez SC, Rees M, Yang C, Pierroz DD. Revised global consensus statement on menopausal hormone therapy. Maturitas. 2016;91:153–5.
26. Riecher-Rössler A. Sex and gender differences in mental disorders. Lancet Psychiatry. 2017;4:8–9.
27. Riecher-Rössler A, Kulkarni J. Estrogens and gonadal function in schizophrenia and related psychoses. Curr Top Behav Neurosci. 2011;8:155–71.

Suggested Reading

Pasquali R. Obesity and androgens: facts and perspectives. Fertil Steril. 2006;85:1319–40.
Pasquali R, Gambineri A. Glucose intolerance states in women with the polycystic ovary syndrome. J Endocrinol Invest. 2013;36:648–53.
Pasquali R, Vicennati V, Gambineri A, Pagotto U. Sex-dependent role of glucocorticoids and androgens in the pathophysiology of human obesity. Int J Obes. 2008;32:1764–79.

Urogenital and Reproductive Disorders 21

Giulia Gava, Renato Seracchioli,
and Maria Cristina Meriggiola

Key Points

- Biological and social gender differences should always be acknowledged when considering the presentation, the severity, the treatment, and the consequences of both reproductive and general health diseases. Gender has a significant impact on health, and it should be considered in the development of strategies for prevention and treatment of health conditions.
- Biological differences can make women more prone than men to certain medical conditions during reproductive years. Women are more susceptible to HIV and other sexually transmitted infections with potential long-term consequences.
- Even if a large number of men would welcome the opportunity to use male contraceptive methods and recognize that sharing family planning should be an individual right other than responsibility, family planning continues to be demanded to women because options available for male contraception are still obsolete and affected by high failure rates. Women are still often stigmatized and blamed in case of infertility even if infertility can have also a male factor.

G. Gava · R. Seracchioli · M. C. Meriggiola (✉)
Gynecology and Physiopathology of Human Reproduction, Department of Medical and Surgical Science, S. Orsola-Malpighi Hospital, University of Bologna, Bologna, Italy
e-mail: giulia.gava@studio.unibo.it; renato.seracchioli@aosp.bo.it; cristina.meriggiola@unibo.it

I. Tarricone, A. Riecher-Rössler (eds.), *Health and Gender*,
https://doi.org/10.1007/978-3-030-15038-9_21

- Also after menopause, biological differences make women more susceptible to certain medical conditions such as genital organ prolapse, urinary incontinence, and vaginal atrophy with related sexual dysfunction.
- In certain societies women continue to face discrimination or gender prejudice limiting their access to knowledge and health resources and making them more susceptible to diseases. In rural and poor communities, women's healthcare needs are barely addressed, and also in countries with a higher progress, there is still a need for continuous investment in greater gender equality.

21.1 Introduction

Gender has a significant health impact, and it should be always considered in the development of strategies for the prevention and treatment of health conditions related to reproductive and urogenital disorders. Biological differences can make women more prone to certain medical conditions. Furthermore, women's health can be severely influenced by social vulnerability in societies where women continue to face discrimination or are victims of violence and social or cultural gender prejudice as these conditions can limit women's access to health resources, information, and services [1].

Globally, women have less education, and they are more unemployed or paid less and less protected in their work environment. Women usually face higher health costs than men related to a greater use of healthcare for reproductive or urogenital conditions. At the same time, they are more likely to be poor, unemployed, or part-time workers, and for this reason in some countries, they have no health benefits. In rural and poor communities, often healthcare needs of women are barely addressed, and even in places with higher progress, there is still a need for continuous investment in great equality [1].

Biological and social gender differences should always be acknowledged when considering the presentation, the severity, the treatment, and the consequences of both reproductive and general health diseases.

Reproductive health and gender issues are closely related, and there is also a deep connection between reproductive health and human rights and women's and men's empowerment, equity, and dignity.

Reproductive years for many women represent an opportunity for personal fulfillment and empowerment. However, these years can also be characterized by risks correlated with sex and reproduction that can bring a burden of mortality and disability. It should also be considered that women's health during reproductive years not only is relevant to women themselves but also has an impact on the health and development of the next generation. Pattern of diseases related to reproductive issues are very different between low- and high-income countries. In low-income countries, main causes of mortality and morbidity are maternal conditions and HIV/

AIDS, while in high-income countries, causes of female deaths during fertile years are the traumatic incidents, suicide, and breast cancer [1].

Also after menopause, biological differences make women more susceptible to certain medical conditions such as genital organ prolapse, urinary incontinence, and vaginal atrophy with related sexual dysfunction.

21.2 Sexually Transmitted Diseases (STDs)

HIV is a leading cause of death and disease in women of reproductive age [2]. Women's vulnerability to HIV infection derives from a combination of biological predisposing factors and gender inequality conditions as limited women's knowledge, inability to negotiate safer sex, and, in certain situations violence by intimate partners and sexual violence [3].

The same combination of social and biological factors that makes women more prone to HIV also makes them more vulnerable to other sexually transmitted infections, in particular to chlamydia and trichomonas. STDs are a major public health problem especially in women as they disproportionately bear the long-term consequences of these diseases. Women are severely affected by STDs for several reasons. First of all, the anatomy of the female genital tract is more prone to infection than male anatomy because the mucosa of the vagina is thinner and the vaginal environment can easily promote microorganism growth.

Women with STDs are very often asymptomatic: they are less likely to have symptoms of common STDs, such as chlamydia and gonorrhea, compared to men. And even if they have symptoms, they are more likely to confuse vaginal discharge or itching to yeast infection, while men usually notice symptoms like discharge because they are more unusual for them.

STDs are more common among young women, and almost half of all infected persons worldwide are between 15 and 24 years of age [4].

Delays in diagnosis and treatment, coupled with women's greater vulnerability to complications from untreated infection, result in more serious health complications in women than men. STDs in women can affect future reproductive plans as untreated STDs can lead to pelvic inflammatory disease, which can result in infertility and ectopic pregnancy [5]. For example, chlamydia trachomatis is a sexually transmitted gram-negative bacterium that is a common cause of urethritis in men and cervicitis in women. Chlamydia is more prevalent among women than men [6]. The prevalence is consistently higher among young women, whereas rates peak among men at a slightly older age. Its sequelae can be much more severe for women affecting women's and infants' health during pregnancy and the postnatal period. The infection can result in scarring of the pelvic organs in women (tubes, ovaries, endometrial lining, and perineum) leading to an increase in the risk of future tubal infertility and ectopic pregnancy [6].

Testing and treatment are keys to reducing disease and infertility associated with undiagnosed STDs. Available treatments for STDs can prevent these serious health consequences. Other treatable infections, such as gonorrhea, syphilis, and trichomoniasis, not only present with acute symptoms but can also provoke chronic infection and longer-term consequences of sexually transmitted infections such as infertility, ectopic pregnancy, as well as increased vulnerability to HIV infection. Furthermore, if the woman is pregnant, STDs can affect also the baby causing adverse pregnancy outcomes such as stillbirth, low birth weight, neonatal death, brain damage, blindness, and deafness [5].

Another sexually transmitted infection, the human papillomavirus (HPV), is significant to women's health as it is the main cause of cervical cancer and other genital cancers [7]. It is the most common sexually transmitted infection in women. Whereas most HPV infections are short-lived and benign, persistent genital infection with certain genotypes of the virus can lead to the development of anogenital precancers, cancers, and genital warts. Even if it is common also in men, cases of cancer due to HPV in men are more uncommon than in women.

Cervical cancer is common among women worldwide. The incidence and mortality rates are related to the presence of screening and HPV vaccination programs. Most cases of cervical cancer occur in developing countries, where cervical cancer screening and prevention services are inconsistent [8]. In fact, cervical cancer can be prevented through regular screening and treatment of precancerous lesions, but these services are rarely available in most developing countries. Up to now also highly effective vaccine against HPV exists, but its accessibility is very limited in undeveloped countries.

21.3 Infertility

Infertility is a medical condition that involves a couple rather than a single individual. According to the WHO glossary "infertility is a disease characterized by the failure to establish a clinical pregnancy after 12 months of regular, unprotected sexual intercourse" [9]. Infertility is estimated to affect between 8% and 12% of reproductive-aged couples worldwide [10], reaching higher percentages in some populations in South Asia, Middle East and North Africa, Central and Eastern Europe, and Central Asia [11].

The World Health Organization Task Force on Diagnosis and Treatment of Infertility reported that in developed countries, the female factor infertility is present in 37% of infertile couples, male factor infertility in 8%, and both male and female factor infertility in 35%.

Although infertility can have also a male factor, the female partners are more often stigmatized and blamed when couples fail to reproduce [12, 13]. Male infertility is a chronic reproductive health condition affecting millions of men worldwide, even if it is under recognized and under diagnosed and difficult to treat, lasting over the course of a man's lifetime [14].

In high-income countries, infertility is often linked to a late start of childbearing and often addressed through infertility treatments. In low-income countries, a great majority of infertility cases are caused by sexually transmitted and other infections as well as postpartum and post-abortion infections, which are a major cause of secondary infertility in women [11]. For example, in 47 developing countries in 2004, among 187 million couples affected by infertility, 18 million were said to have primary infertility and the remaining 169 million secondary infertility [15].

For this reason the first approach to infertility should be prevention mainly through reproductive health specialists and public health educators. Infertility prevention should comprehend early detection and treatment of STDs and prevention and effective treatment of postpartum and post-abortion infections.

21.4 Contraception

Various forms of contraception, including the pill, injections, subdermal implants, and intrauterine contraceptives, have been widely available for women since the 1960s (Table 21.1). On the other side, options available for male contraception are obsolete and affected by high failure rate and low efficacy such as condoms and difficulty to reverse such as vasectomy (Table 21.1). For these reasons, family planning continues to be demanded to women even if a large number of men would welcome the opportunity to use male contraceptive methods recognizing that the possibility of sharing family planning should be an individual right other than responsibility.

A large number of men surveyed internationally are interested and would welcome the opportunity to use male contraceptive methods [16–18]. The availability of male hormonal contraceptives would give men the chance to gain control over their own fertility and to share the responsibility of family planning. Among the different approaches to control male fertility, hormonal contraception is the closest to a possible clinical application. However, despite the significant progress showing efficacy, feasibility, and acceptability of hormonal regimens, research in this field has not led to a product approved for clinical use.

Table 21.1 Available female and male contraceptive methods and their effectiveness

Female contraceptive methods	Typical use (%)	Perfect use (%)	Male contraceptive methods	Typical use (%)	Perfect use (%)
Condom	21	5	Condom	18	2
Diaphragm plus spermicide	12	6	Vasectomy	0.15	0.10
Oral contraceptives	9	0.3			
Transdermal patch	8	0.3			
Vaginal ring	8	0.3			
Injectable	6	0.2			
Cu-IUC	0.8	0.6			
Implant	0.05	0.05			
LNG-IUC	0.2	0.3			
Surgical sterilization	0.5	0.5			

The percentages indicate the number out of every 100 women who experienced an unintended pregnancy within the first year of typical or perfect use of each contraceptive method
Adapted from [27]

21.5 Menopause

With increasing life expectancy, the menopausal and postmenopausal phases are becoming more significant events in women's lives, and the postmenopausal phase represents one-third of the total life expectancy. Menopause can bring health, psychological, and cultural changes to a woman's life, sometimes with negative consequences. And certain health risks in women can be associated with menopause (osteoporosis, cardiovascular disease, cognitive impairment, etc.).

Management of menopause should include a full medical evaluation, assessment of woman's opinions and feelings on menopause, and individual concerns. Healthcare provider should advise women about available treatments and set realistic goals from a prescribed management plan. Hormone therapy has been the principal treatment of menopause-related symptoms for over 50 years as an option for women with distress caused by vasomotor and urogenital symptoms as well as an option for some women at risk for bone fractures. Anyway levels of access to menopause-dedicated health facilities and preventive measures are largely influenced by education, social environment, and attitude toward aging. Furthermore, there is an evident close relationship between the acceptance of hormonal therapy and education and social status.

Only in recent years, more attention has been paid to the andropause, that is, the decline of serum concentrations of testosterone in the aging man. However, unlike menopause, where complete estrogen deficiency with known clinical consequences occurs, the decline in testosterone in aging men is more slow, it is modest, and the possible clinical consequences have not been well established.

It can be associated with certain symptoms such as fatigue, tiredness, reduced muscle mass and bone density, diminished hematopoiesis, oligospermia, sexual dysfunction, anxiety, irritability, sleeping disorders, diminished memory, and cognitive function. Anyway the causal link between reduced testosterone levels and these symptoms has not yet been totally defined, and the impact of testosterone replacement in older men with hypogonadal symptoms is still unclear.

21.6 Sexual Health

Sexual dysfunction is highly represented both in men and women, but it is still very often an underdiagnosed condition especially in women.

Normal male sexual function and the causes of sexual dysfunction are very well understood, and there are plenty of effective treatments available. Sexual dysfunction is common in men and increases with age. Sexual dysfunction in men includes decreased libido, erectile dysfunction (ED), sexual pain disorders, and ejaculatory disorders including premature and delayed ejaculation and anejaculation. Diseases involving the central nervous system (brain or spinal cord) and nerves such as the cavernous or pudendal nerves are associated with ED. The major risk factors of ED are diabetes mellitus [19], heart disease, hypertension, dyslipidemia, lower urinary tract symptoms (LUTS), and cigarette smoking. For these reasons, sexual dysfunction in men can be a sign of a possible underlying severe disease giving an opportunity to address greater comorbid disease. In particular, ED and cardiovascular disease share many risk factors as both their origins involve endothelial dysfunction: ED may be an early warning sign of future cardiovascular events and can be used as a warning sign to prevent cardiovascular events [20, 21].

Sexual dysfunction in women is very common as sexual complaints are reported by approximately 40% of women worldwide, and it is very often a distressing condition that has a negative impact on the quality of life [22]. FSD includes lack of sexual desire, impaired arousal, inability to achieve orgasm, or pain with sexual activity. Female sexual dysfunction (FSD) is often underdiagnosed because underreported by the women and because doctors rarely ask the woman about her sexual health.

The female sexual response is still not completely understood even if more studied in recent years. Female sexual function is characterized by a complex interaction of physical, psychosocial, and hormonal factors requiring careful listening and inquiry by clinicians during evaluation. And for this reason, it is still much less well understood and studied. Even if some similarities exist in the physiology and pathophysiology of male and female sexual function, the differences explain the difficulty in finding effective treatments for women. In fact, although there are a multitude of drugs available for male sexual dysfunctions, there are few approved drugs for women with FSD.

Sexual dysfunction is also a very common problem after menopause. Physical examination may be particularly helpful in diagnosing atrophic vaginal changes, which frequently result in dyspareunia after menopause. In fact, in postmenopausal women declining estrogen levels affects vaginal function leading to dryness, burning, dyspareunia, and urinary dysfunction with a negative effect on sexual function. For women with symptomatic vulvovaginal atrophy who do not improve with vaginal lubricants and moisturizers, there are local and systemic therapies available [23]: vaginal estrogen therapy (insert, ring, or cream), ospemifene which is a selective estrogen receptor modulator (SERM) effective in treating dyspareunia and vaginal dryness in menopausal women, and vaginal laser therapy.

21.7 Lower Urinary Tract Disorders and Pelvic Organ Prolapse

The organs composing the lower urinary tract (LUT) in men and women are the bladder and the urethra. Gender-specific differences in the anatomy of LUT are responsible for different health' problems: the urethra in women is shorter making them more susceptible to urinary tract infections and urinary incontinence. The male urethra is much longer and has four parts (the penile urethra, bulbous urethra, membranous urethra, and the prostatic urethra) being more prone than the female one to traumatic injury and stricture formation.

As men and women age, the prevalence of lower urinary tract symptoms (LUTS) increases. Women are more prone to urinary incontinence than men. Urinary incontinence is the involuntary leakage of urine. About 50% of women experience urinary incontinence while only 25–61% of symptomatic women seek care [24, 25].

Women are reluctant to initiate discussions about urinary symptoms due to embarrassment, lack of knowledge about treatment options, and fear. The epidemiology of urinary incontinence has been less studied in men compared to women, but the prevalence of urinary incontinence in men is esteemed from 11% to 34% in men older than 65 years.

Urinary incontinence is not associated with increased mortality; however, it has a significant impact on many aspects of a patient's health, impairing quality of life and sexual function and increasing morbidity (perineal infections, healthcare costs, and in older women with urinary urgency or urge incontinence increasing falls risk). The major clinical types of urinary incontinence are stress incontinence (leakage with maneuvers that increase intraabdominal pressure), urgency incontinence (sudden urgency followed by leakage), mixed incontinence (symptoms of both stress and urgency), and overflow incontinence. After evaluation, initial treatment includes lifestyle modifications and pelvic floor muscle exercises. Further therapies with drugs or surgical therapies should be proposed depending on the type of urinary incontinence.

The anatomic support of the pelvic organs in women is provided by the interaction between the muscles of the pelvic floor and connective tissue attachments to the bony pelvis. Differently from men, this anatomic conformation of the pelvis combined with the trauma given by pregnancies and deliveries makes women and not men prone to pelvic organ prolapse (POP), that is, herniation of the pelvic organs to or beyond the vaginal walls. This condition is very common, and POP's related symptoms usually impact daily activities, sexual function, and exercise. The presence of POP can also have a negative impact on body image and self-esteem. POP when defined by symptoms has a prevalence of 3–6% and up to 50% when based upon medical examination [26]. The most common symptom of prolapse is a sensation of pelvic heaviness or protrusion of tissue from the vagina. Women with prolapse commonly have other pelvic floor disorders, including urinary, bowel, and sexual complaints. Treatment of POP requires significant healthcare resources through ambulatory activity and surgery. Symptomatic women can be managed expectantly, treated with conservative therapy (vaginal pessaries and pelvic floor exercises) or with surgical therapy (vaginal and abdominal open, laparoscopic, or robotic approaches, with and without graft materials).

21.8 Summary

Biological and social gender differences should always be acknowledged when considering the presentation, the severity, the treatment, and the consequences of both reproductive and general health diseases. Biological differences can make women more prone than men to certain medical conditions during reproductive years: they are more prone to HIV and other sexually transmitted infections. The female partners are still often stigmatized and blamed in case of infertility even if infertility can have also a male factor. Family planning continues to be demanded to women because options available for male contraception are still obsolete and affected by high failure rate. But also after menopause, biological differences make women more susceptible to certain medical conditions such as genital organ prolapse, urinary incontinence, and vaginal atrophy with related sexual dysfunction. It should also be considered that in certain societies, women continue to face discrimination or gender prejudice limiting their access to knowledge and health resources making them even more susceptible to diseases. But also in countries with a higher progress, there is still a need for continuous investment in greater gender equality.

References

1. World Health Organization. Gender, women and primary health care renewal: a discussion paper. Geneva: WHO; 2010.
2. Ribeiro PS, Jacobsen KH, Mathers CD, Garcia-Moreno C. Priorities for women's health from the Global Burden of Disease study. Int J Gynaecol Obstet. 2008;102:82–90. https://doi.org/10.1016/j.ijgo.2008.01.025.
3. Chersich MF, Rees HV. Vulnerability of women in southern Africa to infection with HIV: biological determinants and priority health sector interventions. AIDS (London, England). 2008;22(Suppl 4):S27–40. https://doi.org/10.1097/01.aids.0000341775.94123.75.
4. Weinstock H, Berman S, Cates W Jr. Sexually transmitted diseases among American youth: incidence and prevalence estimates, 2000. Perspect Sex Reprod Health. 2004;36:6–10. https://doi.org/10.1363/3600604.
5. Glasier A, et al. Sexual and reproductive health: a matter of life and death. Lancet. 2006;368:1595–607. https://doi.org/10.1016/S0140-6736(06)69478-6.
6. Davies B, Turner KM, Frølund M, Ward H, May MT, Rasmussen S, Benfield T, Westh H, Danish Chlamydia Study Group. Risk of reproductive complications following chlamydia testing: a population-based retrospective cohort study in Denmark. Lancet Infect Dis. 2016;16(9):1057.
7. Committee on Practice Bulletins—Gynecology. Practice Bulletin No. 168: Cervical cancer screening and prevention. Obstet Gynecol. 2016;128(4):e111–30. https://doi.org/10.1097/AOG.0000000000001708.
8. Jemal A, Bray F, Center MM, Ferlay J, Ward E, Forman D. Global cancer statistics. CA Cancer J Clin. 2011;61(2):69–90. https://doi.org/10.3322/caac.20107. Epub 2011 Feb 4. Erratum in: CA Cancer J Clin. 2011;61(2):134.
9. Zegers-Hochschild F, Adamson GD, Dyer S, Racowsky C, de Mouzon J, Sokol R, Rienzi L, Sunde A, Schmidt L, Cooke ID, Simpson JL, van der Poel S. The international glossary on infertility and fertility care, 2017. Hum Reprod 2017;32(9):1786–1801. doi: https://doi.org/10.1093/humrep/dex234.
10. Ombelet W, Cooke I, Dyer S, Serour G, Devroey P. Infertility and the provision of infertility medical services in developing countries. Hum Reprod Update. 2008;14(6):605–21. https://doi.org/10.1093/humupd/dmn042. Epub 2008 Sep 26. Review.
11. Mascarenhas MN, Flaxman SR, Boerma T, Vanderpoel S, Stevens GA. National, regional, and global trends in infertility prevalence since 1990: a systematic analysis of 277 health surveys. PLoS Med. 2012;9(12):e1001356. https://doi.org/10.1371/journal.pmed.1001356. Epub 2012 Dec 18.
12. Inhorn MC. Global infertility and the globalization of new reproductive technologies: illustrations from Egypt. Soc Sci Med. 2003;56(9):1837–51.
13. Wischmann T, Thorn P. (Male) infertility: what does it mean to men? New evidence from quantitative and qualitative studies. Reprod Biomed Online. 2013;27(3):236–43. https://doi.org/10.1016/j.rbmo.2013.06.002. Epub 2013 Jun 19.

14. Kamischke A, Nieschlag E. Update on medical treatment of ejaculatory disorders. Int J Androl. 2002;25(6):333–44. Review.
15. WHO. Women and health: today's evidence tomorrow's agenda. Geneva: WHO; 2009.
16. Zhang L, Shah IH, Liu Y, Vogelsong KM, Zhang L. The acceptability of an injectable, once-a-month male contraceptive in China. Contraception. 2006;73(5):548–53. Epub 2006 Jan 20.
17. Meriggiola MC, Cerpolini S, Bremner WJ, Mbizvo MT, Vogelsong KM, Martorana G, Pelusi G. Acceptability of an injectable male contraceptive regimen of norethisterone enanthate and testosterone undecanoate for men. Hum Reprod. 2006;21(8):2033–40. Epub 2006 May 26.
18. Wang C, Swerdloff RS. Hormonal approaches to male contraception. Curr Opin Urol. 2010;20(6):520–4. https://doi.org/10.1097/MOU.0b013e32833f1b4a. Review.
19. McCulloch DK, Campbell IW, Wu FC, Prescott RJ, Clarke BF. The prevalence of diabetic impotence. Diabetologia. 1980;18(4):279–83.
20. Sullivan ME, Keoghane SR, Miller MA. Vascular risk factors and erectile dysfunction. BJU Int. 2001;87(9):838–45. Review.
21. Chiurlia E, D'Amico R, Ratti C, Granata AR, Romagnoli R, Modena MG. Subclinical coronary artery atherosclerosis in patients with erectile dysfunction. J Am Coll Cardiol. 2005;46(8):1503–6. Epub 2005 Sep 28.
22. Shifren JL, Monz BU, Russo PA, Segreti A, Johannes CB. Sexual problems and distress in United States women: prevalence and correlates. Obstet Gynecol. 2008;112(5):970–8. https://doi.org/10.1097/AOG.0b013e3181898cdb.
23. ACOG Practice Bulletin No. 141: management of menopausal symptoms. Obstet Gynecol. 2014;123(1):202–16. https://doi.org/10.1097/01.AOG.0000441353.20693.78. Erratum in: Obstet Gynecol. 2016;127(1):166.
24. Harris SS, Link CL, Tennstedt SL, Kusek JW, McKinlay JB. Care seeking and treatment for urinary incontinence in a diverse population. J Urol. 2007;177(2):680–4.
25. Minassian VA, Yan X, Lichtenfeld MJ, Sun H, Stewart WF. The iceberg of health care utilization in women with urinary incontinence. Int Urogynecol J. 2012;23(8):1087–93. https://doi.org/10.1007/s00192-012-1743-x. Epub 2012 Apr 12.
26. Barber MD, Maher C. Epidemiology and outcome assessment of pelvic organ prolapse. Int Urogynecol J. 2013;24(11):1783–90. https://doi.org/10.1007/s00192-013-2169-9. Review.
27. Trussell J. Contraceptive failure in the United States. Contraception. 2011;83:397–404.

Suggested Reading

DeLancey JO. What's new in the functional anatomy of pelvic organ prolapse? Curr Opin Obstet Gynecol. 2016;28(5):420–9.

Gava G, Lantadilla C, Martelli V, Fattorini A, Seracchioli R, Meriggiola MC. Hot issues in female and male hormonal contraception. Minerva Ginecol. 2016;68(1):78–89.

Harper DM, DeMars LR. HPV vaccines - a review of the first decade. Gynecol Oncol. 2017;146(1):196–204.

Lukacz ES, Santiago-Lastra Y, Albo ME, Brubaker L. Urinary incontinence in women: a review. JAMA. 2017;318(16):1592–604.

Monteleone P, Mascagni G, Giannini A, Genazzani AR, Simoncini T. Symptoms of menopause - global prevalence, physiology and implications. Nat Rev Endocrinol. 2018;14(4):199–215.

Unemo M, Bradshaw CS, Hocking JS, de Vries HJC, Francis SC, Mabey D, Marrazzo JM, Sonder GJB, Schwebke JR, Hoornenborg E, Peeling RW, Philip SS, Low N, Fairley CK. Sexually transmitted infections: challenges ahead. Lancet Infect Dis. 2017;17(8):e235–79.

Weinberger JM, Houman J, Caron AT, Anger J. Female sexual dysfunction: a systematic review of outcomes across various treatment modalities. Sex Med Rev. 2018. https://doi.org/10.1016/j.sxmr.2017.12.004

Central and Peripheral Nervous Disorders

22

Francesca Pastorelli, Valentina Favoni, Sabina Cevoli, and Roberto Michelucci

Key Points

- The incidence of stroke is higher in adult men than in women. However, incidence rates of stroke rise in older female population and reverse above the seventh decade of life. Biological and physiological cofactors, such as the hormonal changes in the different ages of life and comorbidities, like migraine and hypertension, may play an important role. Reperfusion treatment is a time-dependent therapy that can be performed just in the very first hours from the onset of symptoms: women seem to arrive at hospital later than men, and once they are in the emergency room, women experience greater delays than do men. When compared with men, women have worse functional outcomes and lower quality of life after stroke. Sex differences in stroke severity, treatment, and functional outcome may be influenced by demographics and social factors.
- Alzheimer's disease has a higher prevalence in women than men, while vascular dementia is more frequent in males. Both genetic and hormonal factors may play a role to explain sex differences in the prevalence of

F. Pastorelli (✉) · R. Michelucci
IRCCS Institute of Neurological Sciences of Bologna, UOC Neurologia, Bologna, Italy
e-mail: roberto.michelucci@ausl.bo.it

V. Favoni
Department of Biomedical and NeuroMotor Sciences (DiBiNeM), Alma Mater Studiorum - University of Bologna, Bologna, Italy
e-mail: valentina.favoni2@unibo.it

S. Cevoli
IRCCS Institute of Neurological Sciences of Bologna, UOC Clinica Neurologica, Bologna, Italy
e-mail: sabina.cevoli@isnb.it

I. Tarricone, A. Riecher-Rössler (eds.), *Health and Gender*,
https://doi.org/10.1007/978-3-030-15038-9_22

dementia. Exposure to risk factors for the development of dementia, such as alcohol intake, cigarette smoking, systolic hypertension, elevated body mass index, and physical inactivity may be different in men and women, in different cultural and social environments. Education, primary occupation in earlier life, and cognitively stimulating leisure activities in midlife or later life have been combined into the concept of lifetime intellectual enrichment. Access to school education, job opportunities, and social behaviors may influence the lifetime intellectual enrichment in a gender-related fashion, which may have a dimorphic effect on the risk of dementia.

- The majority of primary headache disorders have a higher prevalence in females than males. Migraine represents a common disorder that is disproportionately prevalent in women. The higher prevalence in women was found at all ages, although the differences varied across the life-span. Women report more severe, more frequent, and longer duration of attacks than men. Men have longer periods of remission compared to women. A possible explanation of sex difference is genetic factors. However, migraine is a polygenic disease with strong modulation by environmental factors. Strong evidence links migraine with the hormonal status of women: timing and frequency of migraine attacks are influenced by hormone-related events such as menarche, menstruation, pregnancy, and menopause. Migraine comorbidity must be taken into account in the choice of hormonal contraception.
- The incidence and prevalence of MS is growing worldwide, and the incidence and relapse rate seems to be increasing in females more than in males. On the contrary, men who develop MS exhibit a more rapid decline in disability and cognitive function than women. It is not clear why sex-related factors which mediate the incidence of the disease and the relapse rate should play different roles in disease progression and disability. Sexual dimorphism in prevalence and clinical course of MS seem to be related to a complex interplay between genetic and biological background and different environmental exposures and modern lifestyles of men and women. Much more study is needed to understand sex and gender differences in the natural history of MS, the response to disease-modifying treatments, and the influence of the disease on the quality of life of MS patients.
- Women with epilepsy (WWE) show distinct specificities in terms of diagnosis and management, particularly during the fertile phases of life. There are a number of issues to be addressed, particularly catamenial epilepsy, hormonal interactions with antiepileptic drugs (AEDs), sexual dysfunction, contraception, pregnancy, menopause, and bone health. Exacerbation of seizures during different phases of the menstrual cycle can affect women with preexisting epilepsy (catamenial epilepsy). There

exist complex and reciprocal interactions between female hormones, seizures, and AEDs. Many AEDs are known to affect the metabolism of estrogen and progesterone, thereby reducing the efficacy and effectiveness of the oral contraceptive pill. The management of WWE during pregnancy should include monitoring of serum levels of AEDs. In fact, the serum concentration of many drugs is prone to decline during pregnancy, affecting the rate of seizures. The major issues of pregnancy in WWE concern the potential of teratogenic effects of AEDs. Evidence-based recommendations include the avoidance of valproate and AED polytherapy during pregnancy, especially during the first trimester, and preconception folic acid supplementation.

22.1 Introduction

"Dimorphic neurology" focuses on differences between men and women in the causes, manifestations, response to treatments, and outcomes of neurological diseases [1]. Moreover, there is increasing attention on determinants of health including not only the genetic and biological differences between males and females defining what we usually call "sex" but also psychological, environmental, and sociocultural factors that define what is commonly called "gender" and which may affect disproportionally men's and women's health [2–4]. Women differ from men in many ways, including genetic differences in immunity, coagulation, hormonal factors, reproductive life including pregnancy and childbirth, and social factors, all of which can influence the risk for disease and impact disease outcomes (AHA guideline). When we talk about "gender and medicine," we should consider many different aspects of the topic and try to answer specific questions:

1. *Do we know any gender-related difference in risk factors for the disease?* We must distinguish between "non-modifiable risk factors" and "modifiable risk factors," as the correction of the last ones can play a key role in disease prevention. Association of more than one risk factor may increase the power of single disease modifiers. Age and race can be considered non-modifiable cofactors. Gender implicates biological and physiological non-modifiable peculiarities but leads also to differences in comorbidity, life habits, and cultural approach to diseases that give food for preventive medicine.
   (a) Genetic risk factors
      - Physiological differences between males and females
      - Genetic diseases: gender-related differences in the incidence, prevalence, and phenotypic expression of the disease
   (b) Acquired risk factors
      - Comorbidity
      - Exposure to environmental agents

- Lifestyle
- Work activity

2. *Do we know any gender-related difference in the access to diagnostic process?*
   (a) Due to differences between men and women in onset and clinical manifestation of the disease
   (b) Due to everyday life habits and cultural, social, and/or economical biases
3. *Do we know any gender-related difference in availability of therapeutic tools?*
4. *Do we know any gender-related difference in compliance to therapy or in clinical response to therapy?*
5. What are the consequences of the disease on the patient's family life and work life? What are the consequences on social integration of the patient? Can we underlie any gender-related difference?

These pages are far from being a complete review about the implications of sex, gender, and neurologic diseases. They want to give students some food for thought about the topic resuming the main aspects of gender differences in neurologic diseases.

22.2 Stroke

Stroke is the second leading cause of death worldwide, and gender-related differences are well known, in incidence, prevalence, and outcome.

The incidence of stroke is higher in adult men than in women. However, incidence rates of stroke rise in older female population and reverse above the seventh decade of life [5]. Estrogen may act a protecting role during the childbearing age, as stroke risk in women increases after menopause, coinciding with a decline in sex hormones. However, animal studies about the role of extradiol, a natural gonadotropic hormone, on cerebral vascular disease are conflicting [6]. Early physiological or iatrogenic menopause (i.e., before the age of 45 years) is related to a higher risk of ischemic stroke. However, also intrinsic biological differences must be taken into account when we try to explain age- and gender-related variability in stroke risk.

The risk for stroke is higher in pregnant than in nonpregnant young women, with the highest stroke risk occurring in the third trimester and postpartum. The incidence of ischemic stroke is about 3.8–18/100,000 childbirths, the incidence of cerebral hemorrhage is 9/100,000, and the incidence of cerebral venous thrombosis is 12/100,000 childbirths [7]. Rare causes of stroke are responsible for 5–12% of maternal deaths during pregnancy. A consensus on the etiology and the level of increased stroke risk during pregnancy has not been achieved; however, hormonal changes occurring during pregnancy should be regarded as a cofactor. The physiological changes of pregnancy, specifically venous stasis, edema, and hypercoagulability, make pregnancy and the postpartum period a time of increased risk for stroke [8].

Pregnancy-related hypertension is the leading cause of both hemorrhagic stroke and ischemic stroke in pregnant and postpartum women. The obstetric anamnesis of a woman can be looked at as a window on the future risk of cardio- and cerebrovascular disease: in fact, it is well known that there is a relationship between the occurrence of obstetric complications such as hypertension or diabetes during pregnancy, preeclampsia, and preterm delivery and higher risk of cardio- and cerebrovascular disease during the woman's lifetime [8].

More than 70% of patients with stroke have blood pressure greater than 140/90 mmHg. In the >64 age population, far more women than men have hypertension, and blood pressure control rate is lower in older women compared to men. It is demonstrated that controlling blood pressure reduces the incidence of ischemic stroke. Additionally, lower rates of recurrent stroke have been associated to lower blood pressure [9].

A complex association between migraine and stroke has been discussed for over four decades [10]. Migraine is a primary headache disorder, and women are affected two to three times more often than men. Recent meta-analysis studies indicate a consistent link between migraine and cardiovascular disease events: migraine increases the risk of myocardial infarction, stroke, angina/coronary revascularization procedures, and cardiovascular mortality [11]. Up to a third of migraineurs experience transient neurologic symptoms called aura, before or during headache: migraine with aura has been consistently associated with increased risk of stroke, especially the ischemic subtype. The correlation between migraine and the risk of hemorrhagic stroke is still under debate. Smoke habits are linked to elevated stroke risk among women with migraine. The role of contraceptive therapy on the course of migraine and stroke risk is still under debate. Current evidence demonstrates that new, low-dose oral contraceptives (25 μg of ethynylestradiol or less) do not enhance vascular risk in migraine women [10].

In terms of clinical presentation, women seem to have a higher frequency of total anterior circulation stroke than men, a lower frequency of posterior circulation strokes, as well as higher frequency of nontraditional onset symptoms, such as impaired consciousness and altered mental status. Onset of stroke with nontraditional symptoms is often associated with a significant delay in the identification of stroke and thus inability to provide treatment promptly.

Reperfusion treatment is the gold standard for acute ischemic stroke, but it is possible if the patient reaches hospital early enough. Thrombolysis and mechanical thrombectomy are time-sensitive treatments: the earlier they are initiated, the better is the chance of a positive outcome. Intravenous thrombolysis can be performed within 4.5 h from the onset of symptoms and intra-arterial thrombolysis and mechanical thrombectomy within 6 h. It is therefore important to identify stroke as soon as possible. There is some evidence of sex differences in prehospital and inhospital delay, that is, time from stroke onset to arrival in the emergency department and treatment: women seem to arrive later than men, and once they are in the emergency room, women experience greater delays than do men. There is also evidence that women are less likely to receive thrombolysis with intravenous recombinant tissue plasminogen activator (IV rt-PA) than men. IV rt-PA is effective for both men and women, but women may be even more likely to benefit from treatment than men: in fact treatment nullified the expected gender gap in outcome, while among patients not treated with rt-PA, women may have worse outcomes than men [12]. Sex disparities in the treatment of stroke remain a concern. Prehospital times are shorter for witnessed stroke events. When a person lives alone, it is less likely for the onset of stroke symptoms to be witnessed by another person. One can assume that clinical factors such as pre-stroke disability and physical or cognitive impairment and social factors, such as residence status (i.e., living alone or in a family environment), may influence prehospitalization times and prevent women from being treated if presentation is outside of the treatment time window [13]. Even stroke clinical presentation may influence prehospital and inhospital times: nontraditional stroke symptoms, which seem to be more common in women, are related to treatment delay [14].

When compared with men, women have worse functional outcomes and lower quality of life after stroke. However, sex differences in stroke severity and functional outcome may be influenced by demographics and social factors: at stroke onset women are older than men and present a high rate of pre-stroke disability. Some studies underlay the importance of social, environmental, and legal gender inequalities to explain poorer outcomes in women after stroke [15]: in countries with lower rights for women compared to men, women seem to have the higher stroke mortality. In particular, indices like lower access to job opportunities, lack of domestic violence legislation, and inequalities in property ownership rights are related to lower health outcome and higher poststroke mortality.

22.3 Dementia

Dementia and mild cognitive impairment are characterized by a progressive decline of cognitive functions. In dementia, the decline affects activities of daily living or social functioning. In mild cognitive impairment, the patient can still engage in complex activities, such as paying bills or taking medication, but greater effort or new strategies might be required to complete tasks successfully. The boundary between mild cognitive impairment and dementia is gray [16]. Dementia is more common in elderly, with exponential increases in incidence over the age of 65. It does not mean that cognitive decline should be considered the inevitable consequence of getting older: prevention is possible, and that means reducing risk factors (cardiovascular disease, cerebrovascular disease, metabolic and psychiatric factors, diet, lifestyle, and education) and improving resilience and brain cognitive reserve. There are many different types of dementia, and Alzheimer's disease (AD) is the most common. AD is a neurodegenerative disorder characterized by progressive loss of memory and overall decline of cognitive function. AD is associated with neuropathologic hallmarks, neurofibrillary tangles, beta-amyloid plaques, loss of connections, inflammation, and eventual death of brain cells, leading to cortical and subcortical atrophy.

Vascular dementia (VaD) is the next most common. VaD refers to the heterogeneous group of clinical syndromes, which include dementia, resulting from ischemic, hemorrhagic, anoxic, or hypoxic brain damage. Ischemic VaD may be due to a combination of macrovascular or microvascular cerebral disease. The combination of AD and cerebrovascular pathologies corresponds to a type of dementia called mixed dementia [17]: pure cerebrovascular disease and pure Alzheimer's disease represent the two extremes of a broad spectrum of clinical and neuropathological patterns [18].

Some studies underlie a higher prevalence of AD in women than men, while VaD is more frequent in males [19]. Many different factors, that is, genetic and hormonal factors, may play a role to explain sex differences in the prevalence of dementia.

Genetic studies examined the association between single-nucleotide polymorphisms and AD.

The E4 allele of the apolipoprotein E gene (APOE) is the strongest known susceptibility variant for AD. There are three major isoforms of the ApoE protein (ApoE2, ApoE3, and ApoE4) that are encoded by three alleles of the APOE gene (E2, E3, and E4). Carriers of one E4 allele are three to four times more likely to develop AD than noncarriers. Carriers of the E4 allele also have an earlier age of onset of AD. The effects of the E4 allele are more pronounced in women than in men, but, interestingly, sex differences in E4 carriers seem to be reduced after the age of 85. Sex-related factors, such as hormonal levels in women and men, or the interaction with other genes hosting in chromosome X and Y, as well as gender-related factors may explain such difference in E4 allele effects.

The estrogen produced by the ovaries in a woman before menopause has a protective effect on the brain: apolipoprotein E may have a critical role in the neuroprotective actions of estrogen. Early physiological or iatrogenic menopause causes an abrupt deficiency of estrogen, progesterone, and testosterone and a disruption of the hypothalamic-pituitary-ovarian axis. However, the impact of estrogen loss and of hormone replacement therapy (HRT) on the risk of AD in women remains controversial. On the other hand, it is possible that apolipoprotein E interacts synergistically with known risk factors for dementia, such as alcohol intake, cigarette smoking, systolic hypertension, elevated body mass index, and physical inactivity. The exposure to protective and risk factors may be different in men and women in different cultural and social environments.

Lower education is one of the strongest risk factors for dementia and AD. However, subjects who are involved in mentally stimulating activities at work and in leisure activities may reduce their initial risk due to lower education. It means that education, primary occupation in earlier life, and cognitively stimulating leisure activities in midlife or later life have been combined into the concept of lifetime intellectual enrichment. It has been hypothesized that lifetime intellectual enrichment may provide an important brain reserve mechanism to delay the onset of cognitive decline and dementia [20]. The protective effect of intellectual enrichment is comparable in men and women. On the other hand, the access to school education, job opportunities, and social behaviors may be looked at as gender-related and historically contingent variables that may have a dimorphic effect on the risk of dementia, when it is observed in different countries and social contexts.

22.4 Headache

Headache is the commonest neurological condition worldwide, and sex-specific differences are widely observed. With few exceptions, it is well established that the majority of primary headache disorders have a higher prevalence in females than males. Among primary headache disorders, migraine represents a common disorder that is disproportionately prevalent in women. Migraine has two major subtypes: migraine without aura (MO) and migraine with aura (MA). MO is a clinical syndrome characterized by headache attacks lasting 4–42 h, characterized by generally unilateral location, pulsating quality, moderate or severe intensity, aggravation by routine physical activity, and association with nausea and/or photophobia and phonophobia. MA is primarily characterized by transient focal neurological symptoms that usually precede or sometimes accompany a headache with migrainous features. Visual aura is the most common type of aura, occurring in over 90% of patients with MA. It often occurs as a fortification spectrum or a scintillating scotoma and lasts less than 60 min. Around one in four people with migraine have an aura [21].

Worldwide, migraine prevalence is two to three times higher in females compared to men (18% of women vs. 6% of men) and stable over time [22]. The higher prevalence in women was found at all ages, although the differences varied across the life-span. The National Health Interview Survey found that the 1-year prevalence is similar in girls and boys until puberty, after which the prevalence rises in both sexes [23]. During the reproductive years, there is the greatest difference in prevalence between women and men, with a peak among those aged 30–39. Then the prevalence declines, but migraine remains higher in women than in men [22]. Moreover, lifetime prevalence of migraine without aura is two times greater than migraine with aura in both sexes (15.9% vs. 7.5% in women compared to 7.6% vs. 3.6% in men) [24]. Migraine is a chronic disorder with episodic attacks. Women reported more severe, more frequent, and longer duration of attacks than men. Men have longer periods of remission compared to women. Controversy exists regarding the role of sex as a risk factor for the conversion from episodic migraine to chronic migraine. The Global Burden of Disease Study ranks migraine as the fourth cause of disability in women and the eighth in men. This results in a substantial burden of disease. Studies on sex differences of comorbid diseases report conflicting results. A possible explanation of sex difference is genetic factors. However, migraine is a polygenic disease with strong modulation by environmental factors.

Strong evidence links migraine with the hormonal status of women. Timing and frequency of migraine attacks are influenced by hormone-related events such as menarche, menstruation, pregnancy, and menopause, as well as use of oral contraceptives and hormone replacement therapy (HRT). Usually migraine starts after menarche, occurs more frequently during menstruation, and ameliorates during pregnancy and after menopause. According to the "estrogen withdrawal" hypothesis, migraine is triggered by the sudden decline in estrogen levels occurring immediately before menses and during the transition toward menopause or in the early postmenopausal period [25].

Many women note that their migraine attacks occur in temporal relationship with their menses. Studies show that about 50% of the women with migraine experience a relationship between menstruation and the occurrence of migraine attacks. Menstrual migraine is defined as attacks of migraine that occur regularly in at least two of three consecutive menstrual cycles and occur exclusively on day 1–2 of menstruation, but may range from 2 days before (defined as −2) to 3 days after (defined as +3 with the first day of menstruation as day +1). The menstrual migraine attacks are usually without aura, last much longer, are more often associated with severe nausea, and are more painful than non-menstrual attacks [26].

Pregnancy is associated with an improvement of migraine in 60–70% of women, mainly during the second and third trimester. Women with perimenstrual migraine prepregnancy are more likely to achieve improvement during pregnancy. On the contrary, the migraine type is not a significant prognostic factor for improvement. However, migraine with aura is more likely to continue or develop for the first time in pregnancy. After childbirth, just over half of the women with migraine have recurrence of migraine in the first month. Migraine occurrence may be delayed by breastfeeding, with most studies supporting breastfeeding as protective against migraine [25].

During fertile years, a significant number of women with migraine have to face the choice of reliable hormonal contraception. Combined hormonal contraceptives (CHCs) may be used in the majority of women with migraine. Historically, CHCs are associated with an aggravation of migraine. Migraine with aura worsens more (56.4%) than migraine without aura (25.3%). A specific "window" of vulnerability to migraine is triggered by the days of hormone-free interval. Furthermore, women can present migraine with aura for the first time during the initiation of CHCs. However, migraine with aura, and to a lesser extent also migraine without aura, may increase vascular risk. Migraine with aura is associated with a twofold increased risk of ischemic stroke, but the absolute risk associated with CHC use is very low in healthy young women with no additional risk factors (smoking, hypertension, diabetes, hyperlipidemia, and thrombophilia, age over 35 years) and mostly related to the estrogen dose. In this context, it is very important to remember that the World Health Organization Medical Eligibility Criteria for Contraceptive Use stated that migraine with aura at any age is an absolute contraindication to the use of CHCs [27]. Guidelines recommend progestogen-only contraception as an alternative safer option because it does not seem to be associated with an increased risk of venous thromboembolism and ischemic stroke.

During the transition to menopause, migraine attacks can become more severe and frequent due to fluctuating and changing estrogen and progesterone levels in this period. The achievement of hormonal stability on menopause is positively associated with migraine improvement. Migraine improvement after menopause is a widely accepted notion. Reported migraine prevalence during menopause ranges from 10% to 29%. However, the type of menopause has a substantial effect on migraine. In spontaneous menopause, migraine improves in 50–60% of women. On the contrary, surgically induced menopause (i.e., oophorectomy with or without hysterectomy) appears to be associated with worsening of migraine in two-thirds of women. The reason for the worsening is still unclear, but it may be related to the abrupt, large change in hormones and/or the use of supplementary estrogen following surgery. The effect of HRT on migraine is unpredictable. Either the usual contraceptive regimens or estrogen supplements can be used during the perimenopause. HRT may have variable effects depending on the route of administration, type of estrogen, and type of administration (cyclical vs. continuous). Transdermal preparations may be less likely to exacerbate migraine. Progesterone supplementation may be effective for treating menstrual migraine by suppressing menstruation. In general, progesterone dosing does not seem to change migraine frequency, duration, or severity. From a clinical perspective, no specific therapies can be indicated for menopausal migraine. To date, migraine does not represent a contraindication for HRT [28].

From a therapeutic point of view, acute and prophylactic management of migraine is the same in women and men. In menstrual migraine, rizatriptan has the best overall evidence for acute treatment and for short-term prevention; frovatriptan, zolmitriptan, or naratriptan, as well as magnesium, estrogen, naproxen sodium, or dihydroergotamine, may be useful [29]. For women planning a pregnancy, the potential benefits must overweigh the potential risks for the fetus. Management of migraine during pregnancy should first focus on avoiding potential triggers and to use non-pharmacologic therapies as biofeedback and acupuncture. If pharmacologic treatment becomes necessary, acetaminophen is a safe fist-line abortive agent; ASA and NSAIDs (ibuprofen, naproxen) can be used as a second choice, but not for long periods of time, and they should be avoided during the last trimester. On the contrary, metoclopramide should be restricted to the third trimester. In some refractory cases, dexamethasone or prednisone can be considered. Should prophylactic treatment become indicated, the beta-adrenergic receptor antagonists (e.g., propranolol) can be used. On the contrary, topiramate and sodium valproate are contraindicated. During lactation, if prophylaxis is needed, beta-adrenergic receptor antagonists, tricyclic antidepressants, and sodium valproate can be used [30].

22.5 Multiple Sclerosis

It is well known that many autoimmune diseases, including multiple sclerosis (MS), predominantly affect women: the female-to-male sex rate for MS is about 3:1. MS is an autoimmune disease mediated by CD4+ T cells reactive against central nervous system (CNS) antigens. Th cells initiate autoimmune inflammatory damage in the CNS, leading to demyelination, neuron degeneration, and progressive disability. The symptoms depend on the disease type and the site of lesions. MS is characterized by a broad heterogeneity of clinical expressions and degree of response to treatment and outcome. Approximately 85% of patients present with a relapsing-remitting course (RRMS), which is characterized by episodes of acute worsening of function followed by partial or complete recovery. RRMS onset typically occurs in early adulthood and may develop secondary progressive MS (SPMS) in about one-half of cases. SPMS is defined as a steady clinical deterioration, independent of relapses. In 10–15% of the MS population, the disease has a rapid and progressive course right from the onset (primary progressive MS (PPMS)). MS is a complex multifactorial disease. A body of literature has provided new insights through the identification of genetic, epigenetic, and environmental factors that may alter the risk of MS by triggering the autoimmune response and/or modulating the vulnerability of neuronal cells and glia to inflammatory insult. Many MS risk factors are sex and/or age specific, and their relative contribution to epidemiology and clinical manifestation of the disease may vary between geographic regions [31].

The incidence and prevalence of MS is growing worldwide, and many recent studies argue for a growing susceptibility of females in MS over the last decades. It is not clear, however, why the incidence of MS seems to be increasing only in women: changing environmental or lifestyle factors may be interacting with female sex to enhance MS risk. In addition, women with MS present more frequent relapsing-remitting MS, while primary progressive (PPMS) affects women and men equally. Moreover, a higher number of relapses are observed in females compared to males with RRMS, at any age. On the other hand, men who develop MS exhibit a more rapid decline in disability and cognitive function than women. MRI studies suggest that gray matter atrophy and white matter damage are more prominent in men than in women with MS, but at the moment, we are far from understanding the reason of sex differences in neurodegeneration. It suggests that sex-related factors which mediate the incidence of the disease and the relapse rate play different roles in disease progression and disability.

Biologic and environmental factors may be the reason for sex differences in the behavior of the disease.

MS is an autoimmune disease, driven principally by Th-cell activity, although recent studies underlay the importance of B cells and autoantibodies in mediating relapses in MS patients. The autoimmune component of MS predominates in the early stages of the disease and contributes to disease susceptibility and relapses. Neurodegenerative components are stronger in later stages and drive progression of permanent disability. One possible explanation of the sex ratio in MS incidence is that women develop more robust autoimmune responses than men.

Genetics have a contributory role, as first-degree relatives of MS patients show up to 15-fold increased risk to develop the disease. Genome-wide association studies (GWAS) identified more than 200 independent regions across the genome associated with susceptibility in MS, including a number of polymorphisms homed within the major histocompatibility complex (MHC) region [32]. The strongest MS genetic determinant is located in the human leucocyte antigen (HLA) class II DRB1 and DQB1 loci. Many other DNA variants related to MS susceptibility lie in close proximity to genes involved in common pathways of antigen presentation, T regulatory function, Th-cell activation, and cytokine production. The incident attack in RRMS and early relapses seem to be brought about when myelin-activated Th cells are primed in the peripheral lymphoid tissue, expand, and cross the blood-brain barrier (BBB) into the CNS to initiate inflammation, demyelination, and axon damage in the acute MS lesion.

Women have higher numbers of Th (CD4+) cells in peripheral blood as compared to men, and female T cells expand more robustly than male cells upon antigenic stimulation. In addition, CD4+ T cells from females show a higher propensity to produce inflammatory cytokines and seem to be better able to support humoral responses than male cells. However, the link between Th1 response and MS incidence is not yet understood. In addition, recent data indicate that even the BBB in females may also be more permissive to the entry of autoreactive lymphocytes [33].

The incidence of RRMS is highest in the reproductive years, with a peak age of onset at 29 years for women and 31 years for men. The female-to-male ratio of MS also presents a boost postpuberty, when females are prone to MS onset two to three times more than males. The F/M ratio is lower after 50 years (F/M 1.4–1.9:1) and is almost 1:1 before the age of 9 years. Puberty, pregnancy, and reproductive aging are characterized by marked hormonal transitions that may influence inflammatory activity and neurodegeneration in MS. Puberty is characterized by dramatic hormonal changes, triggered in both sexes by sustained increase of pulsatile release of gonadotropin-releasing hormone (GnRH). GnRH stimulates the pituitary-luteinizing hormone (LH) and follicle-stimulating hormone (FSH) that in turn act on gonads [34]. The trend of F/M ratio during the life-span suggests that alterations in gonadotrophin or gonadal hormone levels may influence the autoimmune mechanisms, particularly in females. Indeed, an earlier age of menarche increases the risk of RRMS, and women with relapsing-onset MS present a higher relapse rate than male patients. Pregnancy constitutes a well-established protective factor on MS relapse frequency, while the postpartum period is associated with increased relapse risk. The underlying mechanisms are not completely understood. Overall, the protective effect of pregnancy may reflect attempts to balance maternal tolerance for a semi-allogenic fetus with immune protection against infectious pathogens in both mother and fetus [35].

The incidence and prevalence of MS are changing worldwide. Improvements in MS diagnosis, greater awareness of the disease both in the patients and physicians, and a longer life expectancy have been postulated as explanations, but it is also possible that an increasing number of people in the world are developing MS in the last decades. Marked increases in MS rates are detected particularly in young females. The access of women to medical care has increased in many countries in modern times, and recent improvements in the sensitivity of diagnostic criteria and MRI imaging techniques enhanced the diagnostic accuracy of MS in the earliest stages of the disease, when the incidence of the disease is higher in women. However, recent studies on MS in genetic stable populations with a homogeneous rate of medical care provided to men and women suggest an intricate relationship between genetic and environmental factors acting in concert to explain changes in MS epidemiology [36]. The urbanization process may change deeply the living conditions and social habits of a population with protective or predisposing effects on the incidence of the disease.

Many environmental factors have been pointed out to explain the gender-related differentiation in the incidence of MS at a population level: later childhood exposure to Epstein-Barr virus (EBV), cigarette smoking, childhood obesity, low sunlight exposure and reduced circulating vitamin D, and changes in reproductive habits of women [37].

The "hygiene hypothesis" links the rise in allergic and autoimmune diseases to prevention or delay of childhood infections in developed countries. In fact, a lower exposure to infections in the first years of life may enhance the risk of autoimmunity by predisposing the immune system toward a more pro-inflammatory response. At present, EBV is the only pathogen for which there is compelling evidence of a link between infection and increased MS risk. In developing countries, infection occurs in the first years of life, and it is usually asymptomatic, while in developed countries, improved hygienic conditions delay the primary infections in adolescence or adult life, when they are more severe and frequently symptomatic, manifesting in mononucleosis. The serologic evidence of past EBV infection and a history of mononucleosis are consistently associated with an increased risk of MS independently from ethnic group [38]. However, the underlying biology of the relationship between EBV infection, infectious mononucleosis, and MS is still not clear. Moreover, very little is known as to whether EBV infection is related to recent rise in MS risk in females.

There is strong evidence that cigarette smoking is a risk factor for MS [39], with an increase in relative risk of 50% in ever smokers over never smokers. Among smokers, MS risk increases with smoking duration and intensity, and adverse effects seem to be even higher in men compared to women. Coinciding with the rise in MS, the female-to-male ratio of smoking has also been increasing worldwide in the last decades.

Geographical studies reported a positive correlation between the female-to-male sex ratio of MS and latitude in the same geographic areas and a strong correlation between UVR exposure and reduced MS incidence. Women seem to be more sensitive to protective effects of UVR exposure than men. The protective effects of UVR in MS are thought to occur through the enhancement of circulating vitamin D3 levels. Moreover, women who reported a regular intake of vitamin D-containing supplements had a lower risk of MS as compared to those who never supplemented. How vitamin D may be protective on MS risk is not clear, but a growing body of literature suggest an immunomodulatory effect of vitamin D, which may be relevant for MS [40].

A number of large case control and prospective studies found no evidence for an association of MS with oral contraceptive use. On the other hand, many studies describe an association with decreased parity: recent studies found an association between higher parity and reduced risk of a first demyelinating event [41]. It has been documented that in urbanized areas, parity has reduced and childbearing is delayed in the last decades, due to increased presence of women in the workforce and the introduction of oral contraceptives.

In conclusion, sexual dimorphism in prevalence and clinical course of MS seem to be related to a complex interplay between genetic and biological background and different environmental exposures and modern lifestyles of men and women. Much more study is needed to understand sex and gender differences in the natural history of MS, the response to disease-modifying treatments, and the influence of the disease on quality of life of MS patients.

22.6 Epilepsy

Epilepsy, defined as an enduring predisposition to generate seizures, encompasses a number of different conditions in terms of seizure types, etiologies, epilepsy syndromes, and comorbidities. Therefore epilepsy is a heterogeneous condition, and accordingly antiepileptic treatment should be tailored to each individual and epileptic condition. Women with epilepsy (WWE) show distinct specificities in terms of diagnosis and management, particularly during the fertile phases of life. It has long been known that the hormonal changes may play a role in terms of seizure frequency and recurrence, and on the other hand, specific physiological states such as pregnancy may generate a number of problems concerning the use of drugs and their effects on newborns. Overall there are a number of issues to be addressed, particularly catamenial epilepsy, hormonal interactions with AEDs, sexual dysfunction, contraception, pregnancy, menopause, and bone health [42].

Catamenial epilepsy. Catamenial epilepsy refers to exacerbation of seizures during different phases of the menstrual cycle in women with preexisting epilepsy. Catamenial epilepsy can affect one-third to one-half of WWE [43–45]. The occurrence of changes in estrogen and progesterone levels is thought to be a key factor in catamenial epilepsy, with progesterone being considered an anticonvulsant hormone and estrogen a proconvulsant.

Careful assessment of menstrual and seizure diaries and categorization of cycle type (ovulatory versus anovulatory) and duration are important steps in the diagnosis of catamenial epilepsy. There is limited evidence about the use of pharmacotherapy in managing catamenial epilepsy [43]. Increasing the dose of AEDs at the time of anticipated seizure occurrence is a possible treatment option. The use of intermittent clobazam, on days when seizures are anticipated, is the only treatment option shown to have benefit in a randomized controlled trial [46]. Alternative therapies include acetazolamide or progestogens given perimenstrually. Results from a randomized controlled trial [47] showed that WWE who present with the C1 catamenial seizure pattern may benefit from progesterone treatment.

22.6.1 Female Hormones and Contraception

There exist complex and reciprocal interactions between female hormones, seizures, and AEDs.

A number of AEDs, including carbamazepine, oxcarbazepine, topiramate, phenobarbitone, and phenytoin, are known to have cytochrome-inducing properties (CYP3A4 group) and therefore may affect the metabolism of estrogen and progesterone, thereby reducing the efficacy and effectiveness of the oral contraceptive pill (OCP). WWE taking these AEDs together with hormonal forms of contraception should receive counseling about the possible risks. No clinically relevant interaction has been documented between sodium valproate, levetiracetam, ethosuximide, pregabalin, gabapentin, vigabatrin, tiagabine, benzodiazepines, and any form of

OCP. Patients taking the OCP can show reduced concentrations of lamotrigine, and lamotrigine plasma levels should therefore be monitored [48]. There are no reported interactions between lamotrigine and the progestogen-only contraceptive pill [49]. Finally, medroxyprogesterone acetate depot injection, levonorgestrel-releasing intrauterine systems, and copper-containing intrauterine devices are methods of contraception not affected by enzyme-inducing AEDs [50]. Both depot preparations and non-hormonal methods of contraception can be recommended as safe options for WWE on AEDs [51].

22.6.2 Reproductive and Sexual Dysfunction

The most common reproductive endocrine disorder in WWE is PCOS, a condition characterized by hyperandrogenism, multiple ovarian cysts, anovulatory cycles, hirsutism, and obesity. The prevalence of PCOS in WWE has been estimated at between 4% and 19%. Most studies suggest an increased incidence of PCOS in women taking valproate [52, 53] as opposed to carbamazepine or lamotrigine [54]. Women younger than 20 years seem to be especially vulnerable to the effects of valproate [54]. The etiology of sexual dysfunction in WWE is considered to be multifactorial, with contributions from both the physical and psychological domains, including depression [55].

22.6.3 Pregnancy and Lactation

Seizure frequency is not significantly affected by pregnancy, and converging evidence from multiple studies shows that seizure activity during gestation is unchanged from prepregnancy baseline in more than half of cases [56]. The pharmacokinetic profiles of AEDs, however, may play an important role in changes in seizure frequency during pregnancy. The management of WWE during pregnancy should include monitoring of serum levels of AEDs, especially lamotrigine, carbamazepine, and phenytoin. Lamotrigine and oxcarbazepine serum concentrations may be particularly prone to decline as a result of increased glucuronidation during pregnancy. WWE taking these AEDs throughout pregnancy have been found to require more dose increases and to suffer more convulsive seizures [57, 58]. After delivery, doses can be reduced to prepregnancy baseline levels to avoid toxicity but maintain seizure control.

The major issues of pregnancy in WWE concern the potential of teratogenic effects of AEDs. Several AEDs are known to have teratogenic effects on the developing fetus (Table 22.1). In a recent longitudinal, prospective cohort study based on the EURAP International Registry including data from pregnancies in women who were exposed to antiepileptic drug monotherapy at conception, 7355 pregnancies were exposed to one of eight antiepileptic drugs [59]. It was found that the prevalence of major congenital malformations was 142 (10.3%) of 1381 pregnancies for valproate, 19 (6.5%) of 294 for phenobarbital, 8 (6.4%) of 125 for phenytoin, 107 (5.5%) of 1957 for carbamazepine, 6 (3.9%) of 152 for topiramate, 10 (3.0%) of 333 for oxcarbazepine, 74 (2.9%) of

Table 22.1 Most commonly reported teratogenic effects of antiepileptic drugs

Major congenital malformations	AEDs
Congenital heart disease	Phenobarbital, phenytoin, valproate, carbamazepine
Orofacial and craniofacial clefts	Benzodiazepines, phenobarbital, phenytoin, lamotrigine
Neural tube defects	Valproate, carbamazepine
Hypospadias	Valproate, carbamazepine

2514 for lamotrigine, and 17 (2.8%) of 599 for levetiracetam. Interestingly risks of major congenital malformation associated with lamotrigine, levetiracetam, and oxcarbazepine were within the range reported in the literature for offspring unexposed to antiepileptic drugs. On the other hand, the prevalence of major congenital malformations increased with the dose at time of conception for carbamazepine, lamotrigine, phenobarbital, and valproate. For valproate the risk of major congenital malformation was 25.2% with doses >1450 mg/day, 11.6% for doses between 650 and 1450 mg/day, and 6.3% for doses <650 mg/day. These data demonstrate the high potential for teratogenicity of valproate but also the possibility to manage the risk by decreasing the dose in the first trimester if there are no other options.

Evidence-based recommendations include the avoidance of valproate and AED polytherapy during pregnancy, especially during the first trimester, in order to reduce the risk of congenital malformations. Children born to WWE who were taking valproate throughout pregnancy have been found to have significantly lower IQ scores as compared to the children of WWE taking carbamazepine, phenytoin, or lamotrigine [56, 60, 61]. Moreover, available data show that children exposed to valproate in utero are at increased risk of autism spectrum disorder (approximately threefold) and childhood autism (approximately fivefold) compared with the general population [62]. These data furtherly highlight the need to avoid the use of valproate during pregnancy, although the administration of doses <800 mg has been associated with IQ scores similar to those of children unexposed to valproate [63].

Further recommendations include preconception folic acid supplementation in order to prevent congenital malformations in newborns and possibly improve neurodevelopmental outcomes [64].

In clinical practice, most women can be advised to continue their AED therapy, given the risk of seizures in pregnancy and the potential consequences for both mother and baby [60]. With regard to lactation, it is considered generally safe for WWE taking AEDs to breastfeed, given that only very small amounts of these drugs are excreted in breast milk.

22.6.4 Menopause-Related Issues

It is reported that in the menopause, 40% of WWE can experience a worsening of seizure frequency, whereas up to 27% may go into remission [65]. Hormone replacement therapy is significantly associated with increased frequency of seizures in menopausal women [66]. Finally cytochrome-inducing AEDs are known to affect bone mineral density and are associated with bone disorders such as osteoporosis and fractures during and after menopause.

References

1. Rocca WA, Mielke MM, Vemuri P, Miller VM. Sex and gender differences in the causes of dementia: a narrative review. Maturitas. 2014;79(2):196–201.
2. US Public Health Service. Agenda for research on women's health for the 21st century. A report of the Task Force on the NIH Women's Health Research Agenda for the 21st Century, vol. 5. Bethesda, MD: National Institutes of Health; 1999. (DHHS publication no. (NIH) 99-4389).
3. Institute of Medicine. Women's health research: progress, pitfalls, and promise. Washington, DC: The National Academies Press; 2010.
4. Woods NF, Tsui AO. Editorial: Epidemiologic approaches to women's health. Epidemiol Rev. 2014;36:1–4.
5. Ahnstedt H, McCullough LD, Cipolla MJ. The importance of considering sex differences in translational stroke research. Transl Stroke Res. 2016;7(4):261–73.
6. Shekhar S, Travis OK, He X, Roman RJ, Fan F. Menopause and ischemic stroke: a brief review. MOJ Toxicol. 2017;3(4) https://doi.org/10.15406/mojt.2017.03.00059.
7. SPREAD. (Stroke Prevention And Educational Awareness Diffusion) - Ictus cerebrale: linee guida italiane di prevenzione e trattamento - VIII Edizione.
8. Bushnell C, McCullough LD, Awad IA, Chireau MV, Fedder WN, Furie KL, Howard VJ, Lichtman JH, Lisabeth LD, Piña IL, Reeves MJ, Rexrode KM, Saposnik G, Singh V, Towfighi A, Vaccarino V, Walters MR, on behalf of the American Heart Association Stroke Council, Council on Cardiovascular and Stroke Nursing, Council on Clinical Cardiology, Council on Epidemiology and Prevention, and Council for High Blood Pressure Research. Guidelines for the prevention of stroke in women. A statement for healthcare professionals from the American Heart Association/American Stroke Association. Stroke. 2014;45:1545–88.
9. Samai AA, Martin-Schild S. Sex differences in predictors of ischemic stroke: current perspectives. Vasc Health Risk Manag. 2015;11:427–36.
10. Gryglas A, Smigiel R. Migraine and stroke: What's the link? What to do? Curr Neurol Neurosci Rep. 2017;17:22.
11. Kurth T, Winter AC, Eliassen AH, Dushkes R, Mukamal KJ, Rimm EB, Willett WC, Manson JE, Rexrode KM. Migraine and risk of cardiovascular disease in women: prospective cohort study. BMJ. 2016;353:i2610.
12. Reeves MJ, Bushnell CD, Howard G, Gargano JW, Duncan PW, Lynch G, Khatiwoda A, Lisabeth L. Sex differences in stroke: epidemiology, clinical presentation, medical care, and outcomes. Lancet Neurol. 2008;7(10):915–26.
13. Boheme AK, Carr BG, Kasner SE, Albright KC, Kallan MJ, Elkind MSV, Branas CC, Mullen MT. Sex differences in rt-PA utilization at hospitals treating stroke: the national inpatient sample. Front Neurol. 2017;8:500. https://doi.org/10.3389/fneur.2017.00500.
14. Berglund A, Schenk-Gustafsson K, von Euler M. Sex differences in the presentation of stroke. Maturitas. 2017;99:47–50.
15. Kim TD, Jung YH, Caso V, Bushnell CD, Saposnik G, on behalf of the Women's Disparities Working Group. Countries with women inequalities have higher stroke mortality. Int J Stroke. 2017;12(8):869–74.
16. Livingston G, Sommerlad A, Orgeta V, Costafreda SG, Huntley J, Ames D, Ballard C, Banerjee S, Burns A, Cohen-Mansfield J, Cooper C, Fox N, Gitlin LN, Howard R, Kales HC, Larson EB, Ritchie K, Rockwood K, Sampson EL, Samus Q, Schneider LS, Selbæk G, Teri L, Mukadam N. Dementia prevention, intervention and care. Lancet. 2017;390(10113):2673–734.

17. Bannett D. Public health importance of vascular dementia and Alzheimer's disease with cerebrovascular disease. Int J Clin Pract Suppl. 2001;(120):41–8.
18. Rizzi L, Rosset I, Roriz-Cruz M. Global epidemiology of dementia: Alzheimer's and vascular types. BioMed Res Int. 2014;2014:908915, 8 pages.
19. Mielke MM, Vemuri P, Rocca WA. Clinical epidemiology of Alzheimer's disease: assessing sex and gender differences. Clin Epidemiol. 2014;6:37–48.
20. Stern Y. Cognitive reserve. Neuropsychologia. 2009;47(10):2015–28.
21. Headache Classification Committee of the International Headache Society. The international classification of headache disorders, 3rd edition (beta version). Cephalalgia. 2013;33(9):629–808.
22. IHME. Global burden of disease study 2015 (GBD 2015). Seattle, WA: Institute for Health Metrics and Evaluation; 2016.
23. Victor TW, Hu X, Campbell JC, Buse DC, Lipton RB. Migraine prevalence by age and sex in the United States: a life-span study. Cephalalgia. 2010;30:1065–72.
24. Russell MB, Rasmussen BK, Thorvaldsen P, Olesen J. Prevalence and sex-ratio of the subtypes of migraine. Int J Epidemiol. 1995;24:612–8.
25. Vetvik KG, MacGregor EA. Sex differences in the epidemiology, clinical features, and pathophysiology of migraine. Lancet Neurol. 2017;16(1):76–87.
26. Granella F, Sances G, Allais G, Nappi RE, Tirelli A, Benedetto C, Brundu B, Facchinetti F, Nappi G. Characteristics of menstrual and nonmenstrual attacks in women with menstrually related migraine referred to headache centres. Cephalalgia. 2004;24(9):707–16.
27. WHO. Medical eligibility criteria for contraceptive use. 5th ed. Geneva: World Health Organization; 2015.
28. Ripa P, Ornello R, Degan D, Tiseo C, Stewart J, Pistoia F, Carolei A, Sacco S. Migraine in menopausal women: a systematic review. Int J Womens Health. 2015;7:773–82.
29. Maasumi K, Tepper SJ, Kriegler JS. Menstrual migraine and treatment options: review. Headache. 2017;57(2):194–208.
30. Allais GB, Rolando S, Benedetto C. La donna emicranica. In: Bonavita V, Bussone G, Casucci G, Frediani F, Manzoni GC, editors. Le Cefalee- Clinica e Terapia. Milano, Italy: Cortina Editore, press; 2015.
31. Segal BM, Cohen JA, Antel J. Americas Committee for Treatment and Research in Multiple Sclerosis Forum 2017: Environmental factors, genetics, and epigenetics in MS susceptibility and clinical course. Mult Scler J. 2018;24(1):4–5.
32. Canto E, Oksenberg JR. Multiple sclerosis genetics. Mult Scler J. 2018;24(1):75–9.
33. Dunn SE, Lee H, Pavri FR and Zhang MA. Sex-based differences in Multiple Sclerosis (Part I): biology of disease incidence. Curr Topics Behav Neurosci. 2015. https://doi.org/10.1007/7854_2015_371.
34. Waubant E. Effect of puberty on multiple sclerosis risk and course. Mult Scler J. 2018;24(1):32–5.
35. Bove R, Gilmore W. Hormones and MS: risk factors, biomarkers and therapeutic targets. Mult Scler. 2018;24(1):17–21.
36. Kotzamani D, Panou T, Mastorodemos V, et al. Rising incidence of Multiple Sclerosis in females associated with urbanization. Neurology. 2012;78:1728–35.
37. Dunn SE, Lee H, Pavri FR and Zhang MA. Sex-based differences in Multiple Sclerosis (Part II): rising incidence of Multiple Sclerosis in women and the vulnerability of men to progression of this disease. Curr Topics Behav Neurosci. 2015. https://doi.org/10.1007/7854_2015_371.
38. Langer-Gould A, Jun W, Lucas R, Smith J, Gonzales E, Amezcua L, Haraszti S, Chen LH, Quach H, James JA, Barcellos LF, Xiang AH. Epstein-Barr virus, cytomegalovirus and multiple sclerosis susceptibility. A multiethnic study. Neurology. 2017;89:130–7.
39. Degelman ML, Herman KM. Smoking and multiple sclerosis: a systematic review and meta-analysis using the Bradford Hill criteria for causation. Mult Scler Relat Disord. 2017;17:207–16.
40. Shoemaker TJ, Mowry EM. A review of vitamin D supplementation as disease-modifying therapy. Mult Scler J. 2018;24(1):6–11.

41. Ponsonby AL, Lucas RM, van der Mei IA, et al. Offspring number, pregnancy, and risk of a first clinical demyelinating event: the AusImmune Study. Neurology. 2012;78:867–74.
42. Bangar S, Shastri A, El-Sayeh H, Cavanna AE. Women with epilepsy: clinically relevant issues. Funct Neurol. 2016;31(3):127–34.
43. Foldvary-Schaefer N, Falcone T. Catamenial epilepsy: pathophysiology, diagnosis, and management. Neurology. 2003;61(Suppl 2):S2–15.
44. Herzog AG. Menstrual disorders in women with epilepsy. Neurology. 2006;66(Suppl 3):S23–8.
45. Morrell MJ. Epilepsy in women: the science of why it is special. Neurology. 1999;53(Suppl 1):S42–8.
46. Feely M, Gibson J. Intermittent clobazam for catamenial epilepsy: tolerance avoided. J Neurol Neurosurg Psychiatry. 1984;47:1279–82.
47. Herzog AG, Fowler KM, Smithson SD, et al. Progesterone vs placebo therapy for women with epilepsy: a randomized clinical trial. Neurology. 2012;78:1959–66.
48. Sabers A, Ohman I, Christensen J, et al. Oral contraceptives reduce lamotrigine plasma levels. Neurology. 2003;61:570571.
49. Gaffield ME, Culwell KR, Lee CR. The use of hormonal contraception among women taking anticonvulsant therapy. Contraception. 2011;83:16–29.
50. O'Brien MD, Guillebaud J. Contraception for women taking antiepileptic drugs. J Fam Plann Reprod Health Care. 2010;36:239–42.
51. Dutton C, Foldvary-Schaefer N. Contraception in women with epilepsy: pharmacokinetic interactions, contraceptive options, and management. Int Rev Neurobiol. 2008;83:113–34.
52. Hu X, Wang J, Dong W, et al. A meta-analysis of polycystic ovary syndrome in women taking valproate for epilepsy. Epilepsy Res. 2011;97:73–82.
53. Zhou JQ, Zhou LM, Chen LJ, et al. Polycystic ovary syndrome in patients with epilepsy: a study in 102 Chinese women. Seizure. 2012;21:729–33.
54. Morrell MJ, Hayes FJ, Sluss PM, et al. Hyperandrogenism, ovulatory dysfunction, and polycystic ovary syndrome with valproate versus lamotrigine. Ann Neurol. 2008;64:200–11.
55. Zelená V, Kuba R, Soška V, et al. Depression as a prominent cause of sexual dysfunction in women with epilepsy. Epilepsy Behav. 2011;20:539–44.
56. Harden CL, Meador KJ, Pennell PB, et al. Practice parameter update: management issues for women with epilepsy - focus on pregnancy (an evidence-based review): teratogenesis and perinatal outcomes: report of the Quality Standards Subcommittee and Therapeutics and Technology Assessment Subcommittee of the American Academy of Neurology and American Epilepsy Society. Neurology. 2009;73:133–41.
57. EURAP Study Group. Seizure control and treatment in pregnancy: observations from the EURAP epilepsy pregnancy registry. Neurology. 2006;66:354–60.
58. Vajda FJ, Hitchcock A, Graham J, et al. Foetal malformations and seizure control: 52 months data of the Australian Pregnancy Registry. Eur J Neurol. 2006;13:645–54.
59. Tomson T, Battino D, Bonizzoni E, et al. Comparative risk of major congenital malformations with eight different antiepileptic drugs: a prospective cohort study of the EURAP registry. Lancet Neurol. 2018;17:530–8.
60. Bromley R, Weston J, Adab N, et al. Treatment for epilepsy in pregnancy: neurodevelopmental outcomes in the child. Cochrane Database Syst Rev. 2014;10:CD010236.
61. Meador KJ, Baker GA, Browning N, et al. Cognitive function at 3 years of age after fetal exposure to antiepileptic drugs. N Engl J Med. 2009;360:1597–605.
62. Christensen J, Grønborg TK, Sørensen MJ, et al. Prenatal valproate exposure and risk of autism spectrum disorders and childhood autism. JAMA. 2013;309:1696–703.
63. Baker GA, Bromley RL, Briggs M, et al. IQ at 6 years after utero exposure to antiepileptic drugs. Neurology. 2015;84:1–9.
64. Harden CL, Pennell PB, Koppel BS, et al. Management issues for women with epilepsy – focus on pregnancy (an evidence-based review): III. Vitamin K, folic acid, blood levels, and breast-feeding: Report of the Quality Standards Subcommittee and Therapeutics and Technology Assessment Subcommittee of the American Academy of Neurology and the American Epilepsy Society. Epilepsia. 2009;50:1247–55.

65. Crawford P. Best practice guidelines for the management of women with epilepsy. Epilepsia. 2005;46(Suppl 9):117–24.
66. Harden CL, Pulver MC, Ravdin L, et al. The effect of menopause and perimenopause on the course of epilepsy. Epilepsia. 1999;40:1402–7.

Suggested Reading

Johnson EL, Kaplan PW. Caring for transgender patients with epilepsy. Epilepsia. 2017;58(10):1667–72.

Katan M, Luft A. Global burden of stroke. Semin Neurol. 2018;38(2):208–11.

Kuzma E, Lurida I, Moore SF, Levine DA, Okoumunne OC, Llewellyn DJ. Stroke and dementia risk: a systematic review and meta-analysis. Alzheimer's Dement. 2018;14(11):1416–26.

Rankin K, Bove R. Caring for women with Multiple Sclerosis across the lifespan. Curr Neurol Neurosci Rep. 2018;18(7):36.

Sadr SS, Javanbakht J, Javidan AN, Ghaffarpour M, Khamse S, Naghshband Z. Descriptive epidemiology: prevalence, incidence, sociodemographic factors, socioeconomic domains, and quality of life of epilepsy: an update and systematic review. Arch Med Sci. 2018;14(4):717–24.

Vetvik KG, MacGregor EA. Sex differences in the epidemiology, clinical features, and pathophysiology of migraine. Lancet Neurol. 2017;16(1):76–87.

Psychiatric Disorders

23

Simona Tomassi, Ilaria Tarricone, and Sarah Tosato

Key Points

- Significant gender differences in terms of illness incidence and prevalence, mean age at onset, clinical presentation, course, and response to treatment have been reported for several mental disorders including major depression, bipolar disorder, anxiety disorders, and schizophrenia.
- Depression and anxiety are twice more frequent in women than in men, while men present higher incidence rates of early-onset schizophrenia and an earlier onset of obsessive-compulsive disorder.
- Women affected by depression show higher recurrence and atypical features, and more frequently than men, they attempt suicide (although lethal suicide is more likely to happen in men). Bipolar disorder in men is characterized by manic onset and recurrent episodes (versus depressive onset and recurrent episodes in females) and by lower treatment adherence. Schizophrenia also has significant gender differences: affected males, normally younger at the onset than females, present more severe negative symptoms, worse cognitive impairment, more frequent hospitalizations, and are more likely to commit acts of severe violence.

S. Tomassi · S. Tosato (✉)
Section of Psychiatry, Department of Neuroscience, Biomedicine and Movement Sciences, University of Verona, Verona, Italy
e-mail: simona.tomassi@univr.it; sarah.tosato@univr.it

I. Tarricone
Bologna Transcultural Psychosomatic Team (BoTPT), Department of Medical and Surgical Sciences, Alma Mater Studiorum, University of Bologna, Bologna, Italy
e-mail: ilaria.tarricone@unibo.it

I. Tarricone, A. Riecher-Rössler (eds.), *Health and Gender*,
https://doi.org/10.1007/978-3-030-15038-9_23

- Perinatal depression is a quite frequent (one mother out of ten develops postpartum depression) and potentially severe condition.
- Eating disorders in the past were considered as almost exclusively female disorders, but that is changing rapidly. One million men have been shown to suffer from eating disorders. Research and knowledge on the topic are expanding rapidly, and recent literature elucidates differences and similarities in the clinical presentation of eating disorders in men versus women.

23.1 Major Depression, Bipolar Disorder, and Anxiety Disorders

Depression is the fourth leading cause of disability worldwide [1]. Lifetime prevalence of major depressive episode (MDE), including episodes occurring as a part of bipolar disorder, varies from 1.5% (Taiwan) to 19.0% (Beirut) (midpoints at 9.2% in West Germany and 9.6% in Canada) [2]. Twelve-month prevalence estimates of MDE range from 2.2% (Japan) to 10.4% (Brazil), with the midpoints at around 5.0% across all included countries (5.5% for high-income countries and 5.9% for low-middle income countries) [3]. Lifetime prevalence of major depressive disorder (MDD), thus excluding bipolar disorder, varies from 1.0% (Czech Republic) to 16.9% (USA) (midpoints at 8.3% in Canada and 9.0% in Chile), while the 12-month prevalence estimates of MDD range from 0.3% (Czech Republic) to 10.0% (USA) (midpoints at 4.5% in Mexico and 5.2% in West Germany) [4]. Prior to puberty, although major depression is difficult to diagnose at that age, boys and girls seem to show a similar symptom profile with an estimated prevalence of 5.0% [5]. During adolescence, girls and boys are differently exposed to stressors, with girls being more vulnerable, particularly to interpersonal stress. This gender difference in stress exposure has been suggested to partially mediate the later increased prevalence of depression in women [6, 7]. After puberty and until menopause, women experience major depression at twice the rate of men. Differences were found across all age groups [8] and nationalities and were similar in high-income and low-middle income countries [9, 10]. Men and women show differences in depression presentation, course, treatment response, and outcome. With respect to gender differences in symptom profile, women seeking treatment for depression report greater symptom severity and are more likely to experience "atypical" depression with hypersomnia, increased appetite, weight gain, interpersonal sensitivity, and gastrointestinal symptoms [11–13]. Women are also more likely to have a comorbid anxiety, eating, or somatoform disorder. They report more past suicide attempts, although men are more likely to make a lethal attempt [14]. Comorbid alcohol and substance use are also more likely in men [15]. With regard to gender differences in the course of depression, women have generally an earlier-onset, more severe, longer, and recurrent depressive episodes and a lower quality of life than men [16]. A robust body of research on the topic shows that the psychopharmacological treatment of depression also might present significant gender dissimilarities, particularly in terms of antidepressant efficacy. This discrepancy has been associated with several factors: adherence and side effect profile; changes in physiology and hormone levels during puberty, menstruation, pregnancy, and menopause; comorbid diseases; and biological characteristics, among others (body fat and weight distribution, liver metabolism rates, interactions between estrogen and serotonin in the brain, brain monoamine functioning) [16]. Still, there is no clear consensus on whether there are gender-related differences in antidepressant efficacy [16]. In detail, some studies [17–20] showed a better response to antidepressants in women than in men, and some others demonstrated the inverse [21–23]. Several studies suggested better responses to serotonin reuptake-inhibiting antidepressants (SSRIs) in women than in men and better response to tricyclic antidepressants (TCAs) in men and older women [21, 24]. It is worth noting that many studies have not detected gender differences at all in the efficacy of antidepressants: studies on serotonin-norepinephrine reuptake inhibitor (SNRI) venlafaxine, SSRIs [25], TCAs, and monoamine oxidase inhibitors (MAOIs) [26] produced comparable responses in men and women, showing no gender differences in drug efficacy. This inconsistency of evidence might be linked to diverse methodological concerns due to not only the criteria used to define "response" and the study design but also the demographics (age) and nosology and type, amount, regimen, and duration of drug exposure.

Bipolar disorder is a severe mental disorder that affects 1.3% (0.4–1.6% for bipolar disorder type I and 0.5–1.9% for bipolar disorder type II) [27] of the general population. Both genders show a similar prevalence of bipolar disorder type I, while there is a significant gender difference in terms of lifetime prevalence of bipolar disorder type II, with more affected women [28–30]. Bipolar disorder is clinically characterized by the presence of extreme dysregulation in mood and energy levels, and it might severely compromise functioning. It influences familial and social aspects and generally affects negatively a person's quality of life. The onset of illness usually occurs early in adolescence or in young adulthood. Gender differences are more frequently observed in bipolar disorder type I, with reference to clinical presentation, the course of illness, and comorbidity [29, 31]. Women usually have an older age of onset [31], and they typically manifest a depressive polarity at the onset and a predominance of depression phases during lifetime [32]. Women are also more likely to undergo mixed [33] and seasonal [34] episodes and have an increased risk of developing rapid cycling mood disturbances [29]. Conversely, men present more frequently a manic first episode of illness and spend more time in manic phases [29]. Comorbidity of psychiatric (eating and anxiety disorders) and medical (thyroid disease, migraine, obesity) conditions are more common in women, while substance use disorder is more common in men [31]. There is no evidence that women and men suffering from bipolar disorder differ significantly in treatment response to mood stabilizers [33]. However, while women may be more at risk of receiving delayed diagnosis and treatment [34], men typically have a lower adherence to medication [35]. Moreover, a significant gender difference has been proven in terms of prevalence of secondary effects potentially associated with diverse treatment adherence and response [36]. Pregnancy and first weeks postpartum are for women lifetime periods of enhanced vulnerability for manic first [37] or recurrent [38] episodes [39]. Postpartum manic episodes are characterized by a more severe symptomatology than in typical manic episodes: women often manifest severe bizarre and/or disorganized behavior, hallucinations, and persecutory delusion [40]. If delusional thoughts incorporate the infant, women should be considered at risk of infanticide. The health of mothers and babies should be promoted: an individualized risk/benefit assessment of pregnant and postpartum ill women is necessary to evaluate treatment benefits and potential adverse effects of both illness and medication [41]. To summarize, in women the depressive component prevails, both at onset and during lifetime; alongside this they generally experience comorbid anxiety, eating, or medical disorders. Particular attention should be paid to pregnant and postpartum women, whether affected by bipolar disorder or not. Men vice versa usually are likely to have a prevalence of manic phases: they more often have a manic polarity both at onset and during their lifetime. Furthermore, in men the onset often occurs at a younger age, comorbidity of substance use disorder is more frequent, and adherence to medication is lower than in women (Table 23.1).

Regarding anxiety disorders, the 12-month prevalence is 18.1% [42]: 2.7% for panic disorder (PD), 3.1% for generalized anxiety disorder (GAD), and 1.0% for obsessive-compulsive disorder (OCD). In contrast to major depression, an enhanced risk of anxiety disorders in women emerges starting from middle childhood [43].

Table 23.1 Gender differences in major depression and bipolar disorder

Characteristics	Women	Men
Major depression		
Frequence (prevalence/incidence)	↑	↓
Age of onset	Younger	Older
Symptom severity	↑	↓
Recurrency	↑	↓
Atypical depression	↑	↓
Suicide attempt	↑	↓
Lethal suicide	↓	↑
Quality of life	↓	↑
Psychiatric comorbidity	Anxiety, eating, or somatoform disorder	Alcohol and substance use disorder
Treatment response	No clear evidence	
Bipolar disorder		
Frequence (prevalence/incidence)	= for type I ↑ for type II	= for type I ↓ for type II
Age of onset	Older	Younger
Onset episode	Depressive	Manic
Depressive episodes	↑	↓
Manic episodes	↓	↑
Mixed episodes	↑	↓
Psychiatric comorbidity	Anxiety or somatoform disorder	Substance use disorder
Treatment response	=	=
Treatment adherence	↑	↓

= means no significant gender difference

↑ means higher/more frequent

↓ means lower/less frequent

A higher risk for panic disorder and agoraphobia occurs in women starting with adolescence [44], and the prevalence of these disorders during adulthood is to two to three times higher in women than in men [45]. Anxiety sensitivity, or the fear of anxiety-related feelings, has been considered one of the key phenomena, found greater in women than men, independent of age [46, 47]. Consequently, anxiety sensitivity should be taken into consideration in the gender differences observed in panic disorder. In addition, clinical presentation of panic attacks is different in women and men: women frequently fear the physical symptoms of panic, like "shortness of breath," "faintness," and "feeling smothered," while men more often fear the social consequences of anxiety [48].

The lifetime prevalence of GAD is equal to 6.6% and 3.6%, in women and in men, respectively [45], with the enhanced risk for females arising with mid-adolescence [44]. Gender also influences course and presentation of generalized anxiety disorder: women more frequently refer to somatic distress including fatigue, muscle tension, and cardiorespiratory and gastrointestinal symptoms, while men tend more to report difficulties in terms of relationship (among friends and within their respective families), as a consequence of the increased levels of concern, fear, and apprehension. Comorbidity with alcohol and substance pathological use is more frequent in men, while women have higher rates of mood disorder in association with chronic generalized anxiety disorder [49].

The 12-month prevalence and lifetime rates of OCD are quite similar internationally and equal to 1.2% and 2–3%, respectively [42, 50, 51]. There are no significant gender differences in terms of prevalence in adulthood onset of OCD [51]. On the contrary, children receiving a diagnosis of OCD are boys in seven cases out of ten [50]. The childhood onset of OCD has been hypothesized to be a distinct subtype of OCD much more common in men than in women, with a greater family risk in men [52, 53] and with affected boys usually presenting tics and attention deficits [50, 54]. In terms of clinical presentation, checking, contamination obsessions and cleaning compulsions, and obsessions about harming others are more frequent in women, while symmetry and ordering compulsions and intrusive sexual and religious obsessions are more reported by men [55] (Table 23.2).

Table 23.2 Gender differences in anxiety disorders

Anxiety disorders		
Characteristics	Women	Men
Frequence (prevalence/incidence)	↑ for PD and GAD = for late-onset OCD ↓ for early-onset OCD	↓ for PD and GAD = for late-onset OCD ↑ for early-onset OCD
Panic disorder (PD)	↑ physical symptoms	↑ dread the social consequences of anxiety
Generalized anxiety disorder (GAD)	↑ somatic distress	↑ difficulties in terms of relationship
Obsessive-compulsive disorder (OCD)	↑ checking, contamination obsessions and cleaning compulsions, and obsessions about harming others	↑ intrusive sexual and religious obsessions and symmetry and ordering compulsions

= means no significant gender difference
↑ means higher/more frequent
↓ means lower/less frequent

It is an ongoing research challenge to discern the biological and environmental factors, including cultural gender stereotypes, which could contribute to the occurrence of these gender differences in terms of prevalence, symptom pattern, and course. Longitudinal observational studies, preferably with long-term follow-up across periods of hormonal change and incorporating sex-specific biomarkers, genetics, epigenetics, neuroimaging, and neuropsychological testing, are warranted. In addition, cross-cultural comparisons may be effective to disentangle the contribution of cultural expectations and social experiences to the increased vulnerability for depression and anxiety disorders in women. Future studies should also aim to clarify whether cultural gender stereotypes associated with depression are grounded on sex differences in the brain and physiology throughout the life span [56]. Finally, the role of life experiences and cultural expectations in modifying gene expression via epigenetic mechanisms resulting in the development of biologically determined sex-specific traits of vulnerability for depression should be taken in account [57, 58].

23.2 Perinatal Depression and Postpartum Psychosis

Most attention has been paid recently to the health, including mental health, of mothers, fathers, and babies during the perinatal period. Late weeks of pregnancy and early days after the delivery are characterized by significant biological, social, and psychological changes and might be very stressful and demanding. Most future or new parents adjust normally to these changes and face the challenge of becoming parents in a positive manner. However, for some of them, and here evidence focuses near principally on new mothers, a mild depressive symptomatology, known as "maternity blues" [59] might occur, while some others develop perinatal depression, and a minority falls severely ill, affected by postpartum psychosis.

"Maternity blues" [59] is not recognized yet as a disorder by the DMS-5 [60] nor by the ICD-10 [61]; therefore, an internationally validated definition of it does not exist, with all the ensuing consequences in terms of prevalence estimate, clinical detection, and treatment. In terms of incidence, for example, "maternity blues" was found to hit 20.0% [62] up to 84.0% [63] of new mothers. It has been defined, among other definitions, as a transient depressive mood swing, usually occurring in the first days after delivery and resolving itself spontaneously within 1 week [64]. It is clinically characterized by mild depressive symptoms, such as weeping, sadness, unstable mood, lack of concentration, fidgeting, grumpiness, anxiety, and sleep and appetite problems [65, 66]. It has been proven to influence mother and baby attachment style: mothers suffering from blues experience higher levels of anxiety in connecting to their babies [67] and less frequently touch and cuddle them [68]. Vulnerability factors contributing to "maternity blues" are quite debatable, and the research on the topic still lacks of clarity. Nonetheless, mothers, fathers, and their families should be prepared and well informed about the complexities of the postpartum. Mothers should know that during the first days after delivery they could experience mild depressive symptoms and be more reactive, nervous, and fidgety. They should be aware of the fleeting and self-resolving nature of these symptoms, so that any form of blaming themselves as "bad mothers" could be avoided. Moreover, only an informed family will be able to detect a prolonged (longer than 2 weeks) or more severe symptomatology and to seek help in time.

The incidence of major depression in women during the perinatal period is significantly higher than in other periods of their lives [69, 70]. The DSM-5 [60] recognizes a specificity, in terms of timing and psychopathology, for perinatal depressive episodes and includes, as a separated nosology entity, perinatal depression, characterized by an onset of symptomatology occurring during pregnancy or the first 4 weeks postpartum. Others [71] extend up to 1 year the time frame during which it is possible to observe, and diagnose, a perinatal depressive episode. During pregnancy, depression prevalence is equal to 7.4–11.0%, 8.5–12.8%, and 8.5–12.0% in the first, second, and third trimester, respectively [71, 72]. Overall, as many as 18.4% of pregnant women are depressed during their pregnancy (i.e., from conception to birth), with as many as 12.7% having an episode of major depression [71]. After delivery, prevalence of depression is highest in the third month at 12.9%, declines slightly in the fourth through seventh months postpartum, staying in the range of 9.9–10.6%, and later drops to 6.5% in the year postpartum. Overall, as many as 19.2% of new mothers may have depression in the first 3 months after delivery, with as many as 7.1% having major depression [71]. A recent meta-analysis showed that the point prevalence of depression ranges from 8.5% to 11.0% during pregnancy and from 6.5% to 12.9% during the first year postpartum [73].

A recent study [70] showed an incidence rate of 2.2% during pregnancy and 6.8% in the postpartum period. Among those women with a history of depression, 3.7% had a recurrent depressive episode during pregnancy and 7.7% in the postpartum period. Moreover, 1.6% and 5.7% of women without a previous history of depression had a new onset during pregnancy and in the postpartum period, respectively [70]. The relative risk of depression in the perinatal period was about twofold in women with a history of depression compared with those without a history [70].

Previous depressive episodes [70], perinatal or not, [74] and a family history positive for mental illness [75] represent the major risk factors for developing perinatal depression. Numerous psychosocial elements have also been recognized to facilitate the onset of perinatal depression: among them, poverty, disadvantaged social environments, being part of ethnic minorities [76, 77], and being adolescent new mothers [78]. Moreover, domestic violence, poor social support, bereavement, unemployment, and a recent layoff increase the risk of depression during or after pregnancy [75, 79]. Finally, a primary role in determining women's vulnerability to perinatal depression is played by the partner's mental health and his attitude toward the newborn and mother [80]. Depressed pregnant women often experience loss of control, embarrassment, and shame; they may suffer from anxiety, sadness, and low self-esteem; and they can misinterpret these feelings. Women may consider themselves unsuitable, the baby to be an intruder, and the world outside hostile. Thus, they end up secluded at home [81]. Depression in childbearing women is clinically often characterized by changing mood, irritability, panic, and obsessive symptoms [82]. Fathers as well might be more prone to depression during the perinatal period, with the incidence of paternal depression ranging from 1.2% to 25.5% in community samples and from 24.0% to 50.0% among men whose partners were experiencing postpartum depression [80]. Depressed mothers experience the discrepancy between "ideal" and "real" maternity and often see themselves as unfitting, improper, not-good-enough mothers. Moreover, they might consider these feelings unacceptable and desperately try to reach the standard, socially defined, of a good mother. Families and society around are prone to label them as "failed" mothers. Women report a pervasive sensation of loss and, not so rarely, consider death as the only solution to their sufferance: a recent US survey [83] reported a pregnancy-associated suicide rate of 2.0 per 100,000 live births, 45.7% occurred during pregnancy, while 54.3% occurred postpartum.

Postpartum psychosis is rare (1–2 per 1000 live births) [84], and it is a severe psychiatric condition that requires urgent medical attention and mental health care. Several medical conditions might resemble psychosis, and the differential diagnosis should include drug-induced psychosis, infectious diseases (e.g., mastitis, endometritis), eclampsia [85], autoimmune diseases like postpartum thyroiditis [86] and encephalitis [87], metabolic disorders as primary hypoparathyroidism [88] and vitamin deficiency, and stroke [89]. The initial clinical evaluation for postpartum psychosis should exclude organic causes for acute psychosis and include a full medical and psychiatric history, physical and neurological examinations, and comprehensive laboratory analysis. The onset is generally rapid, within 2 weeks of delivery. Insomnia, mood fluctuation (such as mania, depression, or a mixed state), and obsessive thoughts regarding the newborn are often early symptoms, followed by delusions, hallucinations, and disorganized behavior [90]. When identified early and properly treated, postpartum psychoses show rates of remission at 1 year around 95% [90]. Nonetheless, it is noteworthy that postpartum psychosis is associated with the risk of infanticide [91], and therefore proper safety measures must be applied when caring for mothers affected by psychosis.

23.3 Schizophrenic Psychosis

Schizophrenic psychosis, potentially severe psychiatric disorders that affect around 0.5–1.0% of the worldwide population [92], has been described to have gender-related differences [93, 94] related to illness incidence, mean age at onset, clinical presentation, course, and response to treatment [95–97]. Biological processes (mainly neurodevelopmental ones) and social factors are both implicated on gender differences in schizophrenia course and outcomes.

Gender differences in the incidence of schizophrenia have been described [98]. Incidence rate of early onset is higher in males than females, while at older onset, women predominate. In detail, men show an incidence peak in their early 20s (between 18 and 25 years of age), while the peak for women occurs a few years later (between 25 and 35 years of age) [99–102]. Until the mid-30s, rates are estimated to be approximately 1.5–2 times greater in males than females. Later, rates decrease for both sexes, with a narrowing sex ratio, until the mid-40s when there is a minor secondary peak for women. Prevalence rates are instead quite similar in women and men [98].

In terms of clinical presentation, gender-related differences in schizophrenia have been observed and proven since Kraepelin's period. Kraepelin was the first to remark that the classical picture of schizophrenia with early manifestation in late adolescent/early adulthood, poor premorbid adjustment, affective flattening, and social anhedonia more often occurred in males than in females [103]. Since then, both empirical data and evidence seem to confirm some gender differences in schizophrenia clinical presentation.

Male patients are likely to have more cognitive impairment [94] and poorer premorbid functioning [94, 104, 105], more negative symptoms [106–108] and less severe positive symptoms [106], and more severe deterioration over time [109]. Female patients are more severely impaired in ratings of severe positive symptoms [109], with more hallucinations [104], persecutory delusions [94], affective symptoms [94, 109], and greater number of suicide attempts [104]. Women also show a considerably less severe course of the illness [110]: they show a better social functioning [107, 110–112] and have fewer hospitalizations with shorter inpatient stays [110, 113]. Moreover, women are more often married [114–116], are employed [115], and live independently [115], while men frequently live alone and are unemployed [104, 109] and have poorer social networks [104] and poorer functional outcome [106]. In contrast to the evidence summarized above, several studies have shown no gender difference in symptom profile or severity [104, 107, 115, 117], neurocognitive functioning [115, 117], and social functioning [105].

Obstetric complications [118, 119], paternal age at birth [120, 121], cannabis use [122–124], and childhood trauma [125–127] are among the risk factors for developing schizophrenia [128]. Apart from the fact that men are more prone to use cannabis [129, 130] and that women have been demonstrated to be more susceptible to the negative consequences of early traumatic experiences [131], no definitive evidence is available regarding gender difference in schizophrenia risk factors. Similarly, no significant difference was found between men and women with reference to the duration of untreated psychosis, which was found to be similar for both genders [102]. Severe acts of violence are more frequently committed by males with schizophrenia [132, 133]. Conversely, women are more likely to show less severe aggressive behavior, such as verbal threats [134, 135]. Other studies have found no gender differences in aggressive behavior among patients with schizophrenia [136, 137].

Even if evidence is rather inconsistent, it seems that in schizophrenia men present a poorer premorbid adjustment, an earlier onset, worse negative symptoms and cognitive impairment, a poorer functional outcome, and more frequent acts of severe violence.

A variety of theories (like the neurodevelopmental [138] or the neuropathological theory [139]) and hypotheses (as the estrogen protection hypothesis) have been proposed as explanations for gender differences in schizophrenia. Physiological gender-differentiated brain development seems to have significant implications for elucidating gender differences in schizophrenia. Schizophrenia might be considered a neurodevelopmental disorder with early origins (fetal and postnatal), and it seems therefore likely that gender differences in the brain originated during the early sexual differentiation of the brain [140]. Animal studies have demonstrated that differential brain abnormalities and behavioral consequences in males and females depend on the timing of the insult during fetal and early postnatal brain development [141, 142]. Moreover, human studies demonstrated significantly diverse risks for schizophrenia in females and males, given exposure to particular obstetric factors [140]. More structural brain abnormalities in schizophrenia were generally found among men. In detail, larger lateral and third ventricles, smaller medial temporal volumes, greater sulcal volume, smaller thalamic size, more left-lateralized abnormalities, and overall smaller frontal and temporal lobe volumes were demonstrated in men with schizophrenia [93, 143–148].

Gender differences have also been well recognized in the response to antipsychotic treatment, with women being better responders than men [149, 150]. Environmental and biological factors are likely to contribute to this difference. Diverse environmental factors were demonstrated likely to affect treatment outcomes in schizophrenia, among them, pathological substance use [151], poorer premorbid, and lower social functioning [152]. In detail, worse treatment outcomes in men have been associated with substance abuse or dependence. Pathological substance use has been proven more common in both men belonging to the general population (3% vs. 1% of women) and men with schizophrenia (36% vs. 16% of women) [151]. Pathological substance use has a significant negative effect on illness course [153], affecting age of onset, relapse rates, and hospitalizations, and being associated with poor social outcomes [151, 154]. Interestingly, substance use, especially cannabis consumption, has been proven to lowering age of onset also in women [155]. Furthermore, poorer premorbid and social functioning in men with schizophrenia [152] negatively influences illness course by worsening engagement with treatments and services.

Notwithstanding important social considerations, much evidence has accumulated regarding the fact that women and men differ biologically in their response to antipsychotic medication. Firstly, gonadal hormones and their brain receptors are differently distributed in men and women, and they are known to influence brain sex-related anatomy [156] and function [157–159]. This brain sexual dimorphism could influence pharmacodynamic pathways of antipsychotic drugs and thus affect drug response [93]. Secondly, gender differences in response to antipsychotic medications may also reflect differential effects of treatment on particular kinds of symptoms [152] and cognitive dysfunctions [160]. Finally, gender differences in the pharmacokinetics of typical and atypical antipsychotics may explain much of the gender difference in treatment response. Whether and how women and men with schizophrenia differ is one of the most interesting as well as clinically relevant topics in schizophrenia research (Table 23.3).

Table 23.3 Gender differences in schizophrenia

Schizophrenia		
Characteristics	Women	Men
Prevalence	=	=
Incidence	↑ for late-onset schizophrenia	↑ for early-onset schizophrenia
Duration of untreated psychosis (DUP)	=	=
Age of onset	Younger	Older
Positive symptoms	↑	↓
Negative symptoms	↓	↑
Cognitive impairment	↓	↑
Number of hospitalizations	↓	↑
Acts of severe violence	↓	↑
Treatment response	↑	↓

= means no significant gender difference
↑ means higher/more frequent/more severe
↓ means lower/less frequent/more severe

23.4 Eating Disorders

Anorexia nervosa (AN) and bulimia nervosa (BN) lifetime prevalence among women are equal to 4.0% and 2.0%, respectively [161], while 12-month prevalence is approximately 0.4% for AN and 1–1.5% for BN [60]. In the past, eating disorders were thought of as almost exclusively female disorders, significantly more common in females than males (F:M = 20:1) [162]. However, it was recently reported that 1 million men in the USA suffer from eating disorders [163], and it was demonstrated that despite women being significantly more likely than men to report some behaviors, such as body checking, fasting, and vomiting, effect sizes ("Number Needed to Treat") were small to moderate [164]. Males accounted for roughly 10.0% [165] to 25.0% [161] of eating disorder patients, with the number of men struggling from BN being more than those who struggle with AN. Eating disorder literature has focused on females for decades, but that is changing rapidly. Recent literature now elucidates differences and similarities in the clinical presentation of eating disorders in males versus females. Gender-specific issues have been demonstrated in terms of timing of diagnosis [166], age of onset [167, 168], weight history and compensatory exercise behavior [169], frequency of sexual/physical abuse record [170], substance use rates [171], and body image concerns [172]. A delay in diagnosis is much more probable to happen in men, partially as a consequence of the fact that society still sees eating disorders as a female illness [166]. A later age of onset [167, 168], premorbid obesity, and overexercise are more likely in men [169]. Gender significantly influences weight history. Mild to moderate obesity is frequently observed in men before developing an eating disorder, with obese boys at higher risk later in life. Contrastingly, women, despite the fact that they generally feel fat, usually have a premorbid normal weight. Exercise, used as a compensatory behavior, is also more common in men

[169]. Around 30% of subjects suffering from an eating disorder were victims of sexual abuse [173]: one out of three women and one out of seven men [170]. For men, this event is likely under reported as a consequence of the shame and stigmatization that accompanies sexual abuse in men. Bullying instead is much more common in men. A reaction of being bullied might consist in manipulating the body shape with the goal of becoming more "masculine" and try to protect themselves from an ongoing aggression [174]. Substance abuse is generally more frequent in subjects with eating disorder in comparison to the general population [175]. One linking to the pathological use of substances (particularly stimulants) is to manage and control weight. Substance pathological use is also specific to men, particularly the use of steroids and growth hormones. Among young males in general, the frequency of anabolic steroid use is roughly equal to that of eating disorders in young females [171]. Finally, gender difference is significant in body image concerns. The current ideal of the male body, increasingly showed semi-naked in popular magazines over the past 30 years, is becoming more and more unrealistic [176]. Pope et al. showed that models had bodies achievable (in terms of fat-free mass index) only with the use of anabolic steroids [172]. Conversely, gender issues have not been demonstrated in eating disorders regarding the occurrence of medical complication [177] and the level of functioning [178]. Men are in fact equally at risk of developing complications of eating disorders including arrhythmias, osteoporosis, and hepatitis [177]. Furthermore, the level of impairment from eating issues is similar for males and females [178]. Gender difference has not been demonstrated in terms of illness outcome. A common cause of death in AN and BN is suicide [179–181]. According to evidence, the suicide rate for AN and BN is 1.3 and 0.3 per 1000 person-years, respectively, and one in five deaths in AN or BN is the result of suicide [179–180].

23.5 Conclusion

In mental health, significant gender differences in terms of illness incidence and prevalence, mean age at onset, clinical presentation, course, and response to treatment exist. Today, which biological, psychological, and social factors could be involved in determining these differences, to what extent each of them contributes, and how they interplay are a matter of open debate.

References

1. Murray CJL, Lopez AD, World Health Organization, World Bank, Harvard School of Public Health. Burden of disease: a comprehensive assessment of mortality and disability from diseases, injuries, and risk factors in 1990 and projected to 2020. Geneva: World Health Organization; 1996.
2. Weissman MM, Bland RC, Canino GJ, Faravelli C, Greenwald S, Hwu HG, et al. Cross-national epidemiology of major depression and bipolar disorder. JAMA. 1996;276:293–9.
3. Kessler RC, Birnbaum HG, Shahly V, Bromet E, Hwang I, McLaughlin KA, et al. Age differences in the prevalence and co-morbidity of DSM-IV major depressive episodes: results from

the WHO World Mental Health Survey Initiative. Depress Anxiety. 2010;27:351–64. https://doi.org/10.1002/da.20634.
4. Kessler RC, Bromet EJ. The epidemiology of depression across cultures. Annu Rev Public Health. 2013;34:119–38. https://doi.org/10.1146/annurev-publhealth-031912-114409.
5. Altemus M, Sarvaiya N, Neill Epperson C. Sex differences in anxiety and depression clinical perspectives. Front Neuroendocrinol. 2014;35(3):320–30. https://doi.org/10.1016/j.yfrne.2014.05.004.
6. Ge X, Lorenz F, Conger R, Elder G, Simons R. Trajectories of stressful life events and depressive symptoms during adolescence. Dev Psychol. 1994;30:467–83.
7. Hankin B, Mermelstein R, Roesch L. Sex differences in adolescent depression: stress exposure and reactivity models. Child Dev. 2007;78:279–95.
8. Kessler RC, McGonagle KA, Swartz M, Blazer DG, Nelson CB. Sex and depression in the National Comorbidity Survey. I: Lifetime prevalence, chronicity and recurrence. J Affect Disord. 1993;29(2–3):85–96.
9. Bromet E, Andrade LH, Hwang I, Sampson NA, Alonso J, de Girolamo G, et al. Cross-national epidemiology of DSM-IV major depressive episode. BMC Med. 2011;9:90. https://doi.org/10.1186/1741-7015-9-90.
10. Tarricone I, Stivanello E, Poggi F, Castorini V, Marseglia MV, Fantini MP, Berardi D. Ethnic variation in the prevalence of depression and anxiety in primary care: a systematic review and meta-analysis. Psychiatry Res. 2012;195(3):91–106.
11. Young M, Scheftner W, Fawcett J, Klerman G. Gender differences in the clinical features of unipolar major depressive disorder. J Nerv Ment Dis. 1990;178:200–3.
12. Angst J, Gamma A, Sellaro R. Toward validation of atypical depression in the community: results of the Zurich cohort study. J Affect Disord. 2002;72:125–38.
13. Blanco C, Vesga-Lopez O, Stewart J, Liu S, Grant B, Hasin D. Epidemiology of major depression with atypical features: results from the National Epidemiologic Survey on Alcohol and Related Conditions (NESARC). J Clin Psychiatry. 2012;73:224–32.
14. Rudmin F, Ferranda-Nolf M, Skolbekken J-A. Questions of culture, age, and gender in the epidemiology of suicide. Scand J Psychol. 2003;44:373–81.
15. Marcus S, Kerber K, Rush A, Wisniewski S, Nierenberg A, Balasubrami G, et al. Sex differences in depression symptoms in treatment-seeking adults: confirmatory analyses from the Sequenced Treatment Alternatives to Relieve Depression study. Compr Psychiatry. 2008;49:238–46.
16. Sramek JJ, Murphy MF, Cutler NR. Sex differences in the psychopharmacological treatment of depression. Dialogues Clin Neurosci. 2016;18(4):447–57.
17. Berlanga C, Flores-Ramos M. Different gender response to serotonergic and noradrenergic antidepressants. A comparative study of the efficacy of citalopram and reboxetine. J Affect Disord. 2006;95(1–3):119–23.
18. Naito S, Sato K, Yoshida K, Higuchi H, Takahashi H, Kamata M, et al. Gender differences in the clinical effects of fluvoxamine and milnacipran in Japanese major depressive patients. Psychiatry Clin Neurosci. 2007;61(4):421–7.
19. Young EA, Kornstein SG, Marcus SM, Harvey AT, Warden D, Wisniewski SR, et al. Sex differences in response to citalopram: a STAR*D report. J Psychiatr Res. 2009;43(5):503–11. https://doi.org/10.1016/j.jpsychires.2008.07.002.
20. Yang SJ, Kim SY, Stewart R, Kim JM, Shin IS, Jung SW, et al. Gender differences in 12-week antidepressant treatment outcomes for a naturalistic secondary care cohort: the CRESCEND study. Psychiatry Res. 2011;189(1):82–90. https://doi.org/10.1016/j.psychres.2010.12.027.
21. Kornstein SG, Schatzberg AF, Thase ME, Yonkers KA, McCullough JP, Keitner GI, et al. Gender differences in treatment response to sertraline versus imipramine in chronic depression. Am J Psychiatry. 2000;157(9):1445–52.
22. Hamilton JA, Grant M, Jensvold MF. Sex and treatment of depression: when does it matter? In: Jensvold MF, Halbreich U, Hamilton JA, editors. Psychopharmacology and women: sex, gender, and hormones. Washington, DC: American Psychiatric Press, Inc; 1996. p. 241–60.

23. Old Age Depression Interest Group. How long should the elderly take antidepressants? A double-blind placebo-controlled study of continuation/prophylaxis therapy with dothiepin. Br J Psychiatry. 1993;162:175–82.
24. Khan A, Brodhead AE, Schwartz KA, Kolts RL, Brown WA. Sex differences in antidepressant response in recent antidepressant clinical trials. J Clin Psychopharmacol. 2005;25(4):318–24.
25. Entsuah AR, Huang H, Thase ME. Response and remission rates in different subpopulations with major depressive disorder administered venlafaxine, selective serotonin reuptake inhibitors, or placebo. J Clin Psychiatry. 2001;62(11):869–77.
26. Quitkin FM, Stewart JW, McGrath PJ, Taylor BP, Tisminetzky MS, Petkova E, et al. Are there differences between women's and men's antidepressant responses? Am J Psychiatry. 2002;159(11):1848–54.
27. American Psychiatric Association. Diagnostic and statistical manual of mental disorders. 4th ed. Washington, DC: American Psychiatric Press; 1994.
28. Hendrick V, Altsuler LL, Gitlin MJ, Delrahim S, Hammen C. Gender and bipolar illness. J Clin Psychiatry. 2000;61(5):393–6.
29. Arnold LM. Gender differences in bipolar disorder. Psychiatr Clin North Am. 2003;26(3):595–620.
30. Popovic D, Torrent C, Goikolea JM, Cruz N, Sànchez-Moreno J, Gonzàlez-Pinto A, et al. Clinical implications of predominant polarity and the polarity index in bipolar disorder: a naturalistic study. Acta Psychiatr Scand. 2013;129(5):366–74. https://doi.org/10.1111/acps.12179.
31. Nivoli AM, Pacchiarotti I, Rosa AR, Popovic D, Murru A, Valenti M, et al. Gender differences in a cohort study of 604 bipolar patients: the role of predominant polarity. J Affect Disord. 2011;133(3):443–9. https://doi.org/10.1016/j.jad.2011.04.055.
32. Kawa I, Carter JD, Joyce PR, Doughty CJ, Frampton CM, Wells JE, et al. Gender differences in bipolar disorder: age at onset, course, comorbidity, and symptom presentation. Bipolar Disord. 2005;7(2):119–25.
33. Lòpez-Zurbano S, Gonzàlez-Pinto A, Lòpez P. Gender differences in bipolar disorder. In: Sàenz-Herrero M, editor. Psychopathology in women. Switzerland: Springer International Publishing; 2015. https://doi.org/10.1007/978-3-319-05870-2_28.
34. Altshuler LL, Kupka RW, Hellemann G, Frye MA, Sugar CA, McElroy SL, et al. Gender and depressive symptoms in 711 patients with bipolar disorder evaluated prospectively in the Stanley Foundation bipolar treatment outcome network. Am J Psychiatry. 2010;167(6):708–15. https://doi.org/10.1176/appi.ajp.2009.09010105.
35. Vega P, Alonso M, Alberich S. Why do bipolar men not comply with treatment? The Spanish CIBERSAM data. Eur J Psychiatry. 2009;23:63–9.
36. Henry C. Lithium side-effects and predictors of hypothyroidism in patients with bipolar disorder: sex differences. J Psychiatry Neurosci. 2002;27:104–7.
37. Munk-Olsen T, Laursen TM, Meltzer-Brody S, Mortensen PB, Jones I. Psychiatric disorders with postpartum onset: possible early manifestations of bipolar affective disorders. Arch Gen Psychiatry. 2012;69(4):428–34. https://doi.org/10.1001/archgenpsychiatry.2011.157.
38. Sharma V, Pope CJ. Pregnancy and bipolar disorder: a systematic review. J Clin Psychiatry. 2012;73(11):1447–55. https://doi.org/10.4088/JCP.11r07499.
39. Stewart DE, Klompenhouwer JL, Kendell RE, van Hulst AM. Prophylactic lithium in puerperal psychosis. The experience of three centres. Br J Psychiatry. 1991;158:393–7.
40. Brockington IF, Cernik KF, Schofield EM, Downing AR, Francis AF, Keelan C. Puerperal psychosis. Phenomena and diagnosis. Arch Gen Psychiatry. 1981;38(7):829–33.
41. Tosato S, Albert U, Tomassi S, Iasevoli F, Carmassi C, Ferrari S, et al. A systematized review of atypical antipsychotics in pregnant women: balancing between risks of untreated illness and risks of drug-related adverse effects. J Clin Psychiatry. 2017;78(5):e477–89. https://doi.org/10.4088/JCP.15r10483.
42. Kessler RC, Berglund P, Demler O, Jin R, Merikangas KR, Walters EE. Lifetime prevalence and age-of-onset distributions of DSM-IV disorders in the National Comorbidity Survey Replication. Arch Gen Psychiatry. 2005;62(6):593–602.

43. Lewinsohn P, Gotlieb I, Lewinsohn M, Seely J, Allen N. Gender differences in anxiety disorders and anxiety symptoms in adolescents. J Abnormal Psychol. 1998;107:109–17.
44. Beesdo K, Knappe S, Pine DS. Anxiety and anxiety disorders in children and adolescents: developmental issues and implications for DSM-V. Psychiatr Clin North Am. 2009;32:483–524.
45. Kessler R, McGonagle K, Zhao S, Nelson C, Hughes M, Eshleman S, et al. Lifetime and 12-month prevalence of DSM-III-R psychiatric disorders in the United States. Results from the National Comorbidity Survey. Arch Gen Psychiatry. 1994;51:8–19.
46. Deacon B, Abramowitz J, Woods C, Tolin D. The Anxiety Sensitivity Index - Revised: psychometric properties and factor structure in two nonclinical samples. Behav Res Ther. 2003;41:1427–49.
47. Bernstein A, Zvolensky M, Stewart S, Nancy-Comeau M, Leen-Feldner E. Anxiety sensitivity taxonicity across gender among youth. Behav Res Ther. 2006;44:679–98.
48. Sheikh J, Leskin G, Klein D. Gender differences in panic disorder: findings from the National Comorbidity Survey. Am J Psychiatry. 2002;159:55–8.
49. Vegas-Lopez O, Schneier F, Wang S, Heimberg R, Liu S, Hasin D, et al. Gender differences in generalized anxiety disorder: results from the National Epidemiologic Survey on Alcohol and Related Conditions (NESARC). J Clin Psychiatry. 2008;69:1606–16.
50. Ruscio A, Stein D, Chiu W, Kessler R. The epidemiology of obsessive-compulsive disorder in the National Comorbidity Survey Replication. Mol Psychiatry. 2010;15:53–63. https://doi.org/10.1038/mp.2008.94.
51. Weissman M, Bland R, Canino G, Greenwald S, Hwu H, Lee C, et al. The cross national epidemiology of obsessive compulsive disorder: the cross national collaborative group. J Clin Psychiatry. 1994;55(Suppl):5–10.
52. Geller D, Biederman J, Jones J, Park K, Schwartz S, Shapiro S, et al. Is juvenile obsessive-compulsive disorder a developmental subtype of the disorder? A review of the pediatric literature. J Am Acad Child Adolesc Psychiatry. 1998;37(4):420–7.
53. Hemmings S, Kinnear C, Lochner C, Niehaus D, Knowles J, Moolman-Smook J, et al. Early-versus late-onset obsessive-compulsive disorder: investigating genetic and clinical correlates. Psychiatry Res. 2004;128(2):175–82.
54. Leckman JF, Denys D, Simpson HB, Mataix-Cols D, Hollander E, Saxena S, et al. Obsessive-compulsive disorder: a review of the diagnostic criteria and possible subtypes and dimensional specifiers for DSM-V. Depress Anxiety. 2010;27:507–27.
55. Torresan R, Ramos-Cerqueira A, Shavitt R, do Rosario M, de Mathis M, Miguel E, et al. Symptom dimensions, clinical course and comorbidity in men and women with obsessive- compulsive disorder. Psychiatry Res. 2013;209(2):186–95. https://doi.org/10.1016/j.psychres.2012.12.006.
56. Carter R. Sex variations in youth anxiety symptoms: effects of pubertal development and gender role orientation. J Clin Child Adolesc Psychol. 2011;40:730–41.
57. Curley J, Jensen C, Mashoodh R, Champagne F. Social influences on neurobiology and behavior: epigenetic effects during development. Psychoneuroendocrinology. 2011;36:352–71.
58. Springer K, Stellman J, Jordan-Young R. Beyond a catalogue of differences: a theoretical frame and good practice guidelines for researching sex/gender in human health. Soc Sci Med. 2012;74:1817–24. https://doi.org/10.1016/j.socscimed.2011.05.033.
59. Pitt B. Maternity blues. Br J Psychiatry. 1973;122(569):431–3.
60. American Psychiatric Association. Diagnostic and statistical manual of mental disorders. 5th ed. Washington, DC: American Psychiatric Association; 2013.
61. World Health Organization. International statistical classification of diseases and related health problems, 10th Revision (ICD-10). Geneva: WHO; 1992.
62. Bergant AM, Heim K, Ulmer H, Illmensee K. Early postnatal depressive mood: associations with obstetric and psychosocial factors. J Psychosom Res. 1999;46(4):391–4.
63. O'Hara M, Zekoski E, Phillipps L, Wright E. Controlled prospective study of postpartum mood disorders: comparison of childbearing and nonchildbearing women. J Abnorm Psychol. 1990;99:3–15.

64. Scrandis DA, Sheikh TM, Niazi R, Tonelli LH, Postolache TT. Depression after delivery: risk factors, diagnostic and therapeutic considerations. ScientificWorldJournal. 2007;7:1670–82.
65. Kennerley H, Gath D. Maternity blues. I. Detection and measurement by questionnaire. Br J Psychiatry. 1989;155:356–62.
66. Newport DJ, Wilcox MM, Stowe ZN. Maternal depression: a child's first adverse life event. Semin Clin Neuropsychiatry. 2002;7(2):113–9.
67. Nagata M, Nagai Y, Sobajima H, Ando T, Nishide Y, Honjo S. Maternity blues and attachment to children in mothers of full-term normal infants. Acta Psychiatr Scand. 2000;101(3):209–17.
68. Ferber SG. "With sorrow you will have sons": the constructive consequence of maternity blues. Psychoanal Rev. 2006;93(1):117–30.
69. Ross LE, Dennis CL. The prevalence of postpartum depression among women with substance use, an abuse history, or chronic illness: a systematic review. J Womens Health (Larchmt). 2009;18(4):475–86. https://doi.org/10.1089/jwh.2008.0953.
70. Banti S, Mauri M, Oppo A, Borri C, Rambelli C, Ramacciotti D, et al. From the third month of pregnancy to 1 year postpartum. Prevalence, incidence, recurrence, and new onset of depression. Results from the perinatal depression-research & screening unit study. Compr Psychiatry. 2011;52(4):343–51. https://doi.org/10.1016/j.comppsych.2010.08.003.
71. Gavin NI, Gaynes BN, Lohr KN, Meltzer-Brody S, Gartlehner G, Swinson T. Perinatal depression: a systematic review of prevalence and incidence. Obstet Gynecol. 2005;106(5 Pt 1):1071–83.
72. Bennett HA, Einarson A, Taddio A, Koren G, Einarson TR. Depression during pregnancy: overview of clinical factors. Clin Drug Investig. 2004;24:157–79.
73. Gaynes BN, Gavin N, Meltzer-Brody S, Lohr KN, Swinson T, Gartlehner G, et al. Perinatal depression: prevalence, screening accuracy, and screening outcomes. Evidence report/technology assessment no. 119. (Prepared by the RTI-University of North Carolina Evidence-based Practice Center, under contract no. 290-02-0016.) AHRQ publication no. 05-E006-2. Rockville, MD: Agency for Healthcare Research and Quality; 2005.
74. Dietz PM, Williams SB, Callaghan WM, Bachman DJ, Whitlock EP, Hornbrook MC. Clinically identified maternal depression before, during, and after pregnancies ending in live births. Am J Psychiatry. 2007;164(10):1515–20.
75. Johnstone SJ, Boyce PM, Hickey AR, Morris-Yatees AD, Harris MG. Obstetric risk factors for postnatal depression in urban and rural community samples. Aust N Z J Psychiatry. 2001;35(1):69–74.
76. O'Hara MW, Swain Annette M. Rates and risk of postpartum depression-a meta-analysis. Int Rev Psychiatry. 1996;8(1):37–54.
77. Yonkers KA, Ramin SM, Rush AJ, Navarrete CA, Carmody T, March D, et al. Onset and persistence of postpartum depression in an inner-city maternal health clinic system. Am J Psychiatry. 2001;158(11):1856–63.
78. Lanzi RG, Bert SC, Jacobs BK, Centers for the Prevention of Child Neglect. Depression among a sample of first-time adolescent and adult mothers. Child Adolesc Psychiatr Nurs. 2009;22(4):194–202. https://doi.org/10.1111/j.1744-6171.2009.00199.
79. Nielsen Forman D, Videbech P, Hedegaard M, Dalby Salvig J, Secher NJ. Postpartum depression: identification of women at risk. BJOG. 2000;107(10):1210–7.
80. Goodman JH. Paternal postpartum depression, its relationship to maternal postpartum depression, and implications for family health. J Adv Nurs. 2004;45(1):26–35.
81. Bennett HA, Boon HS, Romans SE, Grootendorst P. Becoming the best mom that I can: women's experiences of managing depression during pregnancy--a qualitative study. BMC Womens Health. 2007;7:13.
82. Gao LL, Chan SW, You L, Li X. Experiences of postpartum depression among first-time mothers in mainland China. J Adv Nurs. 2010;66(2):303–12. https://doi.org/10.1111/j.1365-2648.2009.05169.x.
83. Palladino CL, Singh V, Campbell J, Flynn H, Gold KJ. Homicide and suicide during the perinatal period: findings from the National Violent Death Reporting System. Obstet Gynecol. 2011;118(5):1056–63. https://doi.org/10.1097/AOG.0b013e31823294da.

84. Di Florio A, Forty L, Gordon-Smith K, Heron J, Jones L, Craddock N, et al. Perinatal episodes across the mood disorder spectrum. JAMA Psychiat. 2013;70(2):168–75. https://doi.org/10.1001/jamapsychiatry.2013.279.
85. Brockington I. Early postpartum syncope, delirium and stupor. Arch Womens Ment Health. 2006;9(6):347–8.
86. Bergink V, Kushner SA, Pop V, Kuijpens H, Lambregtse-van den Berg MP, Drexhage RC, et al. Prevalence of autoimmune thyroid dysfunction in postpartum psychosis. Br J Psychiatry. 2011;198(4):264–8. https://doi.org/10.1192/bjp.bp.110.082990.
87. Bergink V, Armangue T, Titulaer MJ, Markx S, Dalmau J, Kushner SA. Autoimmune encephalitis in postpartum psychosis. Am J Psychiatry. 2015;172(9):901–8. https://doi.org/10.1176/appi.ajp.2015.14101332.
88. Patil NJ, Yadav SS, Gokhale YA, Padwa N. Primary hypoparathyroidism: psychosis in postpartum period. J Assoc Physicians India. 2010;58:506–8.
89. Brockington I. Parturient delirium and stupor. Arch Womens Ment Health. 2007;10(1):33–4.
90. Bergink V, Burgerhout KM, Koorengevel KM, Kamperman AM, Hoogendijk WJ, Lambregtse-van den Berg MP, et al. Treatment of psychosis and mania in the postpartum period. Am J Psychiatry. 2015;172(2):115–23. https://doi.org/10.1176/appi.ajp.2014.13121652.
91. Chandra PS, Venkatasubramanian G, Thomas T. Infanticidal ideas and infanticidal behavior in Indian women with severe postpartum psychiatric disorders. J Nerv Ment Dis. 2002;190(7):457–61.
92. Wu YC, Hill RA, Gogos A, Van Den Buuse M. Sex differences and the role of estrogen in animal models of schizophrenia: interaction with BDNF. Neuroscience. 2013;239:67–83.
93. Goldstein JM, Seidman LJ, O'Brien LM, Horton NJ, Kennedy DN, Makris N, et al. Impact of normal sexual dimorphisms on sex differences in structural brain abnormalities in schizophrenia assessed by magnetic resonance imaging. Arch Gen Psychiatry. 2002;59:154–64.
94. Leung A, Chue P. Sex differences in schizophrenia, a review of the literature. Acta Psychiatr Scand. 2000;401:3–38.
95. Castle DJ, Abel KM, Takei N, Murray RM. Gender differences in schizophrenia: hormonal effect or subtypes? Schizophr Bull. 1995;21:1–12.
96. Tarricone I, Mimmi S, Paparelli A, Rossi E, Mori E, Panigada S, Carchia G, Bandieri V, Michetti R, Minenna G, Boydell J, Morgan C, Berardi D. First-episode psychosis at the West Bologna Community Mental Health Centre: results of an 8-year prospective study. Psychol Med. 2012;42(11):2255–64.
97. Jongsma HE, Gayer-Anderson C, Lasalvia A, Quattrone D, Mulè A, Szöke A, Selten JP, Turner C, Arango C, Tarricone I, Berardi D, Tortelli A, Llorca PM, de Haan L, Bobes J, Bernardo M, Sanjuán J, Santos JL, Arrojo M, Del-Ben CM, Menezes PR, Velthorst E, Murray RM, Rutten BP, Jones PB, van Os J, Morgan C, Kirkbride JB, European Network of National Schizophrenia Networks Studying Gene-Environment Interactions Work Package 2 (EU-GEI WP2) Group. Treated incidence of psychotic disorders in the multinational EU-GEI study. JAMA Psychiatry. 2018;75(1):36–46.
98. Kirkbride JB, Fearon P, Morgan C, Dazzan P, Morgan K, Tarrant J, et al. Heterogeneity in incidence rates of schizophrenia and other psychotic syndromes: findings from the 3-Center ÆSOP study. Arch Gen Psychiatry. 2006;63(3):250–8.
99. Häfner H, Riecher-Rössler A, Fätkenheuer B, Hambrecht M, Löffler W, An der Heiden W. Sex differences in schizophrenia. Psychiatr Fennica. 1991;22:123–56.
100. Häfner H, Riecher-Rössler A, An Der Heiden W, Maurer K, Fatkenheuer B, Löffler W. Generating and testing a causal explanation of the gender difference in age at first onset of schizophrenia. Psychol Med. 1993;23(4):925–40.
101. Häfner H, Riecher A, Maurer K, Fatkenheuer B, Löffler W, an der Heiden W, et al. Geschlechtsunterschiede bei schizophrenen Erkrankungen. [Sex differences in schizophrenic diseases]. Fortschr Neurol Psychiatr. 1991;59(9):343–60.

102. Häfner H, Maurer K, Löffler W, Fatkenheuer B, an der Heiden W, Riecher-Rössler A, et al. The epidemiology of early schizophrenia. Influence of age and gender on onset and early course. Br J Psychiatry Suppl. 1994;(23):29–38.
103. Kraepelin E. Psychiatrie: Ein Lehrbuch fur Studierende und Artze. [Psychiatry: a textbook for students and physicians]. 4th ed. Leipzig: JA Barth; 1893.
104. Thorup A, Petersen L, Jeppesen P, Ohlenschloeger J, Christensen T, Krarup G, et al. Gender differences in young adults with first-episode schizophrenia spectrum disorders at baseline in the Danish OPUS study. J Nerv Ment Dis. 2007;195:396–405.
105. Cotton SM, Lambert M, Schimmelmann BG, Foley DL, Morley KI, McGorry PD, et al. Gender differences in premorbid, entry, treatment, and outcome characteristics in a treated epidemiological sample of 661patients with first episode psychosis. Schizophr Res. 2009;114:17–24.
106. Moriarty PJ, Lieber D, Bennett A, White L, Parrella M, Harvey PD, et al. Gender differences in poor outcome patients with lifelong schizophrenia. Schizophr Bull. 2001;27:103–13.
107. Shtasel DL, Gur RE, Gallacher F, Heimberg C, Gur RC. Gender differences in the clinical expression of schizophrenia. Schizophr Res. 1992;7:225–31.
108. Morgan J. The invisible man: a self-help guide for men with eating disorders, compulsive exercise, and bigorexia. New York, NY: Routledge; 2008.
109. Tang YL, Gillespie CF, Epstein MP, Mao PX, Jiang F, Chen Q, et al. Gender differences in 542 Chinese inpatients with schizophrenia. Schizophr Res. 2007;97:88–96.
110. Tamminga CA. Gender and schizophrenia. J Clin Psychiatry. 1997;58:33–7.
111. Ochoa S, Usall J, Villalta-Gil V, Vilaplana M, Marquez M, Valdelomar M, et al. Influence of age at onset on social functioning in outpatients with schizophrenia. Eur J Psychiatry. 2006;20:157–63.
112. Ruggeri M, Nosè M, Bonetto C, Cristofalo D, Lasalvia A, Salvi G, et al. Changes and predictors of change in objective and subjective quality of life: multiwave follow-up study in community psychiatric practice. Br J Psychiatry. 2005;187:121–30.
113. Angermeyer MC, Kuhn L, Goldstein JM. Gender and the course of schizophrenia: differences in treated outcomes. Schizophr Bull. 1990;16:293–307.
114. Bertani M, Lasalvia A, Bonetto C, Tosato S, Cristofalo D, Bissoli S, et al. The influence of gender on clinical and social characteristics of patients at psychosis onset: a report from the Psychosis Incident Cohort Outcome Study (PICOS). Psychol Med. 2012;42(4):769–80.
115. Andia AM, Zisook S, Heaton RK, Hesselink J, Jernigan T, Kuck J, et al. Gender differences in schizophrenia. J Nerv Ment Dis. 1995;183:522–8.
116. Gureje O. Gender and schizophrenia: age at onset and sociodemographic attributes. Acta Psychiatr Scand. 1991;83:402–5.
117. Bozikas VP, Kosmidis MH, Peltekis A, Giannakou M, Nimatoudis I, Karavatos A, et al. Sex differences in neuropsychological functioning among schizophrenia patients. Aust N Z J Psychiatry. 2010;44:333–41.
118. Cannon M, Jones PB, Murray RM. Obstetric complications and schizophrenia: historical and meta-analytic review. Am J Psychiatr. 2002;159(7):1080–92.
119. Nosarti C, Reichenberg A, Murray RM, Cnattingius S, Lambe MP, Yin L, et al. Preterm birth and psychiatric disorders in young adult life. Arch Gen Psychiatry. 2012;69(6):E1–8.
120. Buizer-Voskamp JE, Laan W, Staal WG, Hennekam EAM, Aukes MF, Termorshuizen F, et al. Paternal age and psychiatric disorders: findings from a Dutch population registry. Schizophr Res. 2011;129(2–3):128–32. https://doi.org/10.1016/j.schres.2011.03.021.
121. Brown AS, Schaefer CA, Wyatt RJ, Begg MD, Goetz R, Bresnahan MA, et al. Paternal age and risk of schizophrenia in adult offspring. Am J Psychiatr. 2006;159(9):1528–33.
122. Andréasson S, Allebeck P, Engström A, Rydberg U. Cannabis and schizophrenia: a longitudinal study of Swedish conscripts. Lancet. 1987;2:1483–5.
123. Strang J, Witton J, Hall W. Improving the quality of the cannabis debate: defining the different domains. BMJ. 2000;320:108–10.
124. Arseneault L, Cannon M, Poulton R, Murray R, Caspi A, Moffitt TE. Cannabis use in adolescence and risk for adult psychosis: longitudinal prospective study. BMJ. 2002;325(7374):1212–3.

125. Varese F, Smeets F, Drukker M, Lieverse R, Lataster T, Viechtbauer W, et al. Childhood adversities increase the risk of psychosis: a meta-analysis of patient-control, prospective- and cross-sectional cohort studies. Schizophr Bull. 2012;38(4):661–71. https://doi.org/10.1093/schbul/sbs050.
126. Bonoldi I, Simeone E, Rocchetti M, Codjoe L, Rossi G, Gambi F, et al. Prevalence of self-reported childhood abuse in psychosis: a meta-analysis of retrospective studies. Psychiatry Res. 2013;210(1):8–15. https://doi.org/10.1016/j.psychres.2013.05.003.
127. Sideli L, Mule A, La Barbera D, Murray RM. Do child abuse and maltreatment increase risk of schizophrenia? Psychiatry Investig. 2012;9(2):87–99. https://doi.org/10.4306/pi.2012.9.2.87.
128. Tosato S, Lasalvia A. The contribution of epidemiology to defining the most appropriate approach to genetic research on schizophrenia. Epidemiol Psichiatr Soc. 2009;18(2):81–90.
129. Khan SS, Secades-Villa R, Okuda M, Wang S, Pérez-Fuentes G, Kerridge BT, et al. Gender differences in cannabis use disorders: results from the National Epidemiologic Survey of Alcohol and Related Conditions. Drug Alcohol Depend. 2013;130(1–3):101–8. https://doi.org/10.1016/j.drugalcdep.2012.10.015.
130. Wagner FA, Anthony JC. Male-female differences in the risk of progression from first use to dependence upon cannabis, cocaine, and alcohol. Drug Alcohol Depend. 2007;86(2–3):191–8.
131. Myin-Germeys I, Van Os J. Stress-reactivity in psychosis: evidence for an affective pathway to psychosis. Clin Psychol Rev. 2007;27(4):409–24.
132. Wessely SC, Castle D, Douglas AJ, Taylor PJ. The criminal careers of incident cases of schizophrenia. Psychol Med. 1994;24:483–502.
133. Elbogen EB, Johnson SC. The intricate link between violence and mental disorder: results from the national epidemiologic survey on alcohol and related conditions. Arch Gen Psychiatry. 2009;66:152–61.
134. Kiejna A, Janska-Skomorowska M, Baranowski P. Medical procedure with aggressive patients: experiences of the psychiatric clinic in Wroclaw. Psychiatr Pol. 1993;27:501–13.
135. Sebit MB, Siziya S, Acuda SW, Mhondoro E. Use of seclusion and restraint in psychiatric patients in Harare Hospital Psychiatric Unit, Zimbabwe: gender differences. Cent Afr J Med. 1998;44:277–80.
136. Hodgkinson PE, McIvor L, Phillips M. Patient assaults on staff in a psychiatric hospital: a two-year retrospective study. Med Sci Law. 1985;25:288–94.
137. Miller RJ, Zadolinnyj K, Hafner RJ. Profiles and predictors of assaultiveness for different psychiatric ward populations. Am J Psychiatry. 1993;150:1368–73.
138. Woods BT. Is schizophrenia a progressive neurodevelopmental disorder? Toward a unitary pathogenetic mechanism. Am J Psychiatry. 1998;155:1661–70.
139. McDonald C, Murray RM. Early and late environmental risk factors for schizophrenia. Brain Res Rev. 2000;31:130–7.
140. Goldstein JM, Walder D. Sex differences in schizophrenia: the case for developmental origins and etiological implications. Oxford: Oxford University Press; 2006.
141. Goldman PS, Crawford HT, Stokes LP, Galkin TW, Rosvold HE. Sex-dependent behavioral effects of cerebral cortical lesions in the developing rhesus monkey. Science. 1974;186:540–2.
142. Grimm VE, Frieder B. Differential vulnerability of male and female rats to the timing of various perinatal insults. Int J Neurosci. 1985;27:155–64.
143. Flaum M, Swayze VW II, O'Leary DS, Yuh WT, Ehrhardt JC, Arndt SV, et al. Effects of diagnosis, laterality, and gender on brain morphology in schizophrenia. Am J Psychiatr. 1995;152:704–14.
144. Lauriello J, Hoff A, Wieneke MH, Blankeld H, Faustman WO, Rosenbloom M, et al. Similar extent of brain dysmorphology in severely ill women and men with schizophrenia. Am J Psychiatr. 1997;154:819–25.
145. Nopoulos P, Flaum M, Andreasen NC. Sex differences in brain morphology in schizophrenia. Am J Psychiatr. 1997;154:1648–54.
146. Bogerts B, Ashtari M, Degreef G, Alvir JM, Bilder RM, Lieberman JA. Reduced temporal limbic structure volumes on magnetic resonance images in first episode schizophrenia. Psychiatry Res. 1990;35:1–13.

147. Gur RE, Cowell PE, Latshaw A, Turetsky BI, Grossman RI, Arnold SE, et al. Reduced dorsal and orbital prefrontal gray matter volumes in schizophrenia. Arch Gen Psychiatry. 2000;57:761–8.
148. Hirayasu Y, McCarley RW, Salisbury DF, Tanaka S, Kwon JS, Frumin M, et al. Planum temporale and Heschl gyrus volume reduction in schizophrenia. Arch Gen Psychiatry. 2000;57:692–9.
149. Riecher-Rössler A, Häfner H. Schizophrenia and oestrogens - is there an association? Eur Arch Psychiatry Clin Neurosci. 1993;242:323–8.
150. Riecher-Rössler A, Kulkarni J. Estrogens and gonadal function in schizophrenia and related psychoses. Curr Top Behav Neurosci. 2011;8:155–71. https://doi.org/10.1007/7854_2010_100.
151. Jablensky A, McGrath J, Herrman H, Castle D, Gureje O, Evans A, et al. Psychotic disorders in urban areas: an overview of the study on low prevalence disorders. Aust N Z J Psychiatry. 2000;34:221–36.
152. Goldstein JM, Link BG. Gender and the expression of schizophrenia. J Psychiatr Res. 1988;22:141–55.
153. Tosato S, Lasalvia A, Bonetto C, Mazzoncini R, Cristofalo D, De Santi K, et al. The impact of cannabis use on age of onset and clinical characteristics in first-episode psychotic patients. Data from the Psychosis Incident Cohort Outcome Study (PICOS). J Psychiatr Res. 2013;47(4):438–44. https://doi.org/10.1016/j.jpsychires.2012.11.009.
154. Tarricone I, Boydell J, Panigada S, Allegri F, Marcacci T, Minenna MG, Kokona A, Triolo F, Storbini V, Michetti R, Morgan C, Di Forti M, Murray RM, Berardi D. The impact of substance use at psychosis onset on First Episode Psychosis course: results from a 1 year follow-up study in Bologna. Schizophr Res. 2014;153(1–3):60–3.
155. Allegri F, Belvederi Murri M, Paparelli A, Marcacci T, Braca M, Menchetti M, Michetti R, Berardi D, Tarricone I. Current cannabis use and age of psychosis onset: a gender-mediated relationship? Results from an 8-year EFF incidence study in Bologna. Psychiatry Res. 2013;210(1):368–70.
156. Goldstein JM, Seidman LJ, Horton NJ, Makris N, Kennedy DN, Caviness VS Jr, et al. Normal sexual dimorphism of the adult human brain assessed by in vivo magnetic resonance imaging. Cereb Cortex. 2001;11:490–7.
157. McEwen BS. Gonadal steroid influences on brain development and sexual differentiation. In: Greep RO, editor. Reproductive physiology IV, International review of physiology, vol. 27. Baltimore: University Park Press; 1983. p. 99–145.
158. MacLusky NJ, Clark AS, Naftolin F, Goldman-Rakic PS. Estrogen formation in the mammalian brain: possible role of aromatase in sexual differentiation of the hippocampus and neocortex. Steroids. 1987;50:459–74.
159. Ostlund H, Keller E, Hurd YL. Estrogen receptor gene expression in relation to neuropsychiatric disorders. Ann N Y Acad Sci. 2003;1007:54–63.
160. Howard CH, Fiedosewicz H, Patel C, Klegon DA, Bayog R, Berman I. Treatment response and gender in patients with schizophrenia and schizoaffective disorder. Schizophr Res. 2001;49:232.
161. Hudson JL, Hiripi E, Pope HG, Kessler RC. The prevalence and correlates of eating disorders in the national comorbidity survey replication. Biol Psychiatry. 2007;61:348–58.
162. Hoek H, Hoeken D. Review of prevalence and incidence of eating disorders. Int J Eat Disord. 2003;34:383–96.
163. National Institute of Mental Health. Eating disorder statistics. 2008. Retrieved from http://www.gurze.com/client/client_pages/printable_pages/eatingdisorderstats.html.
164. Striegel-Moore RH, Rosselli F, Perrin N, DeBar L, Wilson GT, May A, et al. Gender difference in the prevalence of eating disorder symptoms. Int J Eat Disord. 2009;42(5):471–4. https://doi.org/10.1002/eat.20625.
165. Weltzin T. Eating disorders in men: update. J Mens Health Gender. 2005;2:186–93.
166. Robinson KJ, Mountford VA, Sperlinger DJ. Being men with eating disorders: perspective of male eating disorder service-users. J Health Psychol. 2013;18:176–86. https://doi.org/10.1177/1359105312440298.

167. Gueguen J, Goodart N, Chambry J, Brun-Eberentz A, Foulon C, Divac SM, et al. Severe anorexia nervosa in men: comparison with severe anorexia nervosa in women and analysis of mortality. Int J Eat Disord. 2012;45:537–45.
168. Norris ML, Apisom M, Harrison M, Obeid N, Buchholz A, Henderson KA, et al. An examination of medical and psychological morbidity in adolescent males with eating disorders. Eat Disord. 2012;20:405–15.
169. Andersen A. Eating disorders in males: critical questions. In: Lemberg R, Cohn L, editors. Eating disorders: a reference sourcebook. Phoenix, AZ: Oryx Press; 1999. p. 73–9.
170. Schwartz M, Cohn L. Sexual abuse and eating disorders. New York, NY: Brunner/Mazel; 1996.
171. Schooler D, Ward M. Average Joes: men's relationships with media, real bodies, and sexuality. Psychol Men Masculinity. 2006;7(1):27–41.
172. Pope H, Phillips K, Olivardia R. The Adonis complex: how to identify, treat, and prevent body obsession in men and boys. New York, NY: Touchstone; 2002.
173. Connors ME, Worse W. Sexual abuse and eating disorders: a review. Int J Eat Disord. 1993;13:1–11.
174. Morgan VA, Castle DJ, Jablensky AV. Do women express and experience psychosis differently from men? Epidemiological evidence from the Australian National Study of Low Prevalence (Psychotic) Disorder. Aust N Z J Psychiatry. 2008;42:74–82.
175. Dunn E, Larimer M, Neighbors C. Alcohol and drug-related negative consequences in college students with bulimia nervosa and binge eating disorder. Int J Eat Disord. 2002;32:171–8.
176. Halliwell E, Dittmar H, Orsborn A. The effects of exposure to muscular male models among men: exploring the moderating role of gym use and exercise motivation. Body Image. 2007;4:278–87.
177. Sabel AL, Rosen E, Mehler PS. Severe anorexia nervosa in males: clinical presentations and medical treatment. Eat Disord. 2014;22(3):209–20. https://doi.org/10.1080/10640266.2014.890459.
178. Striegel RH, Bedrosian R, Wang C, Schwartz S. Why men should be included in research on binge eating: results from a comparison of psychosocial impairment in men and women. Int J Eat Disord. 2012;45:233–40. https://doi.org/10.1002/eat.20962.
179. Arcelus J, Mitchell AJ, Wales J, Nielsen S. Mortality rates in patients with anorexia nervosa and other eating disorders. A meta-analysis of 36 studies. Arch Gen Psychiatry. 2011;68:724–31.
180. Preti A, Rocchi MB, Sisti D, Camboni MV, Miotto P. A comprehensive meta-analysis of the risk of suicide in eating disorders. Acta Psychiatr Scand. 2011;124:6–17. https://doi.org/10.1111/j.1600-0447.2010.01641.x.
181. Franko DL, Keshaviah A, Eddy KT, Krishna M, Davis MC, Keel PK, et al. A longitudinal investigation of mortality & in anorexia nervosa and bulimia nervosa. Am J Psychiatry. 2013;170:917–25. https://doi.org/10.1176/appi.ajp.2013.12070868.

Gender and Pain

24

Rita Maria Melotti, Andrea Fanelli,
and Maria Cristina Sorella

Key Points

- Chronic pain afflicts approximately 20% of the adult population worldwide.
- Gender is one of the critical factors influencing the experience of pain.
- Women report more severe levels of pain and chronic pain than men.
- The response to pain therapy appears to be gender-related.
- Sex hormones, endogenous opioid function, genetic factors, and psychosocial mechanisms contribute to gender differences in pain.

24.1 Introduction

Chronic non-cancer pain afflicts approximately 20% of the adult population worldwide representing the most frequent distress faced by physicians of all disciplines [1]. One-third of the patients with chronic pain are in severe pain, and approximately half of them have constant pain leading to diminished quality of life [2].

A broad range of variables, from genotype to psychosocial factors, contribute to the individual pain response. Gender is one of the critical factors influencing the experience of pain. For this reason research related to the correlation between gender and pain has recently proliferated [3].

Population-based research and large-scale epidemiological studies demonstrate that women report more severe level of pain and chronic pain than men [4–7]. In fact, the population prevalence of several common chronic pain conditions is greater

R. M. Melotti · A. Fanelli (✉) · M. C. Sorella
Anesthesia and Pain Therapy Unit, Department of Medical and Surgical Science,
University of Bologna, Bologna, Italy
e-mail: andrea.fanelli@aosp.bo.it

I. Tarricone, A. Riecher-Rössler (eds.), *Health and Gender*,
https://doi.org/10.1007/978-3-030-15038-9_24

Table 24.1 Female sex prevalence of various painful disorders

Migraine headache with aura
Chronic tension headache
Post-dural puncture headache
Hemicrania continua
Cervicogenic headache
Tic douloureux
Temporomandibular joint disorder
Occipital neuralgia
Periapical periodontitis and abscess
Atypical odontalgia
Burning tongue
Carotidynia
Chronic paroxysmal hemicrania
Temporal arteritis
Carpal tunnel syndrome
Raynaud's disease
Chilblains
Causalgia
Reflex sympathetic dystrophy
Hemicrania continua
Chronic venous insufficiency
Fibromyalgia syndrome
Esophagitis
Reflux esophagitis with peptic ulcer
Slipping rib syndrome
12th rib syndrome
Gallbladder disease
Post-cholecystectomy syndrome
Irritable bowel syndrome
Interstitial cystitis
Acute intermittent porphyria
Proctalgia fugax
Chronic constipation
Pyriformis syndrome
Peroneal muscular atrophy
Multiple sclerosis
Rheumatoid arthritis
Pain of psychological origin
Age dependent sex differences

for women than men, including fibromyalgia, chronic pelvic pain, migraine, chronic tension-type headache and temporomandibular disorders (Table 24.1) [4, 8]. Some of the observed differences between males and females in terms of prevalence of these chronic painful syndromes can be related to specific problems occurring over a woman's life such as gynaecological syndromes [7, 9].

Despite that, while chronic pain affects a higher proportion of women than men worldwide, women are less likely to receive an appropriate treatment [10].

24.2 Pain Severity and Treatment

Previous reviews have concluded that women report greater sensitivity to multiple pain modalities and greater temporal summation of pain compared with men. The literature related to the correlation between pain severity and gender is less consistent due to the influence of several methodological variables [11–20]. In order to reduce the confounding factors, quantitative sensory testing was used by researches to explore gender differences in pain response to controlled noxious stimuli. Models of noxious stimulation used to evoke pain include pressure, thermal, mechanical, chemical and ischaemic stimulation [21]. Pain responses have been assessed by a number of different outcome measures including indices of threshold and tolerance and self-report measures of pain intensity and unpleasantness. Despite the standardisation of the noxious stimuli and the outcome evaluated, the results still varied between studies indicating that gender differences in nociception depend on multiple factors including the type of stimulus, testing, end points, body location, age and reproductive status [22].

The response to pain therapy appears to be gender-related. Several studies based on analgesic consumption have demonstrated that women consume and are prescribed more drugs than men. Despite that, in a review published in 2000 by Miaskowski and colleagues [23], a lower opioid consumption was observed in the postoperative period among women. This has not been a consistent result and may be related to the type of surgery or by the increased incidence of side effects in women that can limit the use of opioids [24, 25].

Although a lack of gender-specific effects for opioid analgesics was recently reported by Niesters, a greater analgesic effect was observed for women, restricting the analysis to the administration of opioid through a patient-controlled analgesia (PCA) device [26]. To better understand the clinical impact of the currently available evidence, it is important to note that these studies assessed only opioid consumption rather than pain relief, which may be influenced by factors other than analgesia.

In a study published by Calderone, evaluating the influence of gender on the frequency of pain and sedative medication administered in the postoperative period, women were given sedatives more often for pain after surgery, whereas men were more likely to receive analgesics [27]. This has led many authors to conclude that women are potentially at risk for under-treatment of their pain. Several studies show that the differences in pain treatment and the potential disparities in pain management between women and men are not only related to patients' gender but are mainly influenced by both patient and healthcare provider characteristics [28].

24.3 Mechanism Underlying Sex Differences

It has been suggested that an interaction of biological, psychological and sociocultural factors contributes to gender differences in pain (Fig. 24.1), even though the specific underlying mechanisms are not clear.

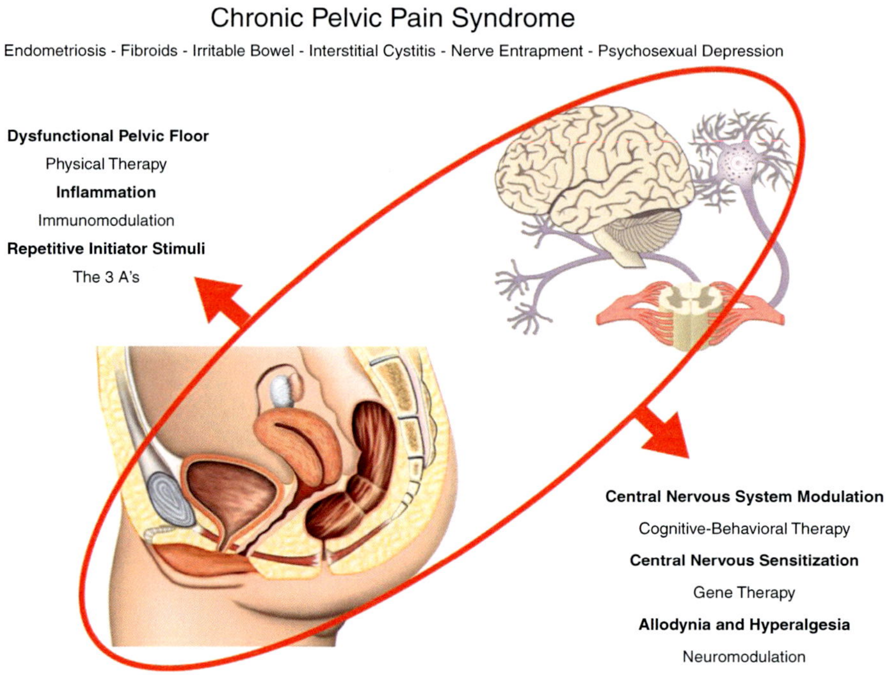

Fig. 24.1 Example of the interaction among those mechanisms which contribute to pain syndromes more commonly reported by females

Sex hormones and their receptor distribution in areas of the peripheral and central nervous system associated with nociceptive transmission suggest that they play an important role in the observed differences between man and women in the response to pain and pain treatments. Estradiol and progesterone show pro-nociceptive effect on pain, while testosterone appears to be more anti-nociceptive, especially given the association between decreased androgen concentration and chronic pain [29–32]. Nevertheless, in a model of neuropathic pain, Vacca et al. recently showed even an anti-nociceptive effect induced by oestrogen [33]. The authors demonstrated that male and female mice react differently to sciatic nerve ligature. Male mice showed a gradual decrease of allodynia and complete recovery, while in females the allodynia and gliosis were still present 4 months after the damage. The administration of estradiol reduced the allodynia and induced a complete recovery also in female mice. Furthermore, the mice treated with estradiol showed a functional improvement of the injured limb, a faster regenerative process of the peripheral nerves and decreased neuropathy-induced gliosis [33].

The use of exogenous hormones increases the risk to develop some types of chronic pain and also reduces the influence of the menstrual cycle on pain sensitivity [34–38]. Contraceptive pills (CP) produce a low endogenous estradiol, low progesterone environment similar to the early follicular phase of the menstrual cycle, with a variable effect on serum androgen levels. Vincent et al. published a study evaluating the response of healthy women to experimental thermal stimuli, in both a natural and CP-induced low endogenous estradiol state [39]. Looking at the results of this study, it seems that, in a low endogenous estradiol state, testosterone may represent a key factor in modulating pain sensitivity. In particular, failure to engage descending inhibition at the level of the rostral ventromedial medulla may be responsible for the reduction in temperature required by CP users with low circulating testosterone to develop pain [39].

Another important determinant of gender-based differences in pain sensitivity may be the interaction between the opioidergic system and the gonadal hormones. In fact, as showed by Smith et al., women in high estradiol/low progesterone states exhibit decreased pain sensitivity and increased brain mu-opioid receptor binding than women in low estradiol states, while decreased endogenous opioid neurotransmission was associated with low estradiol [31].

Genotype is a potential factor able to modulate gender differences in pain perception. One example is the melanocortin-1 receptor (MC1R) gene associated with red hair and fair skin. MC1R has been found to moderate analgesia in a gender-dependent manner. Specifically, women with two variant alleles of the gene demonstrate greater analgesic responses to pentazocine compared to men and women who do not have the variant alleles [40]. In another study the A118G single-nucleotide polymorphism of the mu-opioid receptor gene (OPRM1) was associated with pressure pain sensitivity in men but not women. Furthermore, differential effects on thermal pain sensitivity were observed in women with a rare allele: they exhibited increased pain sensitivity, while the opposite was observed for men with the rare allele [41]. These findings were recently extended to a clinical population, in that women with the rare allele showed poorer recovery from lumbar disc herniation, while the rare allele predicted enhanced recovery among men [42].

Psychosocial mechanisms may play a fundamental role in gender-related differences in pain. For example, pain-coping strategies have been found to differ between men and women. While men usually use behavioural distraction and problem-focused tactics to manage pain, women are likely to use a range of coping techniques including social support, positive self-statements, emotion-focused techniques, cognitive reinterpretation and attentional focus [43, 44]. Catastrophising is a method of pain coping referring to the magnification and rumination of pain-related information. Research has shown that catastrophising is associated with pain and pain-related disability and women engage in catastrophising more often than men. Self-efficacy refers to the belief that one can successfully perform a behaviour to achieve a desirable target. A lower degree of self-efficacy has been found to be associated with higher levels of pain and physical dysfunction. Jackson et al. indicated that men show greater self-efficacy which was associated with lower cold pressor pain sensitivity [45–49].

Gender differences in pain sensitivity may be influenced by gender-related expectations regarding performance, suggesting that gender-related motivation may influence pain expression. For example, in a study by Robinson et al., both men and women believed that men are less prone to report pain than women [50–52]. A study by Fowler and colleagues found that social priming may impact gender differences in pain. When primed with a feminine gender role, men reported increased cold pressor pain [53]. The authors concluded that feminine gender role may alter pain report more than masculine one. Culture-related variability may also play a role in the differences between men and women. A recent study assessing pain sensitivity and gender roles among Israelites and Americans found that both Israelite men and women reported a more masculine role in regard to views of pain sensitivity when compared with Americans, thus implying the importance of cultural differences in pain-related beliefs [54]. Early exposure to environmental stress, such as prior pain and history of abuse, may also contribute to variability in pain report between men and women. Childhood abuse has been linked to adult chronic pain with individuals having pain complaints later in life reporting a history of early-life abuse [55]. Fillingim et al. observed that a history of childhood abuse was associated with decreased pain sensitivity; however, this effect was only observed in women [56]. It has also been observed that a family history of pain is associated with greater pain symptoms and increased pain sensitivity among females relative to men [40, 57, 58].

24.4 Conclusion

Epidemiological and clinical studies show that women are at increased risk for chronic pain and may experience more severe pain than men. Studies evaluating experimentally induced pain showed that women exhibit greater pain sensitivity, enhanced pain facilitation and reduced pain inhibition compared with men. In addition, some evidence suggests gender differences in response to pharmacological treatments.

Several different biopsychosocial mechanisms contribute to gender differences in pain, including sex hormones, endogenous opioid function, genetic factors, pain coping and catastrophising, and gender roles even though the specific underlying mechanisms are not clear.

References

1. Breivik H, Collett B, Ventafridda V, Cohen R, Gallacher D. Survey of chronic pain in Europe: prevalence, impact on daily life, and treatment. Eur J Pain. 2006;10(4):287–333.
2. Turner JA, Franklin G, Heagerty PJ, et al. The association between pain and disability. Pain. 2004;112(3):307–14.
3. Bartley EJ, Fillingim RB. Sex differences in pain: a brief review of clinical and experimental findings. Br J Anaesth. 2013;111(1):52–8.
4. Berkley KJ. Sex differences in pain. Behav Brain Sci. 1997;20(3):371–80.
5. Fillingim RB, King CD, Ribeiro-Dasilva MC, Rahim-Williams B, Riley JL III. Sex, gender, and pain: a review of recent clinical and experimental findings. J Pain. 2009;10:447–85.
6. Gerdle B, Bjork J, Coster L, Henriksson K, Henriksson C, Bengtsson A. Prevalence of widespread pain and associations with work status: a population study. BMC Musculoskelet Disord. 2008;9:102.
7. Pieretti S, Di Giannuario A, Di Giovannandrea R, Marzoli F, Piccaro G, Minosi P, et al. Gender differences in pain and its relief. Ann Ist Super Sanit. 2016;52(2):184–9.

8. Mogil JS. Sex differences in pain and pain inhibition: multiple explanations of a controversial phenomenon. Nat Rev Neurosci. 2012;13:859–66.
9. Meriggiola MC, Nanni M, Bachiocco V, Vodo S, Aloisi AM. Menopause affects pain depending on pain type and characteristics. Menopause. 2012;19(5):517–23.
10. Foreman J. Why millions of women are living in chronic pain. WSJ. 2014.
11. Fillingim RB, Doleys DM, Edwards RR, Lowery D. Clinical characteristics of chronic back pain as a function of gender and oral opioid use. Spine. 2003;28:143–50.
12. Keefe FJ, Lefebvre JC, Egert JR, Affleck G, Sullivan MJ, Caldwell DS. The relationship of gender to pain, pain behavior, and disability in osteoarthritis patients: the role of catastrophizing. Pain. 2000;87:325–34.
13. Barnabe C, Bessette L, Flanagan C, et al. Sex differences in pain scores and localization in inflammatory arthritis: a systematic review and metaanalysis. J Rheumatol. 2012;39:1221–30.
14. Tang YR, Yang WW, Wang YL, Lin L. Sex differences in the symptoms and psychological factors that influence quality of life in patients with irritable bowel syndrome. Eur J Gastroenterol Hepatol. 2012;24:702–7.
15. Edwards RR, Augustson E, Fillingim RB. Differential relationships between anxiety and treatment-associated pain reduction among male and female chronic pain patients. Clin J Pain. 2003;19:208–16.
16. Robinson ME, Wise EA, Riley JLI. Sex differences in clinical pain: a multi-sample study. J Clin Psychol Med Settings. 1998;5:413–23.
17. Turk DC, Okifuji A. Does sex make a difference in the prescription of treatments and the adaptation to chronic pain by cancer and non-cancer patients? Pain. 1999;82:139–48.
18. Paller CJ, Campbell CM, Edwards RR, Dobs AS. Sex-based differences in pain perception and treatment. Pain Med. 2009;10:289–99.
19. Fillingim RB, Maixner W. Gender differences in the responses to noxious stimuli. Pain Forum. 1995;4:209–21.
20. Popescu A, LeResche L, Truelove EL, Drangsholt MT. Gender differences in pain modulation by diffuse noxious inhibitory controls: a systematic review. Pain. 2010;150:309–18.
21. Edwards RR, Sarlani E, Wesselmann U, Fillingim RB. Quantitative assessment of experimental pain perception: multiple domains of clinical relevance. Pain. 2005;114(3):315–9.
22. Holdcroft A, Berkley KJ. Sex and gender differences in pain and its relief. In: McMahon SB, Koltzenburg M, editors. Wall and Melzack's textbook of pain. Philadelphia, PA: Elsevier; 2006.
23. Miaskowski C, Gear RW, Levine JD. Sex-related differences in analgesic responses. In: Fillingim RB, editor. Sex, gender, and pain. Seattle, WA: IASP Press; 2000. p. 209–30.
24. Chang K-Y, Tsou M-Y, Chan K-H, Sung C-S, Chang W-K. Factors affecting patient-controlled analgesia requirements. J Formos Med Assoc. 2006;105:918–25.
25. Fillingim RB, Ness TJ, Glover TL, et al. Morphine responses and experimental pain: sex differences in side effects and cardiovascular responses but not analgesia. J Pain. 2005;6:116–24.
26. Niesters M, Dahan A, Kest B, et al. Do sex differences exist in opioid analgesia? A systematic review and metaanalysis of human experimental and clinical studies. Pain. 2010;151:61–8.
27. Calderone KL. The influence of gender on the frequency of pain and sedative medication administered to postoperative patients. Sex Roles. 1990;23:713–25.
28. Leresche L. Defining gender disparities in pain management. Clin Orthop Relat Res. 2011;469:1871–7.
29. Craft RM. Modulation of pain by estrogens. Pain. 2007;132:S3–S12.
30. Craft RM, Mogil JS, Aloisi AM. Sex differences in pain and analgesia: the role of gonadal hormones. Eur J Pain. 2004;8:397.
31. Smith YR, Stohler CS, Nichols TE, Bueller JA, Koeppe RA, Zubieta JK. Pronociceptive and antinociceptive effects of estradiol through endogenous opioid neurotransmission in women. J Neurosci. 2006;26:5777–85.
32. Cairns BE, Gazerani P. Sex-related differences in pain. Maturitas. 2009;63:292–6.
33. Vacca V, Marinelli S, Pieroni L, Urbani A, Luvisetto S, Pavone F. 17beta-estradiol counteracts neuropathic pain: a behavioural, immunohistochemical, and proteomic investigation on sex-related differences in mice. Sci Rep. 2016;6:18980.

34. LeResche L, Saunders K, Von Korff MR, Barlow W. Use of exogenous hormones and risk of temporomandibular disorder pain. Pain. 1997;69:153.
35. Tedford WH, Warren DE, Flynn WE. Alteration of shock aversion thresholds during the menstrual cycle. Percept Psychophys. 1977;21:193–6.
36. Goolkasian P. Cyclic changes in pain perception: an ROC analysis. Percept Psychophys. 1980;27:499.
37. Dao TT, Knight K, Ton-That V. Modulation of myofascial pain by the reproductive hormones: a preliminary report. J Prosthet Dent. 1998;79:663–70.
38. Hapidou EG, Rollman GB. Menstrual cycle modulation of tender points. Pain. 1998;77:151.
39. Vincent K, Warnaby C, Stagg CJ, Moore J, Kennedy S, Tracey I. Brain imaging reveals that engagement of descending inhibitory pain pathways in healthy women in a low endogenous estradiol state varies with testosterone. Pain. 2013;154(4):515–24.
40. Fillingim RB, Edwards RR, Powell T. Sex-dependent effects of reported familial pain history on recent pain complaints and experimental pain responses. Pain. 2000;86:87–94.
41. Fillingim RB, Kaplan L, Staud R, et al. The A118G single nucleotide polymorphism of the mu-opioid receptor gene (OPRM1) is associated with pressure pain sensitivity in humans. J Pain. 2005;6:159–67.
42. Olsen MB, Jacobsen LM, Schistad EI, et al. Pain intensity the first year after lumbar disc herniation is associated with the A118G polymorphism in the opioid receptor mu 1 gene: evidence of a sex and genotype interaction. J Neurosci. 2012;32:9831–4.
43. Unruh AM, Ritchie J, Merskey H. Does gender affect appraisal of pain and pain coping strategies? Clin J Pain. 1999;15:31–40.
44. Keogh E, Eccleston C. Sex differences in adolescent chronic pain and pain-related coping. Pain. 2006;123:275–84.
45. Sullivan MJ, Thorn B, Haythornthwaite JA, et al. Theoretical perspectives on the relation between catastrophizing and pain. Clin J Pain. 2001;17:52–64.
46. Bandura A. Self-efficacy: toward a unifying theory of behavioral change. Psychol Rev. 1977;84:191–215.
47. Keefe FJ, Brown GK, Wallston KA, Caldwell DS. Coping with rheumatoid arthritis pain: catastrophizing as a maladaptive strategy. Pain. 1989;37:51–6.
48. Somers TJ, Kurakula PC, Criscione-Schreiber L, Keefe FJ, Clowse MEB. Self-efficacy and pain catastrophizing in systemic lupus erythematosus: relationship to pain, stiffness, fatigue, and psychological distress. Arthritis Care Res. 2012;64:1334–40.
49. Jackson T, Iezzi T, Gunderson J, Nagasaka T, Fritch A. Gender differences in pain perception: the mediating role of self-efficacy beliefs. Sex Roles. 2002;47:561–8.
50. Robinson ME, Riley JL III, Myers CD, et al. Gender role expectations of pain: relationship to sex differences in pain. J Pain. 2001;2:251–7.
51. Fillingim RB, Browning AD, Powell T, Wright RA. Sex differences in perceptual and cardiovascular responses to pain: the influence of a perceived ability manipulation. J Pain. 2002;3:439–45.
52. Robinson ME, Gagnon CM, Riley JL III, Price DD. Altering gender role expectations: effects on pain tolerance, pain threshold, and pain ratings. J Pain. 2003;4:284–8.
53. Fowler SL, Rasinski HM, Geers AL, Helfer SG, France CR. Concept priming and pain: an experimental approach to understanding gender roles in sex-related pain differences. J Behav Med. 2011;34:139–47.
54. Defrin R, Shramm L, Eli I. Gender role expectations of pain is associated with pain tolerance limit but not with pain threshold. Pain. 2009;145:230–6.
55. Walsh CA, Jamieson E, MacMillan H, Boyle M. Child abuse and chronic pain in a community survey of women. J Interpers Violence. 2007;22:1536–54.
56. Fillingim RB, Edwards RR. Is self-reported childhood abuse history associated with pain perception among healthy young women and men? Clin J Pain. 2005;21:387–97.
57. Edwards PW, Zeichner A, Kuczmierczyk AR, Boczkowski J. Familial pain models: the relationship between family history of pain and current pain experience. Pain. 1985;21:379.
58. Koutantji M, Pearce SA, Oakley DA. The relationship between gender and family history of pain with current pain experience and awareness of pain in others. Pain. 1998;77:25.

The Brain-Gut Axis and the Gender

25

Giovanni Barbara, Maria Giulia Regazzi, Maria Raffaella Barbaro, Giovanni Dothel, and Ilaria Tarricone

Key Points

- The term brain-gut axis describes an anatomic and functional substrate in which the brain and psychosocial factors influence the GI tract and vice versa.
- The clinical phenotype that we understand as functional gastrointestinal disorders (FGIDs) emerges from the interactions of multiple systems in the periphery and in the brain interacting with each other in bidirectional ways that lead to the FGID phenotype.
- Pain and other symptoms seen in FGIDs may generate in women more than in men a feeling of anger, shame, or silence. These symptoms are often considered typical traits of FGIDs. Furthermore, a certain body of evidence shows enhanced prevalence of FGID-associated symptoms such as urinary urgency, muscle stiffness, and altered taste or smell in women compared to men.
- A large body of evidence suggests a sex-related activity of several pathophysiological factors involved in irritable bowel syndrome (IBS) symptom generation. Interestingly, female patients with IBS showed an enhanced mast cell activity compared to male IBS patients. Recent findings indicate an increased permeability of female patients with IBS.
- Women with FGID appear to respond well to psychological treatment and the newer serotonergic agents, such as 5-HT3 antagonists and 5-HT4 agonists.

G. Barbara (✉) · M. G. Regazzi · M. R. Barbaro · G. Dothel
Department of Medical and Surgical Sciences, St. Orsola-Malpighi Hospital, University of Bologna, Bologna, Italy
e-mail: giovanni.barbara@unibo.it

I. Tarricone
Bologna Transcultural Psychosomatic Team (BoTPT), Department of Medical and Surgical Sciences, Alma Mater Studiorum, University of Bologna, Bologna, Italy

I. Tarricone, A. Riecher-Rössler (eds.), *Health and Gender*,
https://doi.org/10.1007/978-3-030-15038-9_25

25.1 The Brain-Gut Axis

The term brain-gut axis depicts an anatomic and functional substrate in which the brain and psychosocial factors influence the GI tract and vice versa. The hardwiring between the brain and gut is mainly, but not solely, represented by a complex integrated circuitry that exchanges information from emotional and cognitive centers of the brain to the peripheral functioning of the GI tract and vice versa [1]. This communication is mainly based on a dense network of neurons connecting the brain and the gut, composed by afferent and efferent components and functioning via the exchange of neurochemical molecules released at the level of neuronal synapses, namely, neurotransmitters. Structurally, there are direct connections between the central nervous system (CNS) and the myenteric plexus, the muscle layers, and other end-organ structures [2]. Other systems take part in the complex process of communication in the brain-gut axis and include immune, endocrine, and microbial factors. The gut microenvironment of the gastrointestinal tract is a rich source of signals for the brain. The gut is particularly enriched with molecules derived from the microbiome (a complex microbial world composed by not only bacteria but also viruses and fungi), enteroendocrine cells (producing 95% of body's serotonin among other hormonal substances), and a large bulk of immune cells, comprising the largest immune organ of the human body. These substances can communicate with the brain via different modalities. These include a direct signaling of immune, endocrine, and bacterial mediators on specific receptors located on sensory nerve ending conveying information to the brain. Examples of this communication include toll-like receptors located on enteric nerves and sensory afferent fibers sensing substances produced by bacteria (e.g., lipopolysaccharide), viruses, and fungi. Gut microenvironment substances can also communicate to the brain through the bloodstream reaching higher centers through the passage of the blood-brain barrier. This is the case for many food-derived substances but also for microbiota-derived molecules or products deriving from the bacterial fermentation of foods (e.g., short-chain fatty acids). The relevance of the bloodstream pathway and the constant production of gut-derived metabolites, particularly of bacterial origin, with a potential impact on the brain, is clearly revealed in patients with liver failure in whom the normal passage of numerous catabolites produced as a process of bacterial degradation of foods (particularly ammonia) reaches the brain without liver detoxification and generates hepatic encephalopathy of various degrees of severity up to coma. Interestingly, this severe brain dysfunction can be reversed by reducing intestinal bacterial load with laxatives (e.g., lactulose) and nonabsorbable antibiotics (e.g., rifaximin).

25.2 Functional Gastrointestinal Disorders and the Brain-Gut Axis

Disorders of gut-brain interactions formerly known as FGIDs (functional gastrointestinal disorders) are the most common diagnoses in gastroenterology. FGIDs encompass morphological and physiological abnormalities including changes in gastrointestinal motor function, visceral hypersensitivity, increased epithelial permeability, mucosal immune activation, changes in gut microbiota, and altered CNS processing. The Rome

Foundation has played a pivotal role in creating diagnostic criteria, thus operationalizing the dissemination of new knowledge in the field of FGIDs.

Several studies investigated the role of the brain, stress, and emotions such as fear, anxiety, and anger on gut physiology. These studies have demonstrated that emotions, including fear, anger, anxiety, pain, and stress can modify gastrointestinal functions (e.g., delaying gastric emptying, accelerating or delaying gut transit). Partly through these mechanisms, stress can contribute to symptom generation such as visceral pain, defecation, and diarrhea. In addition, stress and other psychological factors can evoke visceral pain via impairment of mucosal secretory and barrier functions, favoring the systemic translocation of bacteria and their products from the gut lumen. These mechanisms have been claimed to participate in the generation of symptoms including nausea, abdominal bloating and pain, diarrhea, and constipation found in functional complaints such as non-cardiac chest pain, functional dyspepsia, and IBS.

Changes in gastrointestinal motility, visceral inflammation, and injury can amplify ascending visceral pathways and affect brain areas, leading to greater pain and contributing to altered mental functioning including anxiety and depression. The relationships between psychosocial distress and painful symptoms are at least in part mediated through impairment in the ability of various brain networks such as the cingulate cortex to process bodily pain. The brain can act as a filter to enhance or block pain by upregulating or downregulating afferent signals through a gate control mechanism. The mechanism of downregulation of pain afferent signals has been claimed to be dysfunctional in patients with functional gastrointestinal disorders, fibromyalgia, and other functional somatic symptoms, leading to increased pain perception. There is also evidence that the anterior cingulate cortex, involved in the affective and motivational components of the emotional arousal and salience network, is defective with IBS and other FGIDs characterized by pain. Experience of stress opens the gate and the pain threshold decreases. Conversely, improvement in pain control can be enabled by cognitive or emotional factors such as focused attention, hypnosis, psychological treatment, and certain antidepressants. In addition, evidence suggests that pain may overstimulate the afferent system leading to neurogenesis as well, possibly contributing to long-lasting effects once the stressful stimuli have ceased [3].

Thus, the current understanding of brain-gut role in the pathophysiology of FGIDs emerges from the bidirectional interactions of different systems, both in the periphery (microbiome, altered mucosal inflammation, visceral hypersensitivity) and in the brain (brain network systems of emotional arousal, sensorimotor function, central autonomic function) leading to the full phenotype of FGIDs.

25.3 Gender and the Brain-Gut Axis

25.3.1 Sex and Gender-Related Impact of Psychological Factors on FGID Symptoms

The term gender refers to psychological and behavioral features characterizing self-perceived identity, therefore not necessarily relating to the corresponding biological sex traits. Unmet expectations from social environment may greatly impact on individual psychology and be often the main cause of chronic features in stress-related disorders. Physical standards of beauty are gradually shrinking to hardly conceivable parameters. In addition, the acquired condition and quality of life of patients with FGIDs may represent a more detrimental factor to women compared to men. As a result, several limitations caused by symptoms of upper and lower GI tract (nausea, vomiting, urgency of defecation, feeling of losing control of bodily function) may in turn enhance hypervigilance and anxiety behaviors with a positive reinforcement of brain-gut axis signaling, leading to a further exacerbation of symptoms. Therefore, pain and other symptoms seen in FGIDs may generate in women more than in men a feeling of anger, shame, or silence. These symptoms are often considered typical traits of FGIDs. Table 25.1 shows the prevalence of FGIDs and symptom generation in females versus male. In general this table provides evidence that for most FGIDs symptoms are more prevalent in females versus males. Figure 25.1 shows that most studies investigating odds ratio for IBS in women vs. men according to geographic origin showed higher prevalence of IBS in women, although this could be related to the geographic provenience of study results [4].

Furthermore, a certain body of evidence shows enhanced prevalence of FGID-associated symptoms such as urinary urgency, muscle stiffness, and altered taste or smell in women compared to men [5]. A cause-effect relationship between peripheral symptoms and psychological distress is often difficult to be determined as the brain can influence negatively body functions and body dysfunction may generate psychological distress. However, the general perception in non-FGID specialists is that patients with FGIDs have a psychological problem that generates a false perception of a bowel dysfunction. “There is nothing wrong with your bowel”, “all the tests are normal”, “it must be stress.” These are typical attitudes toward patients with FGIDs.

Table 25.1 Effect of sex in functional gastroeintestinal disorders

Functional gastrointestinal disorder	Effect of sex
Esophageal globus	F > M
Rumination	F = M
Functional chest pain	F > M
Functional heartburn	F = M
Dysphagia	F > M
Functional dyspepsia	F = M
Aerophagia	F > M
Functional vomiting	F = M
IBS	F > M
Functional constipation	F > M
Functional diarrhea	F > M
Functional bloating	F > M
Fecal incontinence	F > M
Functional anorectal pain	F > M

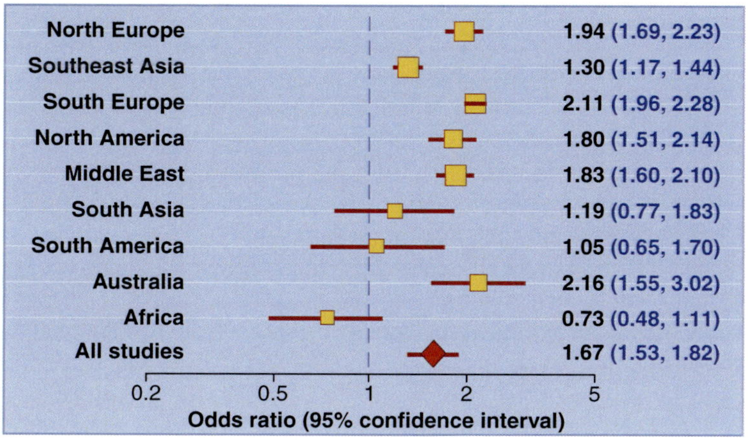

Fig. 25.1 Odd ratios of FGIDs and symptom generation in females versus male

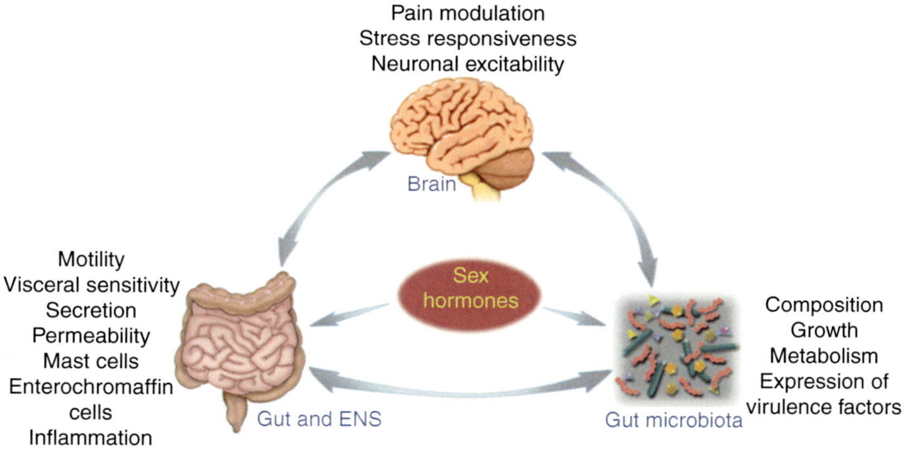

Fig. 25.2 Influence of sex hormones in the brain-gut axis

25.3.2 Sex-Related Pathophysiological Factors in FGIDs

A large body of evidence suggests a sex-related activity of several pathophysiological factors involved in IBS symptom generation. The paragraphs below outline some of the recent findings regarding these major mechanisms, which are summarized in Fig. 25.2.

Brain-gut axis dysregulation: CNS dysfunction and abnormal interaction with peripheral factors contribute to symptom generation in IBS. The alteration between central and peripheral factors is bidirectional. Although in the past FGIDs were considered psychosomatic disorders in which psychological dysfunction was considered the only mechanism leading to symptom perception, novel data suggest that also the periphery contributes substantially to symptom experience. Among people free of FGIDs at baseline, anxiety at baseline was significantly associated with new onset of FGIDs 12 years later. Interestingly, among people free of psychological factors at baseline, FGIDs at baseline were significantly associated with anxiety and depression at follow-up, suggesting that IBS is not "all in the head" in all patients.

Genetic factors: overall, IBS displays features of a complex disorder with interactions between environmental and genetic factors. Several studies evaluated the risk effects of single-nucleotide polymorphisms (SNPs) in IBS candidate genes. A recent study demonstrated in two independent cohorts from Sweden and the USA a strong association between rs4263839 in *TNFSF15* and IBS, particularly IBS-C. The first genome-wide association study (GWAS) in IBS identified a suggestive locus at 7p22.1 with genetic risk replicated in all case-control cohorts. The genes *KDLER2* and *GRIP2IP* map to the associated locus; the latter notably is involved in host-microbiota interactions. In addition, among the candidate loci, *HTR3E* is associated with female IBS-D phenotype.

25.3.3 Role of Endocrine Factors on Symptom Exacerbation

Enteroendocrine alteration: serotonin, or 5-hydroxytryptamine (5-HT), released by a subtype of enteroendocrine cells named enterochromaffin cells in response to mechanical and chemical stimuli regulates gastrointestinal secretory, motor, and sensory functions throughout receptors spread all over the gut. Decreased postprandial 5-HT platelet-depleted plasma levels have been reported in IBS prevalent constipation (IBS-C), while increased plasma levels of 5-HT have been shown under fasting and fed conditions in IBS prevalent diarrhea (IBS-D) (Fig. 25.3).

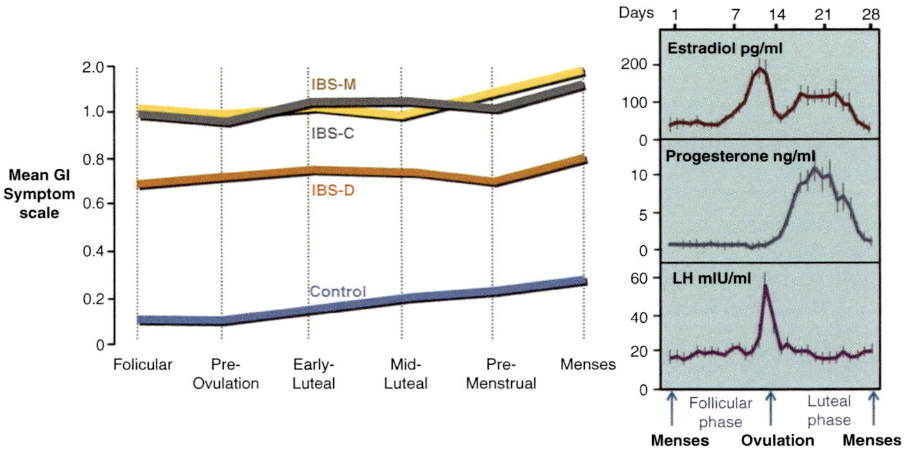

Fig. 25.3 Gastrointestinal symptoms and menstrual cycle

Neuroplastic changes: several studies described neuroplastic changes in patients with IBS. A pioneering study showed that the overall density of mucosal innervation, substance P, and transient receptor potential vanilloid type-1 was increased in patients with IBS. A recent innovative study demonstrated an increased density of mucosal nerve fibers and nerve outgrowth as well as neuronal growth factor (NGF) expression in patients with IBS. Mediators from IBS biopsies evoked neurite elongation and neuronal differentiation in culture neuronal cell lines. NGF of immune cell, particularly mast cell origin, was the main mediator involved in these changes. Interestingly, female patients with IBS showed an enhanced mast cell activity compared to male IBS patients. All together, these data suggest that an abnormal mucosal milieu play a role in the pathophysiology of IBS inducing long-lasting neuroplastic changes.

Increased mucosal permeability: several structures contribute to the intestinal mucosal barrier, including microbiota, mucus layer, enterocytes, and intercellular tight junctions (TJs), adherent junctions, and desmosomes positioned between epithelial cells. All together these components regulate the intestinal permeability. Disruption of the mucosal barrier leads to contact between environmental antigens and mucosal immune system, with subsequent immune activation, stimulation of sensory pain pathways, and, finally, pain perception. Increased mucosal permeability has been shown in patients with IBS irrespective to bowel subtype by means of in vivo (including confocal laser endomicroscopy) and in vitro methods both in the small intestine and in the colon, and it was correlated with the main symptom of IBS, the abdominal pain. In addition, recent findings indicate an increased permeability in female patients with IBS [6]. The trigger factors involved in the increased intestinal permeability of IBS remain elusive, although recent studies suggest the participation of genetic factors, stress, food antigens, gluten, or luminal factors.

Altered intestinal microbiota: the introduction of molecular techniques using high-throughput DNA technologies to investigate gut microbiota has renewed interest in intestinal microbiology. Recent studies indicate a different composition of fecal and intestinal mucosal microbiota in patients with IBS. The most consistent abnormality identified in these subjects includes an increased *Firmicutes/Bacteroides* ratio in all or at least a subgroup of patients with IBS, with decreased levels of *Bifidobacteria* and members of the genus *Faecalibacterium* (which includes *F. prausnitzii*). Interestingly, patients with abnormal *Firmicutes/Bacteroidetes* ratio showed changes in bowel physiology including altered bowel transit times, while those with normal microbiota had more psychological impairment (i.e., anxiety and depression).

A correlation between microbial dysbiosis and expression of several host gene pathways, including cell junction integrity and inflammatory response, was demonstrated in PI-IBS and IBS-D. The role of microbiota in FGIDs including IBS has been the subject of exhaustive recent reviews [7, 8].

25.4 Treatment of FGIDs: Several Gender Differences

Gender-related differences have been described to influence the response to pharmacologic therapy. Nonetheless, only some studies with relatively small numbers of patients have evaluated gender differences. A systematic review of therapy with antidepressants showed that most studies did not conduct separate analyses by gender. Therapies targeting 5-HT receptors showed differential gender-related effects. Alosetron, a 5-HT3 antagonist, showed higher efficacy in women than in men [9]. Alosetron is currently indicated and commercialized in the USA only under restrictions (for the occurrence of severe adverse events) only for women with severe IBS-D not responding to conventional therapy [10]. Three large studies [11] of prucalopride, a selective 5-HT4 agonist, was conducted in 85% female IBS-C patients and showed equal efficacy in both sexes. Some trials suggested that there may be higher efficacy of these drugs in women compared with men with IBS-C [12–14]. For other drugs commonly used to treat motility disorders (domperidone, opioid-based constipating agents, laxatives, probiotics), there is no evidence of a gender-related difference in efficacy [15]. Psychological treatment studies have not always provided evidence of gender-related responses. In general, many of these studies have included more women than men. In a large hypnotherapy study, there were different response patterns in men versus women. Although most IBS patients showed a positive treatment response, women did better than men [16]. In another study, Gonsalkorale et al. reported that men showed a less efficacious long-term outcome after hypnotherapy compared to women (42% versus 25%) [17].

25.5 Conclusions

The brain-gut axis is a key mechanism in homeostasis of body functions, and its dysregulation may lead to meaningful consequences for human health. There are several gender-related differences in both experiences of symptoms related to brain-gut dysfunction and pharmacological response that should be considered both in clinical practice and in research settings.

References

1. Drossman DA. Functional gastrointestinal disorders: history, pathophysiology, clinical features and Rome IV. Gastroenterology. 2016. https://doi.org/10.1053/j.gastro.2016.02.032.
2. Jones MP, Dilley JB, Drossman D, Crowell MD. Brain-gut connections in functional GI disorders: anatomic and physiologic relationships. Neurogastroenterol Motil. 2006;18(2):91–103.
3. Seminowicz DA, Labus JS, Bueller JA, Tillisch K, Naliboff BD, Bushnell MC, et al. Regional gray matter density changes in brains of patients with irritable bowel syndrome. Gastroenterology. 2010;139(1):48–57.e2.
4. Lovell RM, Ford AC. Effect of gender on prevalence of irritable bowel syndrome in the community: systematic review and meta-analysis. Am J Gastroenterol. 2012;107(7):991–1000.
5. Lee OY, Mayer EA, Schmulson M, Chang L, Naliboff B. Gender-related differences in IBS symptoms. Am J Gastroenterol. 2001;96(7):2184–93.
6. Houghton LA, Heitkemper M, Crowell M, Emmanuel A, Halpert A, McRoberts JA, et al. Age, gender and women's health and the patient. Gastroenterology. 2016. https://doi.org/10.1053/j.gastro.2016.02.017.
7. Barbara G, Feinle-Bisset C, Ghoshal UC, Quigley EM, Santos J, Vanner S, et al. The intestinal microenvironment and functional gastrointestinal disorders. Gastroenterology. 2016. https://doi.org/10.1053/j.gastro.2016.02.028.

8. Simren M, Barbara G, Flint HJ, Spiegel BM, Spiller RC, Vanner S, et al. Intestinal microbiota in functional bowel disorders: a Rome foundation report. Gut. 2013;62(1):159–76.
9. Camilleri M, Mayer EA, Drossman DA, Heath A, Dukes GE, McSorley D, et al. Improvement in pain and bowel function in female irritable bowel patients with alosetron, a 5-HT3 receptor antagonist. Aliment Pharmacol Ther. 1999;13(9):1149–59.
10. Miller JL. FDA draws patients into alosetron risk management. Am J Health Syst Pharm. 2000;57(19):1736.
11. Tack J, van Outryve M, Beyens G, Kerstens R, Vandeplassche L. Prucalopride (Resolor) in the treatment of severe chronic constipation in patients dissatisfied with laxatives. Gut. 2009;58(3):357–65.
12. Muller-Lissner SA, Fumagalli I, Bardhan KD, Pace F, Pecher E, Nault B, et al. Tegaserod, a 5-HT(4) receptor partial agonist, relieves symptoms in irritable bowel syndrome patients with abdominal pain, bloating and constipation. Aliment Pharmacol Ther. 2001;15(10):1655–66.
13. Kellow J, Lee OY, Chang FY, Thongsawat S, Mazlam MZ, Yuen H, et al. An Asia-Pacific, double blind, placebo controlled, randomised study to evaluate the efficacy, safety, and tolerability of tegaserod in patients with irritable bowel syndrome. Gut. 2003;52(5):671–6.
14. Nyhlin H, Bang C, Elsborg L, Silvennoinen J, Holme I, Ruegg P, et al. A double-blind, placebo-controlled, randomized study to evaluate the efficacy, safety and tolerability of tegaserod in patients with irritable bowel syndrome. Scand J Gastroenterol. 2004;39(2):119–26.
15. Ouyang A, Wrzos HF. Contribution of gender to pathophysiology and clinical presentation of IBS: should management be different in women? Am J Gastroenterol. 2006;101(12 Suppl):S602–9.
16. Moser G, Tragner S, Gajowniczek EE, Mikulits A, Michalski M, Kazemi-Shirazi L, et al. Long-term success of GUT-directed group hypnosis for patients with refractory irritable bowel syndrome: a randomized controlled trial. Am J Gastroenterol. 2013;108(4):602–9.
17. Gonsalkorale WM, Miller V, Afzal A, Whorwell PJ. Long term benefits of hypnotherapy for irritable bowel syndrome. Gut. 2003;52(11):1623–9.

Infectious Diseases and Gender: Focus on HIV Infection

26

Leonardo Calza

Key Points

- The HIV disease is a global pandemic still today, with about 5000 new infections per day.
- Women show a higher risk of HIV acquisition per heterosexual intercourse than men.
- The disease progression rate is comparable between women and men.
- Women living with HIV have higher levels of systemic inflammation and immune activation than men.
- Clinical studies have shown similar efficacy and tolerability for modern antiretroviral therapies in women and men.

26.1 Introduction

The acquisition, pathogenesis, and clinical features of infectious diseases are influenced by a complex combination of factors depending on environment, host genetics, and microorganisms. Biological sex, with a distinct genetic complement, hormonal profile, and behavioral and social contexts, is certainly an essential contributor to heterogeneity in clinical manifestations of many infectious diseases.

The human immunodeficiency virus (HIV) infection is a global pandemic still today. There were approximately 37 million people worldwide living with HIV infection at the end of 2016, and an estimated 1.8 million subjects worldwide became newly infected with HIV in 2016 or rather about 5000 new infections per day. HIV gradually weakens the human immune system and leads to several

L. Calza (✉)
Department of Medical and Surgical Sciences, Clinics of Infectious Diseases,
S. Orsola-Malpighi Hospital, "Alma Mater Studiorum" University of Bologna, Bologna, Italy
e-mail: leonardo.calza@unibo.it

I. Tarricone, A. Riecher-Rössler (eds.), *Health and Gender*,
https://doi.org/10.1007/978-3-030-15038-9_26

opportunistic diseases (infections and neoplasms) which manifest as the acquired immune deficiency syndrome (AIDS). One million people died from AIDS-related illnesses in 2016, bringing the total number of individuals who have died from AIDS since the beginning of the epidemic to 35 million [1].

The advent of the highly active antiretroviral therapy (HAART) in 1996 has dramatically reduced the mortality and morbidity of AIDS, but approximately 20–30% of people living with HIV are unaware of their HIV status, so they are not receiving HAART, have a detectable HIV viral load in their biological fluids, and can transmit the infection. Therefore, the access to HIV testing to discover the occult infections is an essential gateway to HIV prevention, care, and support services.

The clinical manifestations of HIV infection are conditioned by genetic factors, such as host HLA genotype that has been delineated in several studies, but many other sources of variation are certainly present, and biological sex plays probably a crucial role. Clinical studies to define the effects of biological sex on HIV disease are still limited, but the available data have produced important suggestions.

26.2 Natural History of HIV Infection

The risk of HIV acquisition per heterosexual intercourse is estimated to be about twofold higher for the women compared to men. This higher risk of HIV infection for females descends from multiple factors, including the characteristics of vaginal mucosal surface, inflammation at the cervicovaginal tract, other sexually transmitted infections, alterations in vaginal microbiome, and different hormone exposure, which reduce the barrier to HIV infection [2–5].

Moreover, sex has a potential role in both pathogenesis and disease progression. Several studies have shown in women lower HIV viral loads early during infection, but higher CD8+ T lymphocyte activation at a given level of HIV RNA, and higher expression of interferon-stimulated genes than in men, so the disease progression rate is comparable between women and men. Cohort studies have demonstrated that the prevalence of spontaneous controllers of HIV (or rather subjects who present undetectable plasma HIV RNA in the absence of antiretroviral therapy) is usually greater among females than among males, and sex-specific mechanisms of protection are certainly involved, but determinants of this spontaneous virologic suppression are still unknown [6–8].

The rates of adverse reactions and therapeutic success of the antiretroviral drugs can also show sex variation depending on sex differences in pharmacokinetics, pharmacodynamics, body composition, drug metabolism, and excretion, but data are lacking because of the limited enrollment of women in clinical trials. The most recent clinical studies have shown similar efficacy and tolerability in women and men, consistent with the higher therapeutic index of the modern antiretroviral agents, but some sex differences have been outlined and should be better evaluated [9, 10]. Particularly, some cohort studies have reported discordance in changes in serum inflammation markers after the beginning of cART, with higher baseline values but less change with cART in women. At the same time, some sex differences in residual immune activation may remain after the virologic suppression and can produce different effects on the comorbidity occurrence [11, 12].

26.3 Inflammation and Comorbidities

The observation that women living with HIV have higher levels of systemic inflammation and immune activation than men living with HIV can produce relevant sex differences in the frequency and severity of noncommunicable HIV-associated comorbidities. The mean levels of serum inflammatory markers are usually significantly higher in women with HIV infection than in men with HIV infection and in persons without HIV infection. Moreover, HIV-positive women appear to experience more rapid age-associated changes in monocyte activation and function than HIV-negative ones [13, 14].

A number of epidemiological studies conducted in the USA and Europe have highlighted a 1.5- to 2-fold increased risk of myocardial infarction among HIV-infected patients compared to the general population. Particularly, the relative risk of myocardial infarction among HIV-positive women versus HIV-negative women is significantly higher as compared to that among HIV-positive men versus HIV-negative men. In a large cohort study, women with HIV had a relative risk of 2.98 versus women without HIV, while men with HIV had a relative risk of 1.4 versus men without HIV, after adjustment for traditional cardiovascular risk factors. Moreover, the increased risk of cerebrovascular diseases reported in HIV-infected persons is exaggerated in females [15–17].

Epidemiologic studies from the USA have demonstrated that the prevalence of HIV-associated dementia significantly decreased after the introduction of cART in clinical practice, while the prevalence of mild neurocognitive impairment is increasing. In some cohort studies comparing HIV-infected women and men, women with HIV are more likely to display neurocognitive disorders than men, but severe disorders are very rare in both genders [18, 19].

The available data about sex differences in the frequency of non-AIDS-defining cancers also show a higher incidence of several neoplasms among women with HIV compared to men with HIV, such as cancers of the lung, stomach, kidney, larynx, and large intestine, leukemia, and multiple myeloma [20].

26.4 Reservoirs and Functional Cure

There are very limited data about sex differences in size and dynamics of the viral reservoirs, such as lymphoid tissue and central nervous system. Some cross-sectional studies reported lower levels of HIV DNA in women than in men, but other observational studies did not show any significant difference. In general, conclusions are very approximate because of the low percentage of women enrolled in these trials.

The goal of functional cure has become the essential point for HIV research. Curative interventions are primarily targeting host and not viral factors, and the sex specificity should be considered very carefully in the design of clinical trials, but the exact role of sex differences in cure interventions remains to be explained [21, 22].

To conclude, the understanding of virologic and immunologic differences between women and men living with HIV may suggest effective mechanisms to optimize antiretroviral therapy, management of HIV-associated comorbidities, and functional cure interventions, so further, enlarged studies assessing potential sex differences between women and men with HIV are certainly required.

References

1. UNAIDS. Global AIDS monitoring 2017: indicators for monitoring the 2016 United Nations Political Declaration on HIV and AIDS. Geneva: UNAIDS; 2017. http://www.unaids.org/sites/default/files/media_asset/2017-Global-AIDS-Monitoring_en.pdf.
2. Scully EP. Sex differences in HIV infection. Curr HIV/AIDS Rep. 2018;15:136–46.
3. Masson L, Passmore JA, Liebenberg LJ, et al. Genital inflammation and the risk of HIV acquisition in women. Clin Infect Dis. 2015;61(2):260–9.
4. Naranbhai V, Abdool Karim SS, Altfeld M, et al. Innate immune activation enhances HIV acquisition in women, diminishing the effectiveness of tenofovir microbicide gel. J Infect Dis. 2012;206(7):993–1001.
5. Selhorst P, Masson L, Ismail SD, et al. Cervicovaginal inflammation facilitates acquisition of less infectious HIV variants. Clin Infect Dis. 2016;64:79–82.
6. Madec Y, Boufassa F, Porter K, et al. Spontaneous control of viral load and CD4 cell count progression among HIV-1 seroconverters. AIDS. 2005;19(17):2001–7.
7. Goujard C, Girault L, Rouzioux C, et al. HIV-1 control after transient antiretroviral treatment initiated in primary infection: role of patient characteristics and effect of therapy. Antivir Ther. 2012;17(6):1001–9.
8. Saag M, Deeks SG. How do HIV elite controllers do what they do? Clin Infect Dis. 2010;51(2):239–41.
9. Squires K, Bekker LG, Katlama C, et al. Influence of sex/gender and race on responses to raltegravir combined with tenofovir-emtricitabine in treatment-naïve human immunodeficiency virus-1 infected patients: pooled analyses of the STARTMRK and QDMRK studies. Open Forum Infect Dis. 2017;4(1):ofw047.
10. Squires KE, Young B, Santiago L, et al. Response by gender of HIV-1-infected subjects treated with abacavir/lamivudine plus atazanavir with or without ritonavir for 144 weeks. HIV AIDS (Auckl). 2017;9:51–61.
11. Ticona E, Bull ME, Soria J, et al. Biomarkers of inflammation in HIV-infected Peruvian men and women before and during suppressive antiretroviral therapy. AIDS. 2015;29(13):1617–22.
12. Mathad JS, Gupte N, Balagopal A, et al. Sex-related differences in inflammatory and immune activation markers before and after combined antiretroviral therapy initiation. J Acquir Immune Defic Syndr. 2016;73(2):123–9.
13. Raghavan A, Rimmelin DE, Fitch KV, et al. Sex differences in select non-communicable HIV-associated comorbidities: exploring the role of systemic immune activation/inflammation. Curr HIV/AIDS Rep. 2017;14:220–8.
14. Fitch KV, Srinivasa S, Abbara S, et al. Noncalcified coronary atherosclerotic plaque and immune activation in HIV-infected women. J Infect Dis. 2013;208(11):1737–46.
15. Triant VA, Lee H, Hadigan C, et al. Increased acute myocardial infarction rates and cardiovascular risk factors among patients with human immunodeficiency virus disease. J Clin Endocrinol Metab. 2007;92(7):2506–12.

16. Lang S, Mary-Krause M, Cotte L, et al. Increased risk of myocardial infarction in HIV-infected patients in France, relative to the general population. AIDS. 2010;24(8):1228–30.
17. Freiberg MS, Chang CC, Kuller LH, et al. HIV infection and the risk of acute myocardial infarction. JAMA Intern Med. 2013;173(8):614–22.
18. Simioni S, Cavassini M, Annoni JM, et al. Cognitive dysfunction in HIV patients despite long-standing suppression of viremia. AIDS. 2010;24(9):1243–50.
19. Kabuba N, Menon JA, Franklin DR, et al. HIV- and AIDS-associated neurocognitive functioning in Zambia - a perspective based on differences between the genders. Neuropsychiatr Dis Treat. 2016;12:2021–8.
20. Rubinstein PG, Aboulafia DM, Zloza A, et al. Malignancies in HIV/AIDS: from epidemiology to therapeutic challenges. AIDS. 2014;28(4):453–65.
21. Fourati S, Flandre P, Calin R, et al. Factors associated with a low HIV reservoir in patients with prolonged suppressive antiretroviral therapy. J Antimicrob Chemother. 2014;69(3):753–6.
22. Cuzin L, Pugliese P, Saune K, et al. Levels of intracellular HIV-DNA in patients with suppressive antiretroviral therapy. AIDS. 2015;29(13):1665–71.

Part V

Cure, Organization of Services and Gender

Social Services in Front of Feminine Social Disease

27

Monica Brandoli and Annamaria Nicolini

Key Point

- Homelessness is characterized by complex risk factors, as well as a particular exposure to traumas, violence and diseases. Some aspects are closely related to gender: the individual and social conditions in which women live have a negative influence on their health and the system of services for homeless people developed following a stereotypical male gender. Ongoing experimentations are focused on some strategies: domestic violence prevention and intervention; activities on the community of belonging; education and female entrepreneurship; and healthcare services focused on simplifying the access to healthcare and the doctor-patient relation.

Homelessness is not just an urban phenomenon; it includes various aspects. Nowadays, the primary definition of *homelessness* as "deprivation of a house" tends to be developed into a wider perspective: it is not only the deprivation of a house but also the lack of all those elements that make up the idea of "home". Therefore, besides homeless people in the strict sense, this category now also includes those who have a roof over their head but who are not legally considered "inhabitants" or

M. Brandoli (✉)
Service Against Adult Marginalisation (Servizio Contrasto alla Grave Emarginazione Adulta)—Public Utility: ASP—Personal Care Service, Bologna, Italy
e-mail: Monica.Brandoli@aspbologna.it

A. Nicolini
Beltrame Homeless Shelter—Commnity Lab Belletrame—Social Cooperative: Società Dolce, Bologna, Italy

I. Tarricone, A. Riecher-Rössler (eds.), *Health and Gender*,
https://doi.org/10.1007/978-3-030-15038-9_27

those who do not have a place where to develop normal social relations: for example, those who are hosted by homeless shelters, inmates and so on (houseless[1]). What comes to light is the constant presence of immense pain and solitude, so deeply rooted that they prevent or break up the development of significant relations with oneself, other individuals and society. This condition is characterized by complex risk factors, as well as a particular exposure to traumas, violence and diseases.

Homeless people expose themselves to highly dangerous situations that can generate consequences with troublesome outcomes, which would not occur in safer living conditions.[2] This is proved by the analysis of diseases and the number of entries to the emergency room, which are mainly caused by contusions and injuries. In Italy, the analysis of data shows that the most common diseases among homeless people are tuberculosis, infections, alcoholism, hepatitis and HIV. The most common mental disorders are schizophrenia, mood disorder, depression, anxiety, personality disorder and post-traumatic stress disorders (PTSD). Among other health problems, it is important to mention the dysfunctions of the cardiorespiratory system and those related to malnutrition, as well as diabetes and asthma.

The survival of these people is seriously compromised by living on the streets and in extreme poverty and by environmental factors (wounds, insects bites and complications related to hot or cold weather) because of the lack of hygiene, the attendance of promiscuous places and the impossibility to eat or sleep adequately. Furthermore, the addiction to legal and illegal substances and the misuse of medications are highly frequent.

Among homeless people, rates of diseases and recovery are higher than among ordinary people; life expectancy is shorter; victimization is very frequent; and the percentage of imprisonment and the number of accesses to emergency health services are higher.

It is more difficult for them to benefit from the right to health: for people with no residence, who are forced to live on the street or in a dormitory, the itinerary to access healthcare services is rough, even for basic illnesses, like flu, or in case of a post-acute recovery, after being discharged from the hospital. On the basis of human and legal rights, since living on the street can often lead to premature death, it is evident that these people should have access to basic services, regardless of their legal status, in order to protect their own life, in particular when it is endangered by critical environmental factors (harsh temperatures, etc.). The social determinants and the procedures that facilitate the access to health (from efficacy to efficiency) can only be interpreted as a double-helix model.[3]

---

[1] www.feantsa.org; Amore K. Baker M. Howden-Chapman P. The ETHOS Definition and Classification of Homelessness: An Analysis, in *European Journal of Homelessness*. December, Volume 5, No. 2.

[2] De Maio G., Van den Bergh R., Garelli S., Maccagno B., Raddi F., Stefanizzi A., Regazzo C., Zachariah R., Reaching out to the forgotten: providing access to medical care for the homeless in Italy, Int Health, 2014.

[3] Tarricone I.; Berardi D., La competenza culturale nella relazione medico-paziente, in: P. BRIA E. CAROPPO P. BROGNA M. COLIMBERTI, Trattato italiano di psichiatria culturale e delle migrazioni, ROMA, Società Editrice Universo, 2010. Ed anche Hunter D.J., Health needs more than health care: the need for a new paradigm, in *European Journal of Public Health*, Volume 18.

If we focus on the sphere of homeless women, where the phenomenon shows a lower percentage compared to the men sphere, it appears that some aspects are closely related to gender: the individual and social conditions in which women live have a negative influence on their health; the system of services for homeless people has often developed in order to meet the needs of a stereotypical homeless person of male gender. This proves a lack of attention in the study and in the elaboration of appropriate services for women.[4]

The background of homeless women includes with alarming frequency traumatic migration routes; physical and psychological violence, either domestic or not; being forced into prostitution; being abandoned during their childhood; cultural and emotional deprivation; contexts of origin characterized by deviance and criminality; discrimination against their sexual orientation; addiction; psychological vulnerability; learning impairments that were not promptly diagnosed; workplace injuries; debilitating and/or chronic diseases; and institutionalization.

These social factors trigger consequences that are unlikely reversible and that have a crucial impact on social costs. Added to this, a further complication is the access to safety and intervention measures that are focused on the difficult condition of pregnant women.

Consequently, this picture requires a specific agenda to study the phenomenon and to identify efficient solutions.[5]

The systems for social intervention that are focused on contrasting homelessness are made of fixed services, such as:

- Economic contributions
- Night shelters
- Mobile units
- Support systems for basic needs
- Laboratories focused on socialization and entertainment activities, also open to other citizens
- Daytime facilities focused on educational or work-related activities, to introduce them to employment
- Social secretariat service
- Services of customized support and planning
- Job placement
- Nursing and medical clinics, working on combined actions together with the Italian National Health Service (SSN)
- Specialized legal protection

[4] CFR: Mayock P., Bretherton P., Women's Homelessness in Europe, Springer, 2016; http://www.womenshomelessness.org/.

[5] Laverack G., Improving Health Outcomes through Community Empowerment: A Review of the Literature in http://www.bioline.org.br/pdf?hn06016; Deliberazione AUSL di Bologna n. 156 del 10-05-2017 "Dipartimento di Salute Mentale e Dipendenze Patologiche: istituzione del Programma Integrato Dipendenze Patologiche e Assistenza alle popolazioni vulnerabili e modifiche al Programma Integrato Disabilità e Salute".

- The "housing first" program (direct access to an apartment and support from a team that will follow each individual, until they will earn back their independence and their psychophysical wellbeing)
- Specific support services for victims of violence and trafficking, and for women with children

Ongoing experimentations on homeless women's condition are centred on these thematic focuses: domestic violence prevention and intervention (early detection of warning signs, access to protected apartments, etc.); activities on the community of belonging (programs addressed to violent men and other family members); education and female entrepreneurship (acquiring skills, strengthening and application of their talents, in order to introduce them to employment); and healthcare services focused on simplifying the access to healthcare and the doctor-patient relation.

The keywords are therefore *health* and *gender*. First, they indicate the need for strategies oriented towards the "gender medicine", with respect to the differences that define men and women. And, second, the need for social services to improve the lifestyle of homeless people, with a focus on nutrition, physical activities and sexual, emotional and parental education. In one word, the ability to accept people in their totality.

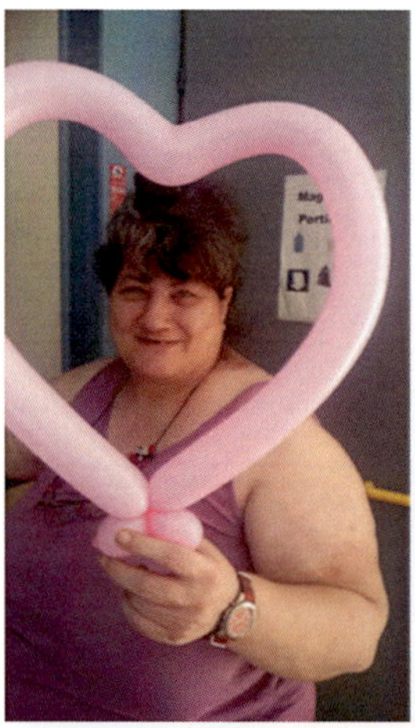

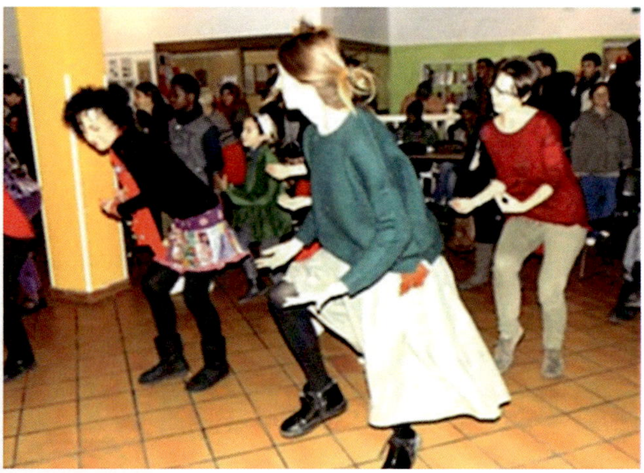

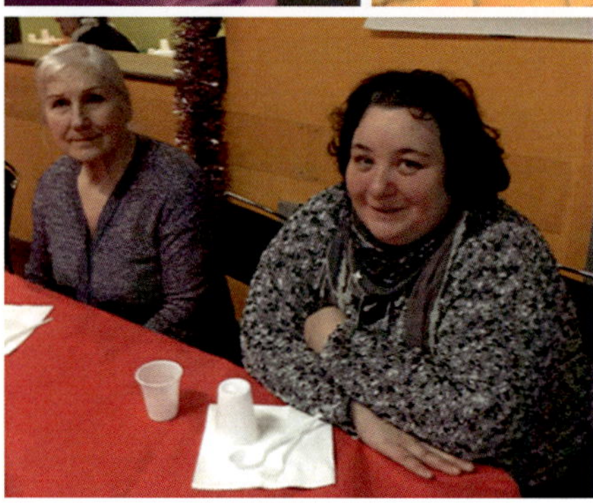

Suggested Reading

Connolly DR. Homeless mothers: face to face with women and poverty. Minneapolis, MN: University of Minnesota Press; 2000.

Cretella C, Sànchez IM. Lessico Familiare. Per un dizionario ragionato della violenza contro le donne. Cagli, Italy: Settenove; 2014.

Freire P. La pedagogia della speranza. Torino: Gruppo Abele; 2008.

Hunter DJ. Health needs more than health care: the need for a new paradigm. Eur J Public Health. 2008;18:217–9.

Linee di Indirizzo per il Contrasto alla Grave Emarginazione Adulta. http://www.fiopsd.org/linee-di-indirizzo-per-il-contrasto-alla-grave-emarginazione-adulta-in-italia/.

Manuzzi P. I corpi e la cura. Pisa, Italy: ETS; 2009.

Primary Care

28

Emanuele Ciotti, Daniele Irmici, and Marco Menchetti

Key Points

- Gender influences the adoption of healthy lifestyles, access and use of the health-care services, and the physicians' approach.
- All professionals working in primary care must carefully consider important challenges for women's health including cardiovascular risk.
- High-prevalence health problems as hypertension, diabetes, osteoporosis, depression, Alzheimer's disease, and urinary disorders are overrepresented in female patients.
- The gender of health professionals is likely to influence the relationship with patient and the choice of treatment.
- Female physicians tend to spend more time with patients and pay more attention to relational aspects of care.

Gender medicine aims to improve the health condition of women and men by intervening both on the disease as a disorder requiring multidimensional care and on lifestyles that represent substantial risk factors. Gender is related to behavior and life experience: it influences the adoption of healthy habits, access and use of the health-care services, and the attitude of medical personnel [1]. The final objective is to reduce the incidence of disabling chronic diseases, such as cardiovascular and respiratory ones, cancer, and diabetes.

In the primary care sector, greater attention to women is needed considering data emerged in the last years. The most important challenges for women's health are

E. Ciotti · D. Irmici
Department of Primary Care, Bologna Local Health Unit, Bologna, Italy

M. Menchetti (✉)
Department of Biomedical and Neuromotor Sciences, University of Bologna, Bologna, Italy
e-mail: marco.menchetti3@unibo.it

I. Tarricone, A. Riecher-Rössler (eds.), *Health and Gender*,
https://doi.org/10.1007/978-3-030-15038-9_28

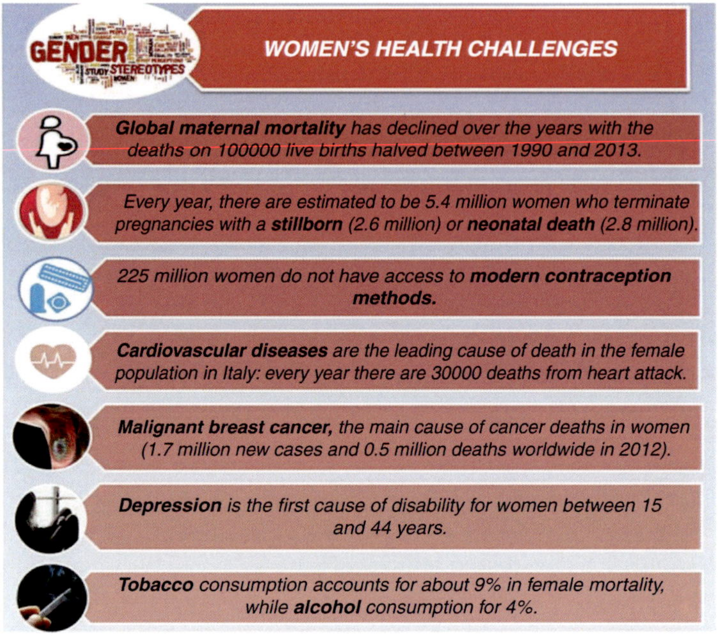

Fig. 28.1 The most important challenges for women's health

shown in Fig. 28.1. Here are some points that seem very relevant to us and which will be briefly mentioned:

1. The so-called women's paradox (higher life expectancy, greater number of diseases) entails more years living in poor health or disability [2]. These data are consistent with several surveys on the health status perception: women complain of a poor health status more frequently than men [3].
2. Biological factors associated to gender also interact with inequalities based on age, sex, ethnicity, social class, education, and allocation of resources. For example, gender norm and social structures may limit mobility and physical activity of girls and women and therefore have a negative effect on their health, well-being, and preventable mortality [4].
3. Global maternal mortality has declined over the years with the deaths on 100,000 live births halved between 1990 and 2013. However, it has not reached the World Health Organization target of a 75% reduction by 2015 [5]. Every year, all over the world, there are estimated to be 5.4 million women who terminate pregnancies with a stillborn (2.6 million) or neonatal death (2.8 million). In addition, 225 million women do not have access to modern contraception methods [6]. Nevertheless, information about this issue and family planning are crucial for the health. Unsafe abortion, practiced by incompetent people in environments without minimum medical standards, favors higher mortality in countries with more restrictive laws, which facilitate the use of illegal practice. This practice, certainly avoidable, is one of the main causes of maternal death and injury.

4. Cardiovascular diseases are the leading cause of death in the female population in Italy [7]: in Italy, every year there are 30,000 deaths from heart attack among women [8]. A key problem is the underestimation of cardiovascular risk for women: the diagnosis is often missed or delayed over time. Therefore, there is a more severe prognosis for the same age group in women suffering from diabetes or obesity than in men [9].
5. Malignant breast cancer, the main cause of cancer deaths in women (1.7 million new cases and 0.5 million deaths worldwide in 2012), is diagnosed too late in low- and middle-income countries, when only palliative care is now possible [10]. The greater attention of the female gender to prevention further opportunities for contact with health systems, but it is not the same everywhere [11]. Inequalities in access to early diagnosis and screening entail large clinical variations in terms of survival after treatment.
6. High-prevalence health problems in primary care such as hypertension, thyroid dysfunction, diabetes, cataracts, osteoporosis, Alzheimer's disease, and urinary disorders are more typically female. In addition, it is well-known the high consumption of drugs in women of older age groups, because of the higher prevalence of pain symptoms [12].
7. Gender is a fundamental determinant also in mental health: women suffer more often from mood and anxiety disorders than men; depression is the first cause of disability for women between 15 and 44 years [13], and suicide is the second cause of death in the same age group [7]. Moreover, women exposed to violence are twice as likely to have depression or alcohol-related disorders and quadruple to commit suicide [14]. As for the pharmacotherapies associated with the most common mental illnesses, it has been often found a greater use of antidepressants in women (Fig. 28.2) and, on equal terms of administrations, a greater number of side effects and adverse drug reactions, due in part to interaction with hormonal therapies [15].

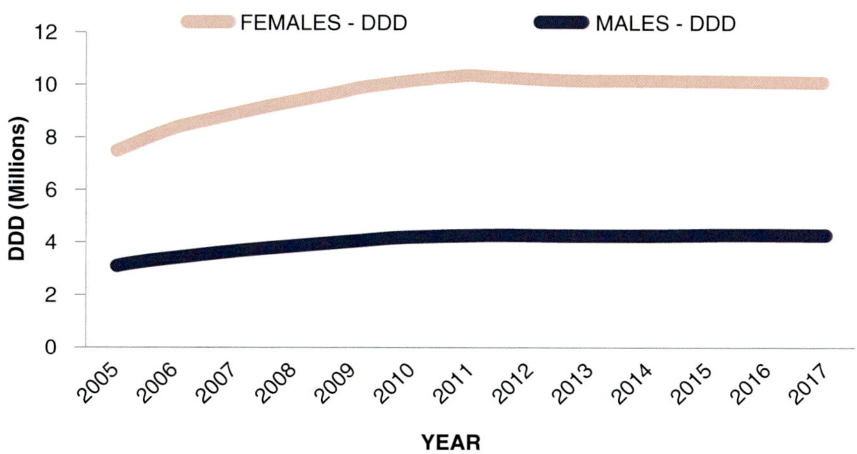

Data collected by AUSL BOLOGNA (Local Health Authorities of province of Bologna) expressed in DDD *(Defined Daily Dose) (2005-2017)*

Fig. 28.2 Use of antidepressants (DDD unit) by gender from 2005 to 2017 in Bologna local health authorities

8. Overall, tobacco consumption accounts for about 9% in female mortality, while alcohol consumption for 4% [16]. Maternal smoking and harmful use of alcohol are associated with risks in pregnancy, preterm births, placental problems, miscarriage, and stillbirths. Use of alcohol, drugs, or other psychoactive agents is increasing in many parts of the world, even during pregnancy.
9. Higher burden was reported by women than men and for health conditions of children and parents [17].

28.1 Focus on Primary Care Services

A gender-specific approach is therefore proposed as an innovative orientation also for general practitioner (GP) and all health professionals working in primary care. These will make the most appropriate choice in the diagnostic-therapeutic pathway paying attention to both gender and clinical severity, although risk factors are often similar for men and women, also in relation to the different efficacy and side effects of drugs or surgical treatments. One of the main problems most frequently faced by the GP is certainly the management of patients with chronic diseases. The meeting with these patients requires continuity of care during the entire life cycle, focusing on the person and his story rather than just on the disease.

The GP can also maintain high attention to sexually transmitted infections (STIs)—among which the human papillomavirus (HPV) is the most common, causing about 70% of cases of cervical cancer in all the world, and affects women and teenage girls disproportionately—and monitor vaccination practices, especially in girls (HPV or rubella) and in fertile women, both to assess coverage and to administer any necessary vaccine as recommended by current accepted standards. Specific prevention interventions in primary care would be desirable, involving above all young people and marginalized people at risk by providing information on the STIs. The instruction on sexuality (comprehensive sexual education) is a key intervention of primary care for improving the promotion and protection of the health of women both young (primarily adolescents) and adults. In 2013, almost 60% of all new HIV infections among young people aged 15–24 occurred in girls and young women.

Another objective concerns the careful monitoring of drug use in fertile women, to limit the use of potentially embryotoxic diagnostic investigations to the maximum. Finally, the phenomenon of violence against women has a strong impact and health relevance. One in three women, aged 15–49, has suffered physical or sexual violence and with short-term and long-term consequences for their health. GPs and other primary care professionals will have to take direct and indirect signals, such as abdominal pain sine causa, which can testify to a violence suffered.

28.2 Attitude and Clinical Behavior of Health Professionals

The attitudes of health professionals are likely to influence relationship with patient, problem identification, and the choice of treatment. With regard to gender differences, literature shows that female physicians tend to spend more time with patients

[18, 19], to pay more attention to relational aspects of care [20], to provide a higher number of follow-up visits for mild and stabilized cases [21], and to be more likely to engage in counseling, education, and conversations about social and family issues [22], compared to male physicians. Otherwise, these latter seemed to pay more attention to technical aspects of care like physical examinations and diagnostic procedures [19, 23].

In a cross-sectional survey promoted by the Emilia-Romagna Regional Programme "G. Leggieri" for the integration between primary care and mental health [24] emerged that female physicians felt less confident in treating anxiety and depressive disorders compared to their male colleagues. In addition, they perceived their knowledge in recognition, diagnosis, and treatment of these disorders as less adequate. Other studies considering different health problems show that female primary care physicians have higher odds of being less confident in identifying and managing medical conditions compared to male [25, 26]. A possible explanation is that the reported evidence-based guidelines' higher influence on female PCPs [27] led them having a high critical perception of their knowledge and their clinical management.

28.3 Conclusions

Gender medicine is a multidisciplinary science that aims to identify and deepen the manifestation of diseases and the consequent therapeutic response keeping in mind gender specificities. This approach allows to set up personalized preventive, diagnostic, and care pathways and to reduce factors that disadvantage female patients, especially for the poorest and most vulnerable. The final intent is to improve the health status of women, families, and, more generally, interpersonal relationships in the community, as well as in society.

References

1. Regitz-Zagrosek V. Sex and gender differences in health. EMBO Rep. 2012;13(7):596–603.
2. Alberts SC, Archie EA, Gesquiere LR, Altmann J, Vaupel JW, Christensen K. The male-female health-survival paradox: a comparative perspective on sex differences in aging and mortality. In: Weinstein M, Lane MA, editors. Sociality, hierarchy, health: comparative biodemography: a collection of papers. Washington, DC: National Academies Press; 2014. p. 339–64.
3. Cavazza G, Malvi C. La fragilità degli anziani [The fragility of the elderly]. Santarcangelo di Romagna, RN: Maggioli Editore; 2014.
4. World Health Organization. Update on the WHO Commission on Ending Childhood Obesity. 2014. http://apps.who.int/gb/ebwha/pdf_files/EB136/B136_10-en.pdf.
5. Save the Children. Surviving the first day: state of the world's mothers. London, UK: Save the Children; 2013.
6. Singh S, Darroch JE, Ashford LS. Adding it up: the costs and benefits of investing in sexual and reproductive health, 2014. New York: Guttmacher Institute; 2014.
7. National Institute of Statistics. Leading causes of death in Italy, year 2012. https://www.istat.it/en/files/2014/12/Leading-causes-of-death.pdf?title=Leading+causes+of+death+in+Italy+-+3+Dec+2014+-+Full+text.pdf.
8. National Institute of Statistics. Annual report 2014 – the state of the Nation. http://www.istat.it/en/files/2014/06/Sintesi-rapp-ann-2014-en1.pdf.

9. Cipriani F, Baldasseroni A, Franchi S. Lotta alla sedentarietà e promozione dell'attività fisica [Fight against sedentariness and promotion of physical activity]. Roma: National System Guidelines; 2011.
10. World Health Organization. Breast cancer: prevention and control. 2011. http://www.who.int/cancer/detection/breastcancer/en.
11. World Health Organization (WHO). Global recommendations on physical activity for health. 2010. http://apps.who.int/iris/bitstream/10665/44399/1/9789241599979_eng.pdf.
12. Fowler RA, Sabur N, Li P, Juurlink DN, Pinto R, Hladunewich MA, et al. Sex-and age-based differences in the delivery and outcomes of critical care. CMAJ. 2007;177:1513–9.
13. Reale E, Carbone U. Il genere nel lavoro. Valutare e prevenire i rischi lavorativi nella donna [The gender in work. Evaluate and prevent work risks in women]. Milano: Franco Angeli Editore; 2009.
14. De Los Angeles CP, Lewis WW, McBain R, Yasamy MT, Olukoya AA, Morris J. Use of mental health services by women in low and middle-income countries. J Pub Ment Health. 2014;13:4.
15. Health Search – Research Institute of Italian Society of General Practice. VIII Report Years 2013/2014. 2014. https://healthsearch.it/documenti/Archivio/Report/VIIIReport_2013-2014/VIII%20Report%20HS.pdf.
16. Nelson D, Jarman DW, Rehm J, Greenfield TK, Rey G, Kerr WC, et al. Alcohol-attributable cancer deaths and years of potential life lost in the US. Am J Public Health. 2013;103:641–8.
17. Shahly V, Chatterji S, Gruber MJ, Al-Hamzawi A, Alonso J, Andrade LH, et al. Cross-national differences in the prevalence and correlates of burden among older family caregivers in the WHO World Mental Health (WMH) Surveys. Psychol Med. 2013;43(4):865–79.
18. Scholle SH, Gardner W, Harman J, Madlon-Kay DJ, Pascoe J, Kelleher K. Physician gender and psychosocial care for children: attitudes, practice, characteristics, identification, and treatment. Med Care. 2001;39(1):26–38.
19. Roter DL, Hall JA, Aoki Y. Physician gender effects in medical communication: a meta-analytic review. JAMA. 2002;288(6):756–64.
20. Levinson W, Lurie N. When most doctors are women: what lies ahead? Ann Intern Med. 2004;141(6):471–4.
21. Fantini MP, Carretta E, Mimmi S, Belletti M, Rucci P, Cavazza G, et al. L'impatto delle caratteristiche e dell'organizzazione dei MMG sulla qualità assistenziali delle malattie croniche [The impact of the characteristics and organization of GPs on the quality of care for chronic diseases]. Mecosan. 2010;73:73–93.
22. Casini F, Sighinolfi C, Tedesco P, Bandieri PV, Bologna M, Colombini N, et al. Primary care physicians' perspective on the management of anxiety and depressive disorders: a cross-sectional survey in Emilia Romagna Region. BMC Fam Pract. 2013;14:75.
23. Bertakis KD, Helms LJ, Callahan EJ, Azari R, Robbins JA. The influence of gender on physician practice style. Med Care. 1995;33(4):407–16.
24. Berardi D, Ferrannini L, Menchetti M, Vaggi M. Primary care psychiatry in Italy. J Nerv Ment Dis. 2014;202(6):460–3.
25. David J, Danielle C, Sharon P, Kim W. Attitudes and practices of general practitioners training to work with drug-using patients. Drug Alcohol Rev. 1999;18(3):287–91.
26. Browne MO, Lee A, Prabhu R. Self-reported confidence and skills of general practitioners in management of mental health disorders. Aust J Rural Health. 2007;15:321–6.
27. Sammer CE, Lykens K, Singh KP. Physician characteristics and the reported effect of evidence-based practice guidelines. Health Serv Res. 2008;43(2):569–81.

Suggested Reading

Amos A, Greaves L, Nichter M, Bloch M. Women and tobacco: a call for including gender in tobacco control research, policy and practice. Tob Control. 2012;21:236–43.

Arganini C, Saba A, Comitato R, et al. Gender differences in food choice and dietary intake in modern western societies. In: Maddock J, editor. Public health social and behavioral health. Croatia: Intech; 2012.

Cancian M, Battaggia A, Celebrano M, et al. The care for chronic heart failure by general practitioners. Results from a clinical audit in Italy. Eur J Gen Pract. 2013;19:3–10.

Doyal L. Sex, gender, and health: the need for a new approach. BMJ. 2001;323:1061–3.

Ferrario M, Chiodini P, Chambless LE, et al. Prediction of coronary events in a low incidence population. Assessing accuracy of the CUORE Cohort Study prediction equation. Int J Epidemiol. 2005;34:413–21.

Fowler RA, Sabur N, Li P, et al. Sex-and age-based differences in the delivery and outcomes of critical care. CMAJ. 2007;177:1513–9.

Franconi F, Campesi I. Sex and gender influences on pharmacological response: an overview. Expert Rev Clin Pharmacol. 2014;7:469–85.

Towards Gender-Sensitive Mental Health Services

29

Carla Comacchio and Mirella Ruggeri

Key Points

- Patterns to care of males and females affected by psychiatric disorders are different, and these differences should be taken into account when delivering services and programmes.
- Female patients with mood disorders and eating disorders make greater use of psychiatric services compared with males.
- Despite evidence of gender differences, there is limited availability of gender-targeted rehabilitation treatments.
- Women-only programmes for people with drug abuse and addiction appear to be more effective than mixed gender programmes for female patients with co-morbid psychiatric disorders.
- Women affected by psychiatric disorders in the perinatal period can be successfully treated in specialised services (Mother and Baby Units (MBUs)) without being separated by their offspring.

29.1 Introduction

The degree of gender equality in a country has been found to be proportional to gender differences in mental health [1, 2], and this has led to great efforts to include gender sensitivity in policy making with a specific focus on mental healthcare delivery and research [3]. Despite this, implementation of gender-specific interventions is slow [4] and research limited.

This chapter is constituted by two parts: in Part 1 we aim to describe gender differences in mental health service use by summarising findings on the main

C. Comacchio · M. Ruggeri (✉)
Section of Psychiatry, University of Verona, Verona, Italy
e-mail: Mirella.ruggeri@univr.it

I. Tarricone, A. Riecher-Rössler (eds.), *Health and Gender*,
https://doi.org/10.1007/978-3-030-15038-9_29

disorders; in Part 2 we report about the available gender-specific mental health services and programmes.

29.2 Gender Differences in Mental Health Service Use

29.2.1 Mood Disorders

Prevalence of major depression is 5–7% among women in the general population [5, 6] and 3–4% among men that however show higher rates of suicide related to mood disorders than women [7–9]. Among individuals affected by depression, women are about twice more likely than men to use mental health services [10–17] even in the presence of suicidal thoughts [18, 19]. This difference can be partly explained by the higher rates of anxiety observed in female patients compared with males, which might be associated with a stronger demand for mental healthcare [1, 20, 21], by the higher compliance with treatment [22] and symptoms awareness in female patients compared with males [23–26] and also by the fact that male patients tend to show higher rates of self-stigmatisation related to viewing mental illness as a consequence of personal weakness than females [27–29].

29.2.2 First Episode Psychosis (FEP) and Longitudinal Outcome of Psychosis

Psychosis affects 1–2% of the general population: its incidence peaks in the early adulthood for both genders and shows a second peak for women in the perimenopausal period [30, 31]. Among female patients with FEP, 73% receive a diagnosis of non-affective psychosis and 27% a diagnosis of affective psychosis [32]. Among male patients with FEP, 86% receive a diagnosis of non-affective psychosis and 14% a diagnosis of affective psychosis. Despite evidence of gender differences in the psychopathological characteristics in FEP patients [33–35], little is known about how gender impacts on the response to the specialised treatments in the early phase [36], as the majority of studies have been conducted prior to the introduction of specialist services for young people with psychosis. As proved in the case of depression, male patients with FEP show less motivation to engage with treatment [33, 37] and greater lack of insight for their illness [33, 38] which may delay treatment efficacy, leading to a poorer prognosis [39]. Regardless of the type of specialised intervention provided, during the first year after psychosis onset, females tend to have higher rates of admission than males. However, males present fewer but longer periods of admission (88.5 days of hospitalisation in males vs. 76.1 in females) [40]. This may be due to females' higher levels of insight, which could allow them seeking effective treatment more often and earlier [41]. Another possible explanation is that women tend to have more affective episodes with greater risk for self-harm which may require more frequent hospitalisation [42]. In fact, females with FEP are more likely to experience a psychosocial stressor at the time of psychosis onset [43] and subsequently to express more depressive symptoms [44] and fewer negative symptoms than males (Table 29.1).

Table 29.1 Gender differences in first episode psychosis (FEP) patients

	Study	Sample size	Females	Males
Diagnosis (NAP vs. AP)[a] %	Bertani et al. [32]	182 F 215 M	73% vs. 27%	86% vs. 14%
Service engagement (Weeks) mean (SD)	Cotton et al. [33]	226 F 435 M	62.6 (35.3)	63.7 (33.6)
Insight (3-pt Likert scale) mean (SD)	Cotton et al. [33]	226 F 435 M	12.6 (28)	6.9 (30)
Hospitalisation (days) mean (SD)	Thorup et al. [40]	231 F 323 M	76.1 (100.5)	88.5 (113.8)
Psychosocial stressors (Diagnostic interview for psychosis) %	Morgan et al. [43]	443 F 647 M	55.7%	32.2%

[a]*NAP* non-affective psychosis, *AP* affective psychosis

29.2.3 Eating Disorders

The prevalence of eating disorders (EDs) in the general population is 3.5% for women and 1–2% for men [45]. EDs are in fact often seen as a "women's disease" [46], with males accounting only for 10% of total ED cases [47]. EDs are associated with increased general health services utilisation [48–50], and patients with undiagnosed EDs appear to be more likely to report higher numbers of primary care visits than patients without ED [48, 51, 52]. It is not clear whether the elevated rate of general services use is due to ED-related co-morbidity, such as obesity [53–56] and depression anxiety [46, 57] or to patients' attempts to receive care without acknowledging the ED to themselves or healthcare providers [58]. Nevertheless, once EDs are diagnosed, rates of services use show an additional increase to both mental health and primary care departments [58]. Due to the higher proportion of females affected by EDs compared with males and the gender stereotypes related to these disorders, the majority of treatments are based on interventions specifically developed for women [59]. Even though treatment in predominantly female environments has shown to be successful also for males [60], male patients appear to be resistant to attend treatment regularly because of stigma and stereotypes [61]. In addition, evidence has suggested that male patients with EDs are less likely to be diagnosed as having an ED than females despite identical symptoms [62] and thus less likely to receive adequate treatment [45, 63].

29.2.4 Drug Abuse and Addiction

Women account for one-third of all substance users [64] and the majority of them are of childbearing age [65]. Women with substance abuse problems are more likely than men to be identified through contacts with child protective services [66] rather than in general healthcare settings [67]. Despite the well-known gender differences in addiction behaviours and treatment needs [68–70], the majority of treatments are not gender-targeted [71, 72].

Women-only (WO) programmes have been developed in the late 1980s [73] to address the barriers that prevent women from entering and staying in treatment [74]. Treatment components in WO programmes include group discussions of addiction, relapse prevention, anger management, HIV education and job training with a focus on how these issues relate to women's recovery, and group discussions utilise a more supportive and less confrontational approach than mixed gender (MG) programmes [71]. The possibility for a substance-abusing mother to be accompanied by her child while on treatment is characteristic of WO specialised treatment. Although some have argued that children in a treatment facility may impact on the mother's ability to attend her programme by delaying or adversely affecting her recovery, available evidence suggests that women who are allowed this provision demonstrate higher rates of retention than women who are not [75]. Findings on the effectiveness of WO programmes are inconsistent [76–79], but some evidence indicates that women, especially those with low self-efficacy [80] or high psychiatric symptom severity [81], are less likely to drop out of WO programmes [77, 82], have better drug outcomes after discharge [83] and have improved criminal justice outcomes [73, 84].

29.2.5 Gender Differences in the Late Period of Life

Historically, in the population over 65-year-old women have always outnumbered men, and this difference persists nowadays despite the decline in males' death rate from other causes [85]. Psychogeriatric is a discipline that has developed in the last 30 years [86] as a consequence of the rapid ageing of the population and the subsequent increased need for psychiatric care in elderly people. It has been estimated that the number of people over the age of 65 will reach 70 million by the year 2030 making up 20% of the population [85]. Even if the majority of elderly people attend regular healthcare visits, they are less likely to use specialised mental services than younger age groups [86], and they tend to seek for psychiatric help in the context of a general medical complaint during a primary care visit [85].

Psychogeriatric units (PGU) are acute hospital units that provide inpatient care to elderly people with mental disorders [87], but their availability is limited [88, 89]. A higher proportion of women is admitted to PGU compared with men [90, 91], mostly for psychosis-related conditions, and women have longer inpatient stay than men. These findings may be explained by the higher incidence of schizophrenia in older women and by the greater female longevity in the older schizophrenic population [92]. By contrast, men show higher readmission rates [87] and better response to rehabilitative intervention targeted for elderly people with psychiatric disorders [93].

29.3 Gender-Specific Mental Health Services

29.3.1 Pregnancy and Postpartum

Depression in pregnancy occurs in 12% of women [94, 95], and in the postpartum period, 10–20% of women develop a major depressive episode [96, 97] and 0.1–0.2% of women a psychotic episode [97–99]. Postpartum is also associated with an increased

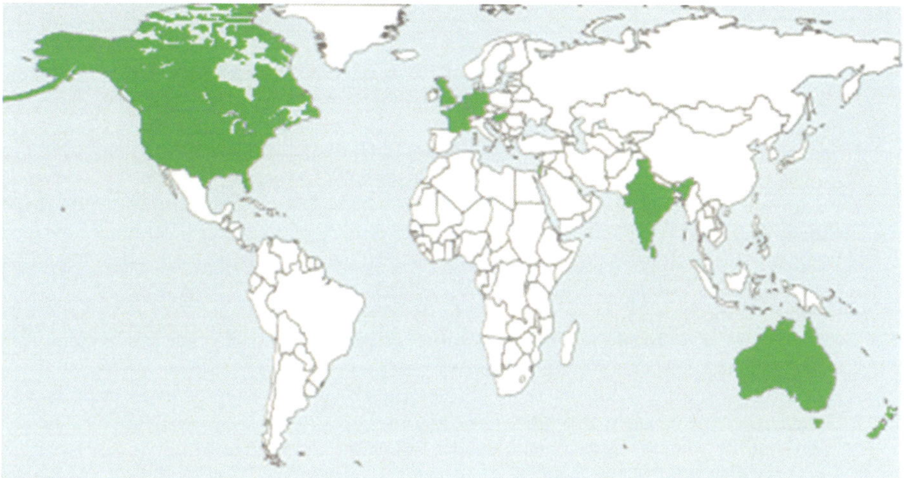

Fig. 29.1 Distribution of MBUs worldwide. MBUs are present in the UK, France, Germany, Belgium, Luxembourg, the Netherlands, Hungary, the USA, Canada, Australia, New Zealand, India, Israel and Sri Lanka [110, 112]

risk of developing bipolar or post-traumatic stress disorder [100] and with relapse and exacerbation of any pre-existing psychiatric condition [101]. Mental disorders in pregnancy and postpartum are associated with a range of adverse outcomes, both for the mother and for the baby [96, 102–105]. However, the perinatal period represents a good chance for mental health professionals, as women are more open to advise and support [106, 107]. Mother and Baby Units (MBUs) have been developed in the late 1950s [108] to respond to the needs of women affected by psychiatric disorders in the perinatal period. MBUs are specialised services in which women can be admitted without being separated from their child—generally under the age of 12 months. Despite the higher rates of patients' preference for treatment in MBUs rather than in acute general wards without their baby and the higher levels of patients' satisfaction [109–111], MBUs are not widespread [110, 112]. Figure 29.1 provides an overview of their localisation worldwide. Specialised interventions for mental disorders in the perinatal period are associated with positive outcomes, both for the mothers and for the babies [112–117], which implies that all women suffering from psychiatric perinatal conditions should have access to this kind of specialised care.

29.4 Conclusion

For a long time, men and women affected by mental disorders have been seen as a homogeneous group, with similar characteristics, needs for care and outcomes [118]. However, men and women differ in relation to prevalence; impact of biological, psychological and social factors; and course of illness [119], and these differences have to be carefully taken into account when planning patient-tailored interventions [120].

References

1. Seedat S, Scott KM, Angermeyer MC, et al. Cross-national associations between gender and mental disorders in the World Health Organization World Mental Health Surveys. Arch Gen Psychiatry. 2009;66(7):785–95.
2. Van de Velde S, Huijts T, Bracke P, Bambra C. Macro-level gender equality and depression in men and women in Europe. Sociol Health Illn. 2013;35(5):682–98.
3. World Health Organisation (WHO). Gender in mental health research. Geneva: World Health Organisation; 2004.
4. Women's Health Council (WHC). Women' s mental health: promoting a gendered approach to policy and service provision. Dublin: Women's Health Council (WHC); 2005.
5. Hasin DS, Goodwin RD, Stinson FS, Grant BF. Epidemiology of major depressive disorder: results from the National Epidemiologic Survey on Alcoholism and Related Conditions. Arch Gen Psychiatry. 2005;62(10):1097–106.
6. Patten SB, Wang JL, Williams JV, et al. Descriptive epidemiology of major depression in Canada. Can J Psychiatry. 2006;51(2):84–90.
7. Ladouceur R. Suicide among men. Can Fam Physician. 2011;57(2):148.
8. Oliffe JL, Ogrodniczuk JS, Bottorff JL, Johnson JL, Hoyak K. "You feel like you can't live anymore": suicide from the perspectives of Canadian men who experience depression. Soc Sci Med. 2012;74(4):506–14.
9. Rutz W. The European WHO mental health programme and the World Health Report 2001: input and implications. Br J Psychiatry. 2003;183:73–4.
10. Addis ME, Mahalik JR. Men, masculinity, and the contexts of help seeking. Am Psychol. 2003;58(1):5–14.
11. Angst J, Gamma A, Gastpar M, et al. Gender differences in depression. Epidemiological findings from the European DEPRES I and II studies. Eur Arch Psychiatry Clin Neurosci. 2002;252(5):201–9.
12. Bertakis KD, Azari R, Helms LJ, Callahan EJ, Robbins JA. Gender differences in the utilization of health care services. J Fam Pract. 2000;49(2):147–52.
13. Burns BJ, Ryan Wagner H, Gaynes BN, Wells KB, Schulberg HC. General medical and specialty mental health service use for major depression. Int J Psychiatry Med. 2000;30(2):127–43.
14. Johnson JL, Oliffe JL, Kelly MT, Galdas P, Ogrodniczuk JS. Men's discourses of help-seeking in the context of depression. Sociol Health Illn. 2012;34(3):345–61.
15. Kovess-Masfety V, Boyd A, van de Velde S, et al. Are there gender differences in service use for mental disorders across countries in the European Union? Results from the EU-World Mental Health survey. J Epidemiol Community Health. 2014;68(7):649–56.
16. Ojeda VD, McGuire TG. Gender and racial/ethnic differences in use of outpatient mental health and substance use services by depressed adults. Psychiatry Q. 2006;77(3):211–22.
17. Rhodes AE, Goering PN, To T, Williams JI. Gender and outpatient mental health service use. Soc Sci Med. 2002;54(1):1–10.
18. Gagné S, Vasiliadis HM, Préville M. Gender differences in general and specialty outpatient mental health service use for depression. BMC Psychiatry. 2014;14:135.
19. Vasiliadis HM, Gagné S, Jozwiak N, Préville M. Gender differences in health service use for mental health reasons in community dwelling older adults with suicidal ideation. Int Psychogeriatr. 2013;25(3):374–81.
20. de Graaf R, ten Have M, van Gool C, van Dorsselaer S. Prevalence of mental disorders and trends from 1996 to 2009. Results from the Netherlands Mental Health Survey and Incidence Study-2. Soc Psychiatry Psychiatr Epidemiol. 2012;47(2):203–13.
21. Vesga-López O, Schneier FR, Wang S, et al. Gender differences in generalized anxiety disorder: results from the National Epidemiologic Survey on Alcohol and Related Conditions (NESARC). J Clin Psychiatry. 2008;69(10):1606–16.

22. Green CA, Pope CR. Gender, psychosocial factors and the use of medical services: a longitudinal analysis. Soc Sci Med. 1999;48(10):1363–72.
23. Hibbard JH, Pope CR. Women's roles, interest in health and health behavior. Women Health. 1987;12(2):67–84.
24. Kovess-Masfety V, Alonso J, Brugha TS, et al. Differences in lifetime use of services for mental health problems in six European countries. Psychiatr Serv. 2007;58(2):213–20.
25. Sevilla-Dedieu C, Kovess-Masfety V, Angermeyer M, et al. Measuring use of services for mental health problems in epidemiological surveys. Int J Methods Psychiatr Res. 2011;20(3):182–91.
26. Wang PS, Aguilar-Gaxiola S, Alonso J, et al. Use of mental health services for anxiety, mood, and substance disorders in 17 countries in the WHO world mental health surveys. Lancet. 2007;370(9590):841–50.
27. Oliffe JL, Ogrodniczuk JS, Gordon SJ, et al. Stigma in male depression and suicide: a Canadian Sex Comparison Study. Community Ment Health J. 2016;52(3):302–10.
28. Pattyn E, Verhaeghe M, Bracke P. The gender gap in mental health service use. Soc Psychiatry Psychiatr Epidemiol. 2015;50(7):1089–95.
29. Schomerus G, Holzinger A, Matschinger H, Lucht M, Angermeyer MC. Public attitudes towards alcohol dependence. Psychiatr Prax. 2010;37(3):111–8.
30. Jackson D, Kirkbride J, Croudace T, et al. Meta-analytic approaches to determine gender differences in the age-incidence characteristics of schizophrenia and related psychoses. Int J Methods Psychiatr Res. 2013;22(1):36–45.
31. Rabinowitz J, Levine SZ, Haim R, Haefner H. The course of schizophrenia: progressive deterioration, amelioration or both? Schizophr Res. 2007;91(1–3):254–8.
32. Bertani M, Lasalvia A, Bonetto C, et al. The influence of gender on clinical and social characteristics of patients at psychosis onset: a report from the Psychosis Incident Cohort Outcome Study (PICOS). Psychol Med. 2012;42(4):769–80.
33. Cotton SM, Lambert M, Schimmelmann BG, et al. Gender differences in premorbid, entry, treatment, and outcome characteristics in a treated epidemiological sample of 661 patients with first episode psychosis. Schizophr Res. 2009;114(1–3):17–24.
34. Hui C, Li A, Chang W-C, Chan S, Lee E, Chen E. Gender specific correlates of neurocognition and functioning in first episode psychosis. Early Interven Psychiatry. 2014;8:74.
35. Ochoa S, Usall J, Cobo J, Labad X, Kulkarni J. Gender differences in schizophrenia and first-episode psychosis: a comprehensive literature review. Schizophr Res Treatment. 2012;2012:916198.
36. Tseliou F, Johnson S, Major B, et al. Gender differences in one-year outcomes of first-presentation psychosis patients in inner-city UK Early Intervention Services. Early Interv Psychiatry. 2017;11(3):215–23.
37. Longenecker J, Genderson J, Dickinson D, et al. Where have all the women gone?: participant gender in epidemiological and non-epidemiological research of schizophrenia. Schizophr Res. 2010;119(1–3):240–5.
38. Malla A, Payne J. First-episode psychosis: psychopathology, quality of life, and functional outcome. Schizophr Bull. 2005;31(3):650–71.
39. McFarlane WR, Lukens E, Link B, et al. Multiple-family groups and psychoeducation in the treatment of schizophrenia. Arch Gen Psychiatry. 1995;52(8):679–87.
40. Thorup A, Albert N, Bertelsen M, et al. Gender differences in first-episode psychosis at 5-year follow-up--two different courses of disease? Results from the OPUS study at 5-year follow-up. Eur Psychiatry. 2014;29(1):44–51.
41. Karow A, Pajonk FG, Reimer J, et al. The dilemma of insight into illness in schizophrenia: self- and expert-rated insight and quality of life. Eur Arch Psychiatry Clin Neurosci. 2008;258(3):152–9.
42. Haro JM, Ciudad A, Alonso J, et al. Remission and relapse in the outpatient treatment of patients with schizophrenia. Outcomes at 3 years. Actas Esp Psiquiatr. 2008;36(4):187–96.

43. Morgan VA, Castle DJ, Jablensky AV. Do women express and experience psychosis differently from men? Epidemiological evidence from the Australian national study of low prevalence (psychotic) disorders. Aust N Z J Psychiatry. 2008;42(1):74–82.
44. Carpenter J, Milne D, Lombardo C, Dickinson C. Process and outcomes of training in psychosocial interventions in mental health: a stepwise approach to evaluation. J Ment Health. 2007;16:505–20.
45. MacCaughelty C, Wagner R, Rufino K. Does being overweight or male increase a patient's risk of not being referred for an eating disorder consult? Int J Eat Disord. 2016;49(10):963–6.
46. Hudson JI, Hiripi E, Pope HG, Kessler RC. The prevalence and correlates of eating disorders in the National Comorbidity Survey Replication. Biol Psychiatry. 2007;61(3):348–58.
47. Muise AM, Stein DG, Arbess G. Eating disorders in adolescent boys: a review of the adolescent and young adult literature. J Adolesc Health. 2003;33(6):427–35.
48. Johnson JG, Spitzer RL, Williams JB. Health problems, impairment and illnesses associated with bulimia nervosa and binge eating disorder among primary care and obstetric gynaecology patients. Psychol Med. 2001;31(8):1455–66.
49. Lewinsohn PM, Striegel-Moore RH, Seeley JR. Epidemiology and natural course of eating disorders in young women from adolescence to young adulthood. J Am Acad Child Adolesc Psychiatry. 2000;39(10):1284–92.
50. Striegel-Moore RH, Dohm FA, Wilfley DE, et al. Toward an understanding of health services use in women with binge eating disorder. Obes Res. 2004;12(5):799–806.
51. Ogg EC, Millar HR, Pusztai EE, Thom AS. General practice consultation patterns preceding diagnosis of eating disorders. Int J Eat Disord. 1997;22(1):89–93.
52. Sansone RA, Wiederman MW, Sansone LA. Healthcare utilization among women with eating disordered behavior. Am J Manag Care. 1997;3(11):1721–3.
53. Evans EJ, Hay PJ, Mond J, et al. Barriers to help-seeking in young women with eating disorders: a qualitative exploration in a longitudinal community survey. Eat Disord. 2011;19(3):270–85.
54. Mond JM, Hay PJ, Rodgers B, Owen C. Health service utilization for eating disorders: findings from a community-based study. Int J Eat Disord. 2007;40(5):399–408.
55. Mond JM, Myers TC, Crosby RD, Hay PJ, Mitchell JE. Bulimic eating disorders in primary care: hidden morbidity still? J Clin Psychol Med Settings. 2010;17(1):56–63.
56. Reidpath DD, Crawford D, Tilgner L, Gibbons C. Relationship between body mass index and the use of healthcare services in Australia. Obes Res. 2002;10(6):526–31.
57. Kraemer HC, Wilson KA, Hayward C. Lifetime prevalence and pseudocomorbidity in psychiatric research. Arch Gen Psychiatry. 2006;63(6):604–8.
58. Striegel-Moore RH, DeBar L, Wilson GT, et al. Health services use in eating disorders. Psychol Med. 2008;38(10):1465–74.
59. National Institute for Health and Clinical Excellence. Core interventions in the treatment and management of anorexia nervosa, bulimia nervosa and related eating disorders. Leicester, UK: British Psychological Society; 2004.
60. Woodside DB, Kaplan AS. Day hospital treatment in males with eating disorders--response and comparison to females. J Psychosom Res. 1994;38(5):471–5.
61. Robinson KJ, Mountford VA, Sperlinger DJ. Being men with eating disorders: perspectives of male eating disorder service-users. J Health Psychol. 2013;18(2):176–86.
62. Currin L, Schmidt U, Waller G. Variables that influence diagnosis and treatment of the eating disorders within primary care settings: a vignette study. Int J Eat Disord. 2007;40(3):257–62.
63. Striegel-Moore RH, Leslie D, Petrill SA, Garvin V, Rosenheck RA. One-year use and cost of inpatient and outpatient services among female and male patients with an eating disorder: evidence from a national database of health insurance claims. Int J Eat Disord. 2000;27(4):381–9.
64. Hepburn M. Drug use and women's reproductive health. London: Routledge; 2002.
65. World Health Organization (WHO). Principles of drug dependence treatment. Geneva: World Health Organisation; 2008.

66. Grella CE, Joshi V. Gender differences in drug treatment careers among clients in the National Drug Abuse Treatment Outcome Study. Am J Drug Alcohol Abuse. 1999;25(3):385–406.
67. Brienza RS, Stein MD. Alcohol use disorders in primary care: do gender-specific differences exist? J Gen Intern Med. 2002;17(5):387–97.
68. Green CA. Gender and use of substance abuse treatment services. Alcohol Res Health. 2006;29(1):55–62.
69. Hser YI, Huang D, Teruya C, Douglas Anglin M. Gender comparisons of drug abuse treatment outcomes and predictors. Drug Alcohol Depend. 2003;72(3):255–64.
70. Robinson EA, Brower KJ, Gomberg ES. Explaining unexpected gender differences in hostility among persons seeking treatment for substance use disorders. J Stud Alcohol. 2001;62(5):667–74.
71. Grella CE, Polinsky ML, Hser YI, Perry SM. Characteristics of women-only and mixed-gender drug abuse treatment programs. J Subst Abus Treat. 1999;17(1–2):37–44.
72. Oser C, Knudsen H, Staton-Tindall M, Leukefeld C. The adoption of wraparound services among substance abuse treatment organizations serving criminal offenders: the role of a women-specific program. Drug Alcohol Depend. 2009;103(Suppl 1):S82–90.
73. Niv N, Hser YI. Women-only and mixed-gender drug abuse treatment programs: service needs, utilization and outcomes. Drug Alcohol Depend. 2007;87(2–3):194–201.
74. Grella CE, Greenwell L. Substance abuse treatment for women: changes in the settings where women received treatment and types of services provided, 1987–1998. J Behav Health Serv Res. 2004;31(4):367–83.
75. Chen X, Burgdorf K, Dowell K, Roberts T, Porowski A, Herrell JM. Factors associated with retention of drug-abusing women in long-term residential treatment. Eval Prog Plann. 2004;27:205–12.
76. Greenfield SF, Back SE, Lawson K, Brady KT. Substance abuse in women. Psychiatr Clin North Am. 2010;33(2):339–55.
77. Greenfield SF, Brooks AJ, Gordon SM, et al. Substance abuse treatment entry, retention, and outcome in women: a review of the literature. Drug Alcohol Depend. 2007;86(1):1–21.
78. Harrison PA, Asche SE. Outcomes monitoring in Minnesota: treatment implications, practical limitations. J Subst Abus Treat. 2001;21(4):173–83.
79. Kaskutas LA, Zhang L, French MT, Witbrodt J. Women's programs versus mixed-gender day treatment: results from a randomized study. Addiction. 2005;100(1):60–9.
80. Cummings AM, Gallop RJ, Greenfield SF. Self-efficacy and substance use outcomes for women in single gender versus mixed-gender group treatment. J Groups Addict Recover. 2010;5(1):4–16.
81. Greenfield SF, Potter JS, Lincoln MF, Popuch RE, Kuper L, Gallop RJ. High psychiatric symptom severity is a moderator of substance abuse treatment outcomes among women in single vs. mixed gender group treatment. Am J Drug Alcohol Abuse. 2008;34(5):594–602.
82. Grella CE. Women in residential drug treatment: differences by program type and pregnancy. J Health Care Poor Underserved. 1999;10(2):216–29.
83. Evans E, Li L, Pierce J, Hser YI. Explaining long-term outcomes among drug dependent mothers treated in women-only versus mixed-gender programs. J Subst Abus Treat. 2013;45(3):293–301.
84. Prendergast ML, Messina NP, Hall EA, Warda US. The relative effectiveness of women-only and mixed-gender treatment for substance-abusing women. J Subst Abus Treat. 2011;40(4):336–48.
85. Bashir M, Holroyd S. Caring for the elderly female psychiatric patient. Psychiatr Clin North Am. 2010;33(2):475–85.
86. Holroyd S, Duryee JJ. Characteristics of persons utilizing a geriatric psychiatry outpatient clinic. J Geriatr Psychiatry Neurol. 1997;10(4):136–41.
87. Dobrohotoff JT, Llewellyn-Jones RH. Psychogeriatric inpatient unit design: a literature review. Int Psychogeriatr. 2011;23(2):174–89.
88. O'Connor D, Melding P. A survey of publicly funded aged psychiatry services in Australia and New Zealand. Aust N Z J Psychiatry. 2006;40(4):368–73.

89. Snowdon J. Psychogeriatric services in the community and in long-term care facilities: needs and developments. Curr Opin Psychiatry. 2007;20(6):533–8.
90. Chiu A, Nguyen HV, Reutens S, et al. Clinical outcomes and length of stay of a co-located psychogeriatric and geriatric unit. Arch Gerontol Geriatr. 2009;49(2):233–6.
91. Draper B, Luscombe G. Quantification of factors contributing to length of stay in an acute psychogeriatric ward. Int J Geriatr Psychiatry. 1998;13(1):1–7.
92. Cohen CI, Cohen GD, Blank K, et al. Schizophrenia and older adults. An overview: directions for research and policy. Am J Geriatr Psychiatry. 2000;8(1):19–28.
93. Mueser KT, Pratt SI, Bartels SJ, et al. Randomized trial of social rehabilitation and integrated health care for older people with severe mental illness. J Consult Clin Psychol. 2010;78(4):561–73.
94. Cantwell R, Clutton-Brock T, Cooper G, et al. Saving mothers' lives: reviewing maternal deaths to make motherhood safer: 2006–2008. The Eighth Report of the Confidential Enquiries into Maternal Deaths in the United Kingdom. BJOG. 2011;118(Suppl 1):1–203.
95. Dennis CL, Dowswell T. Psychosocial and psychological interventions for preventing postpartum depression. Cochrane Database Syst Rev. 2013;(2):CD001134.
96. Friedman SH, Resnick PJ. Postpartum depression: an update. Womens Health (Lond). 2009;5(3):287–95.
97. O'Hara MW, Wisner KL. Perinatal mental illness: definition, description and aetiology. Best Pract Res Clin Obstet Gynaecol. 2014;28(1):3–12.
98. Blackmore ER, Rubinow DR, O'Connor TG, et al. Reproductive outcomes and risk of subsequent illness in women diagnosed with postpartum psychosis. Bipolar Disord. 2013;15(4):394–404.
99. Sit D, Rothschild AJ, Wisner KL. A review of postpartum psychosis. J Womens Health (Larchmt). 2006;15(4):352–68.
100. Munk-Olsen T, Jones I, Laursen TM. Birth order and postpartum psychiatric disorders. Bipolar Disord. 2014;16(3):300–7.
101. Brockington IF, Macdonald E, Wainscott G. Anxiety, obsessions and morbid preoccupations in pregnancy and the puerperium. Arch Womens Ment Health. 2006;9(5):253–63.
102. Beebe B, Jaffe J, Buck K, et al. Six-week postpartum maternal depressive symptoms and 4-month mother-infant self- and interactive contingency. Infant Ment Health J. 2008;29(5):442–71.
103. Davalos DB, Yadon CA, Tregellas HC. Untreated prenatal maternal depression and the potential risks to offspring: a review. Arch Womens Ment Health. 2012;15(1):1–14.
104. Farr SL, Dietz PM, Rizzo JH, et al. Health care utilisation in the first year of life among infants of mothers with perinatal depression or anxiety. Paediatr Perinat Epidemiol. 2013;27(1):81–8.
105. Staehelin K, Kurth E, Schindler C, Schmid M, Zemp Stutz E. Predictors of early postpartum mental distress in mothers with midwifery home care--results from a nested case-control study. Swiss Med Wkly. 2013;143:w13862.
106. Goodman JH. Women's attitudes, preferences, and perceived barriers to treatment for perinatal depression. Birth. 2009;36(1):60–9.
107. Miller L, Shade M, Vasireddy V. Beyond screening: assessment of perinatal depression in a perinatal care setting. Arch Womens Ment Health. 2009;12(5):329–34.
108. Main TF. Mothers with children in a psychiatric hospital. Lancet. 1958;2(7051):845–7.
109. Antonysamy A, Wieck A, Wittkowski A. Service satisfaction on discharge from a psychiatric mother and baby unit: a representative patient survey. Arch Womens Ment Health. 2009;12(5):359–62.
110. Glangeaud-Freudenthal NM, Howard LM, Sutter-Dallay AL. Treatment - mother-infant inpatient units. Best Pract Res Clin Obstet Gynaecol. 2014;28(1):147–57.
111. Neil S, Sanderson H, Wieck A. A satisfaction survey of women admitted to a Psychiatric Mother and Baby Unit in the northwest of England. Arch Womens Ment Health. 2006;9(2):109–12.

112. Cazas O, Glangeaud-Freudenthal NM. The history of Mother-Baby Units (MBUs) in France and Belgium and of the French version of the Marcé checklist. Arch Womens Ment Health. 2004;7(1):53–8.
113. Kahn RS, Zuckerman B, Bauchner H, Homer CJ, Wise PH. Women's health after pregnancy and child outcomes at age 3 years: a prospective cohort study. Am J Public Health. 2002;92(8):1312–8.
114. Minkovitz CS, Strobino D, Scharfstein D, et al. Maternal depressive symptoms and children's receipt of health care in the first 3 years of life. Pediatrics. 2005;115(2):306–14.
115. Nair R, Bilszta J, Shafira N, Salam N, Buist A. Review of patients admitted to a specialist inpatient parent-infant psychiatric service. Australas Psychiatry. 2010;18(6):567–72.
116. Salmon MP, Abel K, Webb R, Warburton AL, Appleby L. A national audit of joint mother and baby admissions to UK psychiatric hospitals: an overview of findings. Arch Womens Ment Health. 2004;7(1):65–70.
117. Wilson DA, Bobier C, Macdonald EM. A perinatal psychiatric service audit in New Zealand: patient characteristics and outcomes. Arch Womens Ment Health. 2004;7(1):71–9.
118. Vlassoff C, Garcia Moreno C. Placing gender at the centre of health programming: challenges and limitations. Soc Sci Med. 2002;54(11):1713–23.
119. Judd F, Armstrong S, Kulkarni J. Gender-sensitive mental health care. Australas Psychiatry. 2009;17(2):105–11.
120. McCormack B, Karlsson B, Dewing J, Lerdal A. Exploring person-centredness: a qualitative meta-synthesis of four studies. Scand J Caring Sci. 2010;24(3):620–34.

Suggested Reading

Anderson KK, Fuhrer R, Malla AK. The pathways to mental health care of first-episode psychosis patients: a systematic review. Psychol Med. 2010;40:1585–97.

Chibber KS, Kaplan RL, Padian NS, et al. A common pathway toward women's health. Glob Public Health. 2008;3(1):26–38.

Claus R, Orwin RG, Kissin W, et al. Does gender-specific substance abuse treatment for women promote continuity of care? J Subst Abus Treat. 2007;32:27–39.

Henderson J, Milligan K, Niccols A, et al. Reporting of feasibility factors in publications on integrated treatment programs for women with substance abuse issues and their children: a systematic review and analysis. Health Res Policy Syst. 2012;10:37.

Moulding N. Disciplining the feminine: the reproduction of gender contradictions in the mental health care of women with eating disorders. Soc Sci Med. 2006;62:793–804.

Vliegen N, Casalin S, Luyten P, et al. Hospitalization-based treatment for postpartum depressed mothers and their babies: rationale, principles, and preliminary follow-up data. Psychiatry. 2013;76(2):150–68.

Wan MW, Warburton AL, Appleby L, et al. Mother and baby unit admissions: feasibility study examining child outcomes 4–6 years. Aust N Z J Psychiatry. 2007;41:150–6.

Woo BJP, Golshan S, Allen EC, et al. Factors associated with frequent admissions to an acute geriatric psychiatric inpatient unit. J Geriatr Psychiatry Neurol. 2006;19:226–30.

Guarantee Committee for Equal Opportunity, Employee Well-Being and Non-discrimination at Work (CUG)

30

Marco Balboni, Sabrina Colombari, and Tullia Gallina Toschi

Key Points

- The Guarantee Committee for Equal Opportunity, Employee Well-being and Non-discrimination at Work (CUG) has been established by the Italian Law in 2010.
- The CUG aims to promote and strengthen equality between workers of the public sector, mainly in the field of gender.
- The CUG has no powers to decide on individual cases.
- The CUG has basically three types of competences: to propose actions in order to promote equality, to give advices to the decision-making bodies on equality policies to be adopted and to assess the results of the actions taken.
- The efficacy of the CUG depends greatly on how their members interpret their role inside the institutions.

M. Balboni
Department of Political and Social Sciences, Alma Mater Studiorum—University of Bologna, Bologna, Italy

S. Colombari
AUSL di Bologna, CUG member and Responsible HR Development and Workplace Well-Being, Bologna, Italy

T. G. Toschi (✉)
Department of Agricultural and Food Sciences, Rector Delegate for the Well-being at Work, Alma Mater Studiorum—University of Bologna, Bologna, Italy
e-mail: tullia.gallinatoschi@unibo.it

I. Tarricone, A. Riecher-Rössler (eds.), *Health and Gender*,
https://doi.org/10.1007/978-3-030-15038-9_30

30.1 Structure of the Governing Body

The Guarantee Committee for Equal Opportunity, Employee Well-being and Non-discrimination at Work (CUG) was established in Italy by Law 183 of 4 November 2010, which amended previous laws on equal opportunity.[1] Its formation can be considered as the implementation, by Italian legislators, of a series of EU directives that oblige to fight various types of discrimination in the workplace using a number of tools, including social dialogue.

The CUG is only foreseen in the public administration and is the same body valid for all personnel. The functioning is regulated by specific guidelines issued by the Minister of Public Administration in March 2011.[2] The Guidelines can be adapted to the needs of various administrations in exercising their autonomy.

One aspect of this autonomy concerns determination of the number of members, which is decided by the individual administration and, however, must comply with criteria of equal representation, designating an equal number of representatives of the administration and trade union organisations, and balanced in terms of gender. The appointment is of a managerial nature, has no political implications, lasts for 4 years and is renewable once.

The location of the CUG in the framework of its administration is important in order to allow the body to operate effectively. There are no specific requirements in this regard, but experience does provide some indications. The CUG does not need to be placed at the top of the organisation, but it should be in close connection with the governance to ensure continuous exchange and access to the resources (e.g. a sufficient budget) needed to carry out its tasks. Moreover, the committee should be part of a network together with those subjects and bodies operating in the same or similar areas.[3] At the same time, the network can be either internal (subjects of the administration operating in the same sector or in contiguous sectors) or external (subjects that operate outside the administration to which they belong). Among these bodies or subjects, the Equality Counsellor,[4] the Independent Assessment Bodies (OIV) and the National Anti-Discrimination Office (UNAR) should be mentioned.

30.2 Objectives and Areas of Interest

The goals of the CUG are not easy to summarise. It can perhaps be easier to start with what the CUG is not intended to be, and in particular the CUG does not function as a body for the protection of individuals. The CUG cannot, therefore, be contacted to intervene in single cases. However, this does not mean that individual situations

[1] In particular, art. 21 of Law 183 amended previous art. 57 of Legislative Decree 165 of 30 March 2001 on equal opportunities.

[2] Minister for Public Administration and Innovation and Minister for Equal Opportunities (2011), Guidelines for "Guarantee Committee for Equal Opportunity, Employee Well-being and Non-discrimination at Work", Rome.

[3] See point 3.4 of the Guidelines, which states that the CUG should regulate "the methods of consultation with other bodies".

[4] Refers to art. 21 of Law 183/2010, point 3.

cannot be voiced at the CUG or that the latter cannot take any action in individual situations. Any action, however, must always focus on the overall objectives. This means that the CUG will, at most, if it is deemed useful, raise awareness among the competent offices or use individual situation to implement general actions.[5] In positive terms, it can be said that the goal of the CUG is to ensure a healthy and peaceful work environment. In this regard, it is important to understand the reason why the European Union first, and Italian legislators in succession, felt that it was important to form a specific body with such an objective. The concern is not only to protect those who work but also to guarantee the results of the work were carried out. Guaranteeing a healthy and serene environment is, in fact, considered to be an indispensable condition for securing effectiveness and efficiency in the workplace. There is therefore a direct relationship between individual well-being and collective results, which views discomfort in the workplace as a dysfunctional element.[6] The relationship between a collective result and individual well-being thus implies that the theme of equal opportunities will be also used to evaluate the overall performance of the body.[7]

[5] By way of example, these include the proposal for a Code of Conduct and connection with a Confidential Counsellor. Both the Codes of Conduct and the Confidential Counsellor were initially foreseen in the European Commission Recommendation 92/131/EEC on the protection of the dignity of women and men at work and subsequently enriched and modified by regulations from European origin. The Code of Conduct is a guarantee instrument, a self-regulatory act by which the employer promotes and protects a work context that respects the dignity of people. It aims to perform a preventive action against behaviours that may damage the psychophysical integrity of workers. According to the Code model envisaged by the aforementioned recommendation, the structure and the minimum contents of the Code are the declaration of values, principles and purposes of the Code itself, the tools and figures working for prevention and protection and the guarantees that the employer intends to adopt when behaviours that damage dignity occur. The Confidential Counsellor is a professional who is internal or external to the organisation and who has the task of preventing and managing cases of harassment, bullying and discrimination. It is up to the Confidential Counsellor to implement the Code of Conduct through activities such as information, training and self-training, listening to staff, applying the procedure provided for by the Code of Conduct, evaluating the results of the activity carried out and annual reporting to the employer and the CUG. The Confidential Counsellor can be contacted by all people who, for whatever reason, work within the organisation and who consider themselves to be victims of compromised situations and/or those that can lead to harassment or discrimination. The Counsellor promotes mediation between the conflicting parties and proposes measures aimed at ending a situation of proven harassment.

[6] The Guidelines specify that "the efficiency and effectiveness of administrative action and productivity should take place through improvement in work organisation. A work context based on the well-being of workers is, in fact, an essential element to guarantee the best contribution in terms of productivity and work. It is known that a work environment where there are episodes of discrimination or mobbing is almost inevitably associated with reduction and deterioration of performance. In addition to the inconvenience caused to both male and female workers, there are negative repercussions on the image of a public administration and its efficiency".

[7] Another problem is obviously that of its measurability. The annual publication of a Gender Equality Report plays a role in this sense. The aspect under examination, however, struggles to make headway. For example, art. 9.3. of the Statute of the University of Bologna relating to the University Evaluation Unit provides that "the choice of the components must be made (…) respecting the principle of gender equality", but it does not seem that gender equality is taken into consideration as an evaluation criterion in the work of the Unit. More generally, the issue of equal opportunities, whatever the risk factor, should be integrated into evaluation criteria, including personnel.

Considering this as the general objective of the CUG, three areas of intervention can be identified: equal opportunities and non-discrimination, well-being at the workplace and reconciliation between life and work.

The area of equal opportunities and non-discrimination involves the fight against all forms of discrimination (direct or indirect, multiple, gender and any other risk factor) and the promotion of positive actions, i.e. actions formally discriminatory, but aiming at removal of deep-rooted and/or historical discriminations.

The area of well-being in the workplace concerns removal of all forms of mental and/or physical discomfort, from the less serious, such as work-related stress,[8] to more serious ones, such as bullying, and promotion of occupational safety, which can have several different aspects that depend on the factors to be protected.

In the past, the area of reconciliation between life and work was characterised by gender, meaning that it was conceived as the adoption of policies allowing women workers to perform functions of care at home. This connotation is still very strong on a cultural level, but in reality the reconciliation between life and work should be gender neutral, as adoption of policy should occur on the assumption that tasks of care at home should be undertaken by men and women alike. This area includes organisational aspects that affect the place and time of work, services related to the care of vulnerable individuals and typical long-term situations, such as returning to work after an extended absence.

30.3 Powers and Functions

The most important aspect concerns identification of the powers that the CUG has in order to realise the above-mentioned objectives. In this regard, paragraph 3.2 of the guidelines identifies three types of tasks, as summarised in Table 30.1, which identify what the CUG can do proposals, consultations and verifications. Firstly, the CUG can make proposals within the areas of its competence. This power is not irrelevant if used appropriately, since the administration is required to take the CUG's proposals into consideration and to direct them as appropriate. The power of proposal is usually expressed by proposing specific initiatives, such as the publication of the gender annual report,[9] by drawing up a positive action plan and promoting training and awareness.

The advisory power seeks to ensure that the CUG has adequate participation in decision-making processes to allow aspects falling within its competence to be properly integrated into administrative action. The consultation must therefore have as much systematic and preventive character as possible, because every type of provision, whatever the subject, can effect aspects that are relevant to the CUG, so

[8] See European Commission (2000), Work-related stress guide, "Hallows of life or deadly poison?" Luxembourg. Available at http://europa.eu.int.

[9] http://www.unibo.it/en/university/who-we-are/gender-budgeting.

Table 30.1 Powers/functions and activities/tasks of the CUG

Powers—functions	Activities—tasks
Proposals	Plan of positive actions (4 years of durations) Promotion of policies for a better life-work balance Actions for the well-being at workplace Plan of training to promote a dignified, secured and healthy working environment
Consultations	Participation in decision-making process Assessment and elaboration of preventive actions *Areas of specific concern*: – Work organisation; – Staff appraisal methods and procedures; – Leave and career progression; – Part-time work; – Teleworking, telecommuting.
Verifications	Evaluation of the results of positive actions Elaboration of well-being at work surveys Assessment of data on discrimination and harassment at work

that evaluation by the body can be adequately taken into account.[10] If this is true in general, there are areas for which the exercise of power in question is more relevant, such as in the areas of organisation, training, hours, staff appraisal, leave and career progression.

With the power of verification, the CUG is called upon to ascertain whether or not the desired results have been achieved. Therefore, the CUG has the important task of verifying the results of its actions. In the event that its proposals have not been adopted, the CUG can ask the administration why its requests were not followed.

30.4 Conclusions

The CUG in Italy is a body with a very broad and flexible spectrum of actions that depends greatly on how its role is interpreted by its members. Its prepositive, advisory and verification role can be extremely relevant for the publication and adoption of positive actions in public organisations (e.g. publication and implementation of a gender equality plan, political pressure for the provision of a budget and a number of months person for the realisation of a gender budget annual report). On the other hand, the CUG has no powers to intervene in individual situations, neither of conciliation nor of an extra-jurisdictional nature. The lack of an organism with these types of power, independent but internal to the administration to which it belongs, is felt very much by those to whom it remains, in these cases, the onerous (and in many ways impractical) recourse to ordinary jurisdictional procedures.

[10] The preventive nature implies that the request for an opinion is carried out in such a way that gives the CUG adequate time to adopt an appropriate resolution. The guidelines foresee that the methods to consult the CUG are predetermined by the administration with specific internal regulations.

Prevention of Violence and Emergency Services

31

Alberto Amadasi, Maria Carla Mazzotti, Maria Caterina Manca, and Susi Pelotti

Key Points

- In the prevention of violence, evidence points toward the need to implement a multidisciplinary approach.
- Adequate training and education of healthcare providers are imperative, and scientific research has a crucial role.
- A balanced combination of clinical and forensic medicine is needed.
- Different steps in the management of violence in emergency are herein discussed.
- For an accurate collection of forensic samples, the Italian Forensic Association of Forensic Genetics (GeFI) guidelines should be followed.

In the field of violence, most research on violence focuses on risk factors, rather than protective factors [1], but evidence points toward a need to implement a multidisciplinary collaboration [2], the cornerstone of prevention [3, 4].

The first step is the knowledge of risk factors, which occur at individual, family, community, and wider society levels. According to the data provided by the World Health Organization (WHO) [5], risk factors among intimate partner and sexual violence include low levels of education, previous child maltreatment, witnessing violence, antisocial personality disorder, alcohol addiction, and multiple partners. Factors associated with intimate partner violence include past history of violence, marital dissatisfaction, difficulties in communication, and controlling behaviors.

A. Amadasi · M. C. Mazzotti · S. Pelotti (✉)
Unit of Legal Medicine, Department of Medical and Surgical Sciences (DIMEC), University of Bologna, Bologna, Italy
e-mail: susi.pelotti@unibo.it

M. C. Manca
Medicina Legale Centro Azienda USL di Bologna—Azienda USL di Bologna, Bologna, Italy

I. Tarricone, A. Riecher-Rössler (eds.), *Health and Gender*,
https://doi.org/10.1007/978-3-030-15038-9_31

Finally, those associated with sexual violence are beliefs in family honor, ideologies of male sexual entitlement, and weak legal sanctions for sexual violence.

More resources are needed to strengthen prevention of response to intimate partner and sexual violence, including primary prevention. There is some evidence from high-income countries that advocacy and counselling interventions to improve access to services for survivors of intimate partner violence may be strongly effective. Health workers outreach is also crucial. However, these have yet to be assessed for use in resource-poor settings, where promising prevention strategies include economic and social empower of woman toward gender equality or communication and relationship skills within couples and communities.

It is therefore crucial to develop and implement policies that promote gender equality by ending discrimination against women in marriage, divorce, and custody laws or improving women's access to paid employment.

In such a scenario, the health sector has a crucial role in order to make violence against women unacceptable and felt as a public health problem with a focus on the prevention of recurrence. Thus, the training and education of healthcare providers is of utmost importance, and scientific research can have a role in preventing violence against women through population-based demographic and health surveys, as well as in surveillance and health information systems, and multisectoral responses to address interpersonal violence, in particular, against women and girls.

Therefore, the role of emergency management of the victim is fundamental. According to the Italian ISTAT data, the number of anti-violence centers has increased over the years from 351 in 2013 to 554 in 2017, with an increase of 57.8%. However, uniformity is lacking among individual regions, since the presence of these services has increased in some, while in others it is strongly diminished [6, 7].

The management of violence in emergency is crucial to "unveil" the violence occurred, cope with emotions and needs of victims, and provide information on prevention and anti-violence network. Therefore, reception is the most complex phase of the relationship between health professionals and victims of violence. For these reasons, the management of the victim leads to the activation of a network of specialized physical and psychological services to allow adequate protection. Moreover, a correct approach relies upon a balanced combination of clinical and forensic medicine. Medical assistance is priority, but also the collection and detailed documentation of forensic evidence is of utmost importance. Therefore, health personnel must be adequately trained. Victims may present with repeated injuries, medical complications, and psychological problems, and healthcare professionals, whether not trained, may fail in assessing correctly.

31.1 The Story Told by the Victim

The first part concerns the collection of the story. This is the first step in contact between the victim and the health workers. It must be carried out in a suitable and protected environment; physicians and other practitioners should be able to recognize one or more risk factors [8], but information can only be obtained with the consent and collaboration of the patient. The story of the aggression must be heard and reported in detail and, possibly, with the words of the victim.

31.2 The Physical and Genital Examination

It must be performed in all cases of sexual violence, regardless of the time after violence [9]. It must be performed carefully, examining the whole body of the victim, from head to toe, with a thorough description of the details of all the injuries (place, shape, dimensions, and morphological features), along with graphical and photographic reports.

The presence of physical symptoms must be recorded (i.e., pain, genital and perianal disorders, and psychic symptoms such as fear, agitation, and absence of emotional reactions). Frequently, signs of injuries are unspecific or blurred, and their interpretation may be really tough [10–12]: many violence may totally lack of physical or genital signs, as well as even a consensual relationship can cause genital or physical injuries. Many studies report that less than 30% of premenopausal and 50% postmenopausal women have visible injuries to the naked eye after a non-consensual relationship [13, 14].

Another important step is the compilation of the general and gynecological anamnesis.

31.3 Patient Treatment

The first objective is to provide the best diagnostic and therapeutic assistance to the victim (i.e., radiological investigations, surgery, suturing), in consideration of the type of violence and time elapsed.

Blood collection for medical purposes (pregnancy, sexually transmitted diseases) should therefore be performed along with collection of samples for forensic purposes (drug research, alcohol), as well as samples (i.e., oral or genital) for the search of biological material. Moreover, vaginal or cervical swab sampling for sexually transmitted diseases should be performed along with blood tests for HIV, HCV, HBsAg, VDRL, and pregnancy and toxicological tests [15]. Prophylaxis for sexually transmitted diseases [16] and postcoital contraception is best performed within 72 h.

Moreover, it may be appropriate to request further examinations by other health professionals, according to symptoms and diseases, as well as planning a hospitalization or placement in a host community.

31.4 Forensic Sampling

The DNA analysis for forensic identification is powerful tool, but it requires correct procedures for samples collection and storage ensuring the compliance of chain of custody of the items. Actually, a correct procedure can avoid the contamination events among different items and between the operator or environment and the items. The correct storage avoids DNA degradation events that could interfere with DNA profiling and influence the interpretation of the results. In addition evidence must be properly labeled and packaged also to ensure the validity of the proof in courts of law. Nevertheless, professionals must be aware that in sexual assault cases, the victim's body may be the most important part of the crime scene [17, 18].

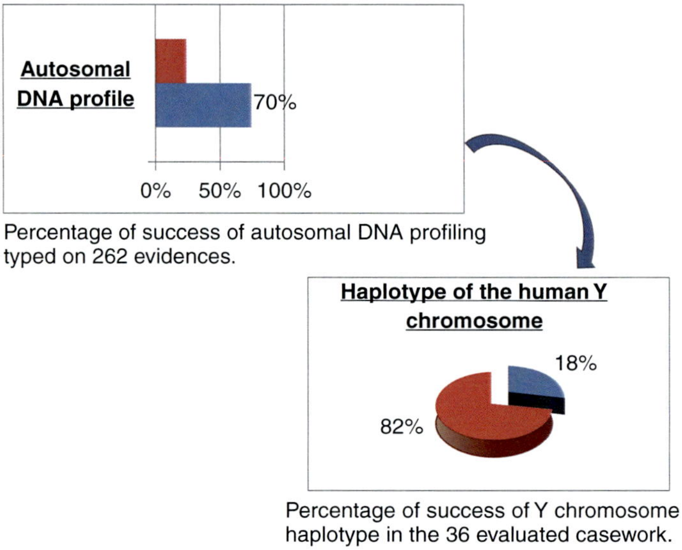

Fig. 31.1 Percentage of success of autosomal DNA profile and Y chromosome haplotype of a sexual violence casework analyzed by the forensic genetics laboratory of the University of Bologna

For the correct management of forensic samples in cases of sexual violence and maltreatment, the Italian Forensic Association of Forensic Genetics (GeFI) published specific guidelines [19].

Blood, urine, hair, nail, skin and vaginal, cervical, anal, and oral swab sampling must be performed according to the victim's story and with the utmost respect for the patient.

A review of 36 sexual violence casework analyzed by the forensic genetics laboratory of the University of Bologna showed that autosomal DNA profiling was successful in 70% of 262 items, and Y chromosome haplotype was useful in 82% of the 36 casework (Fig. 31.1).

As signs of violence (especially in genital and anal regions) tend to disappear with healing process, documentation and collection have to be performed as soon as possible [9, 20]

31.5 Consent of the Patient

Firstly, it is necessary to clearly explain to the patient the different phases of the medical examination [20–22]. Informed consent is crucial: the rationale of every clinical and forensic procedure has to be accurately explained in order to let the victim know what the healthcare staff is doing. This should help in regaining life and rebuilding a physical integrity which may be strongly disturbed by violence.

The patient must know that he can refuse any procedure at any time and can avoid answering the questions about the abuse, if experienced as invasive.

All this, integrated with the information of the subsequent events and the time spent by the abuse, allows to have greater possibilities to find evidence of violence and to evaluate its compatibility with the story. The inconsistency may be due to the attempt to hide the reality of the facts, especially when it comes to domestic violence or, sometimes, to a wrong collection of samples, and can have very significant repercussions on the outcome of a possible trial. Particular attention should be paid to the use of contraceptive methods, and the last consensual sexual relationship, to determine whether to do or not to do postcoital contraception.

31.6 Follow-Up of the Patient

For the prevention of violence, it is essential to activate a multidisciplinary process involving mainly social workers, psychologists, and lawyers, aimed at the full protection of women and their follow-up.

The different phases of the emergency care of the victim of violence are briefly summarized in Table 31.1.

Therefore, the training function of health workers is crucial [23, 24], and clinical forensic medicine has a key role: it is therefore necessary to increase the theoretical knowledge of health professionals in terms of sexual violence with specific reference to the dimension of the phenomenon, to its peculiarities in the case of individuals belonging to different social/cultural/religious groups, to the recognition of violence, to the approach to the victim, and to the family members to whom must be added the essential medical–legal bases in terms of information, consent, privacy, treatment of sensitive data, and report to the judicial authority [25, 26]. Furthermore, it is appropriate to provide practical skills in relation methods for the collection and custody of biological samples useful for judicial purposes, the relationship with police officers and the judicial authorities, and the use of common protocols for the management of the victim. A primary objective is to stimulate the development of

Table 31.1 Objectives of the procedures among the physician-victim relationship

Part of the physician–victim relationship	Objectives
1. The story told by the victim	First contact health professional/victim
	Create a comfortable environment
	Evaluate reliability and associated symptoms
2. The physical and genital examination	Detection and documentation of symptoms and injuries
3. Patient's treatment	Diagnosis and treatment
	Prophylactic treatment
4. Forensic sampling	Genetic investigations
	Search for any type of forensic evidence
5. Consent of the patient	Trust relationship health personnel/victim
	Protection of freedom and rights of the victim
6. Follow-up of the patient	Path of social recovery
	Violence prevention

common operating procedures for the correct management of the phenomenon and for the development of a dedicated information system within the context of a multidisciplinary approach and work in synergy between the individual professional figures (first aid physician, coroner, nurse, psychiatrist, social worker, psychologist). Even more, the need for an adequate preparation of health personnel should be highlighted, through courses having specific training objectives in order to make known the extent of the phenomenon and the consequences of health in the short and long term [8].

References

1. Stith SM, Smith DB, Penn CE, Ward DB, Tritt D. Intimate partner physical abuse perpetration and victimization risk factors: a meta-analytic review. Aggress Violent Behav. 2004;10:65–98.
2. Sims C, Sabra D, Bergey MR, Grill E, Sarani B, Pascual J, et al. Detecting intimate partner violence: more than trauma team education is needed. J Am Coll Surg. 2011;212:867–72. https://doi.org/10.1016/j.jamcollsurg.2011.01.003.
3. Istat – Istituto Nazionale di Statistica. La violenza e i maltrattamenti contro le donne dentro e fuori la famiglia. 2006. http://www.istat.it/it/files/2011/07/testointegrale.pdf. Accessed 17 Dec 2016.
4. Jewkes R. Intimate partner violence: causes and prevention. Lancet. 2002;359:1423–9.
5. WHO – World Health Organization. Global and regional estimates of violence against women: prevalence and health effects of intimate partner violence and non-partner sexual violence. 2013. http://www.who.int/reproductivehealth/publications/violence/9789241564625/en/. Accessed 17 Dec 2016.
6. Istat – Istituto Nazionale di Statistica. La violenza contro le donne. Indagine multiscopo sulle famiglie "Sicurezza delle donne". 2006. http://www3.istat.it/dati/catalogo/20091012_00/Inf_08_07_violenza_contro_donne_2006.pdf. Accessed 17 Dec 2016.
7. Istat – Istituto Nazionale di Statistica. La violenza contro le donne dentro e fuori la famiglia. 2014. https://www.istat.it/it/files/2015/06/Violenze_contro_le_donne.pdf?title=Violenza+contro+le+donne+-+05%2Fgiu%2F2015+-+Testo+integrale.pdf. Accessed 17 Dec 2016.
8. Andersson N, Ho-Foster A, Mitchell S, Scheepers E, Goldstein S. Risk factors for domestic physical violence: national cross-sectional household surveys in eight southern African countries. BMC Womens Health. 2007;16:7–11.
9. Wiley J, Sugar N, Fine D, Eckert LO. Legal outcomes of sexual assault. Am J Obstet Gynecol. 2003;188:1638–41.
10. Slaughter L, Brown CR, Crowley S, Peck R. Patterns of genital injury in female sexual assault victims. Am J Obstet Gynecol. 1997;176(3):609–16.
11. Biggs M, Stermac LE, Divinsky M. Genital injuries following sexual assault of women with and without prior sexual intercourse experience. CMAJ. 1998;159:33–7.
12. Palmer CM, McNulty AM, D'Este C, Donovan B. Genital injuries in women reporting sexual assault. Sex Health. 2004;1(1):55–9.
13. De Munnynck K, De Houwer L, Bronselaer K, Hanssens M, Van de Voorde W. Medico-legal approach to sexual assault victims: the Belgian situation. J Clin Forensic Med. 2006;13:211–4.
14. Poulos CA, Sheridan DJ. Genital injuries in postmenopausal women after sexual assault. J Elder Abuse Negl. 2008;20(4):323–35.
15. Gibelli D, Mazzarelli D, Rizzi A, Kustermann A, Cattaneo C. Persistence of spermatozoa on decomposing human skin: a scanning electron microscopy study. Int J Legal Med. 2013;127:975–9. https://doi.org/10.1007/s00414-013-0817-8.
16. Turillazzi E. Gli accertamenti medico-legali nella valutazione della violenza sessuale: proposta di un protocollo operativo. Riv It Med Leg. 2005;3:483–513.

17. Magalhães T, Dinis-Oliveira RJ, Silva B, Corte-Real F, Nuno Vieira D. Biological evidence management for DNA analysis in cases of sexual assault. ScientificWorldJournal. 2015;2015:365674. https://doi.org/10.1155/2015/36567.
18. Mollen CJ, Goyal MK, Frioux SM. Acute sexual assault: a review. Pediatr Emerg Care. 2012;28(6):584–90; quiz 591–3.
19. GeFi – Genetisti Forensi Italiani. Linee guida per la repertazione di tracce biologiche per le analisi di genetica forense nel percorso assistenziale delle vittime di violenza sessuale e/o maltrattamento. http://www.gefi-isfg.org/temp/2202201374428.pdf. Accessed 10 Dec 2016.
20. Riggs N, Houry D, Long G, Markovchick V, Feldhaus KM. Analysis of 1,076 cases of sexual assault. Ann Emerg Med. 2000;35(4):358–62.
21. Grossin C, Sibille I, Lorin de la Grandmaison G, Banasr A, Brion F, Durigon M. Analysis of 418 cases of sexual assault. Forensic Sci Int. 2003;131:125–30.
22. Santos JC, Neves A, Rodrigues M, Ferrão P. Victims of sexual offences: medicolegal examinations in emergency settings. J Clin Forensic Med. 2006;13(6–8):300–3. Epub 2006 Aug 23.
23. Sundborg E, Törnkvist L, Wändell P, Saleh-Stattin N. Impact of an educational intervention for district nurses about preparedness to encounter women exposed to intimate partner violence. Scand J Caring Sci. 2017. https://doi.org/10.1111/scs.12521.
24. Sundborg E, Törnkvist L, Saleh-Stattin N, Wändell P, Hylander I. To ask, or not to ask: the hesitation process described by district nurses encountering women exposed to intimate partner violence. J Clin Nurs. 2017;26(15–16):2256–65. https://doi.org/10.1111/jocn.12992. Epub 2015 Sep 30.
25. Williams DJ, Donnelly PD. Is violence a disease? Situating violence prevention in public health policy and practice. Public Health. 2014 Nov;128(11):960–7.
26. Hyman I, Vahabi M, Bailey A, Patel S, Guruge S, Wilson-Mitchell K, et al. Taking action on violence through research, policy, and practice. Glob Health Res Policy. 2016;1:6. https://doi.org/10.1186/s41256-016-0006-7.

Suggested Reading

Black MC, Breiding MJ. Adverse health conditions and health risk behaviors associated with intimate partner violence – United States, 2005. MMWR Morb Mortal Wkly Rep. 2008;57:113–7.

Campbell JC. Health consequences of intimate partner violence. Lancet. 2002;359:1331–6.

Coker AL, Smith PH, Bethea L, King MR, McKeown RE. Physical health consequences of physical and psychological intimate partner violence. Arch Fam Med. 2000;9:451–7.

Ellsberg M, Heise L, Pena R, Agurto S, Winkvist A. Researching domestic violence against women: methodological and ethical considerations. Stud Fam Plann. 2001;32:1–16.

García-Moreno C, Jansen HA, Ellsberg M, Heise L, Watts CH. Prevalence of intimate partner violence: findings from the WHO multi-country study on women's health and domestic violence. Lancet. 2006;368:1260–9.

Gray K, Seaberg DC, Wears RL. The prosecution of sexual assault cases: correlation with forensic evidence. Ann Emerg Med. 2002;39:39–46.

Heise L. What works to prevent partner violence? An evidence overview. London: Crown Copyright; 2011. https://assets.publishing.service.gov.uk/media/57a08abde5274a31e0000750/60887-PartnerViolenceEvidenceOverview.pdf. Accessed 24 Feb 2018.

Howard LM, Trevillion K, Khalifeh H, Woodall A, Agnew-Davies R, Feder G. Domestic violence and severe psychiatric disorders: prevalence and interventions. Psychol Med. 2010;40:881–93.

Plichta SB, Falik M. Prevalence of violence and its implications for women's health. Womens Health Issues. 2001;11:244–58.

United Nations Entity for Gender Equality and the Empowerment of Women. Ending Violence against women: from words to action. Study of the Secretary-General. UN Women. 2006. http://www.unwomen.org/-/media/headquarters/media/publications/un/en/englishstudy.pdf?la=en&vs=954. Accessed 24 Feb 2018.

32 When the Woman Is the Mother: The Work of Pediatrician for Caring Mothers and Children

Marcello Lanari, Monia Gennari, and Carlotta Biagi

Key Points

- Intimate partner violence (IPV) during pregnancy and children's exposure to violence are important public health issues and human right violations with serious adverse health consequences for both mother and children.
- The impact of IPV during pregnancy on newborn includes higher risk of preterm labor, intrauterine growth retardation, perinatal death, and potential emotional problems.
- Children exposed to domestic violence can develop emotional, behavioral, physical, social, and academic problems; in extreme cases they can be involved in physical violence between caregivers or experience the multiple losses when a parent kills the other one.
- Different forms of violence (domestic, community, and media violence) often co-occur leading to children's desensitization to violence and to behavioral or emotional problems.
- Pediatricians, educators, and other professionals who work with youth should be aware of the health consequences of IPV during pregnancy and children's exposure to violence to promote the necessary interventions and services for caring mothers and their children.

M. Lanari · M. Gennari · C. Biagi (✉)
Pediatric Emergency Unit, S. Orsola-Malpighi Hospital, University of Bologna, Bologna, Italy
e-mail: carlotta.biagi2@unibo.it

I. Tarricone, A. Riecher-Rössler (eds.), *Health and Gender*,
https://doi.org/10.1007/978-3-030-15038-9_32

32.1 Intimate Partner Violence During Pregnancy

Intimate partner violence (IPV) during pregnancy is an important public health issue with serious adverse health consequences for both mother and newborn. IPV includes physical aggression, frequently focused on the abdomen during pregnancy, together with sexual coercion, emotional abuse, and controlling behaviors [1].

Potential risk factors for IPV among pregnant women are similar to those for IPV in general: less than secondary education, mental disorders, lack of employment, partner's harmful use of alcohol, young age, and male control/authority over women [2]. Moreover, having an unintended pregnancy is a potential risk factor for domestic violence. According to a US population-based survey, women with unintended pregnancies had 2.5 times the risk of experiencing physical abuse compared with those whose with intended pregnancies [3].

The phenomenon of IPV during pregnancy is underestimated, and its prevalence reported in literature varies widely from 3% [4] to 30% [5–7]. These differences may depend on the survey methods employed (face-to-face, telephone, computer-based interviews), the time periods evaluated, and the countries analyzed (high-income versus low-income countries). Globally prevalence appears to be higher in Africa and Latin America compared to Europe and Asia, although estimates within countries were highly variable. Data carried out between 1998 and 2007 from the Demographic and Health Surveys and the International Violence Against Women Survey found a prevalence of IPV in pregnancy of 4–9% in most of the countries, with a maximum of 13.5% in Uganda [8]. A recent meta-analysis confirmed that the prevalence of IPV in Africa is one of the highest reported worldwide: 23–40% for physical, 3–27% for sexual, and 25–49% for emotional IPV among pregnant women [9].

The health consequences of IPV during pregnancy include both maternal and neonatal outcomes (Table 32.1) [10]. Regarding the effects on newborn health, IPV can lead to intrauterine growth restriction (IUGR), low birth weight (LBW), and preterm birth (PTB), which are well-established leading causes of neonatal morbidity and mortality [11, 12]. In a large meta-analysis including 30 studies, LBW (adjusted OR 1.53, 95% CI 1.28–1.82) and PTB (adjusted OR 1.46, 95% CI 1.27–1.67) were significantly increased among women exposed to domestic violence [13]. Similarly, a recent prospective longitudinal study conducted in Baltimore found that after adjusting for education, marital status, income, and substance abuse, IPV in pregnancy was associated with over five times increased odds for any adverse neonatal outcome (e.g., LBW, PTB, and IUGR). In particular women who experienced IPV had four times the odds of having a small for gestational age (SGA) neonate [14]. Moreover several studies have found an increased risk of perinatal death in pregnant abused women [15, 16].

There is a growing need to better clarify how IPV may contribute to the negative newborn outcomes. Direct physical trauma, maternal high-risk behaviors, stress, and neglect are postulated mechanisms. The reported increased use of alcohol and drug and smoking in pregnant abused women together with the delayed prenatal care are well-known risk factors for adverse neonatal outcomes [10, 11]. Moreover, psychological stress may exacerbate maternal hypertension and gestational diabetes and lead to pregnancy complications as preeclampsia and PTB [15].

Table 32.1 Health consequences of IPV during pregnancy

Maternal health consequences	Fatal outcomes	Homicide Suicide
	Nonfatal outcomes	Negative health behavior: • Alcohol and drug abuse during pregnancy • Smoking during pregnancy • Delayed prenatal care
		Physical health: • Injury • Physical impairment
		Mental health: • Depression • Anxiety • Difficulties or lack of attachment to the child
		Reproductive health: • Sexually transmitted infections • Miscarriage • Obstetric complications
Newborn health consequences	• Preterm births • Perinatal death • Low birth weight babies • Behavioral problems	

Furthermore, IPV may directly affect birth outcomes by physiological alterations involving epigenetically mediated changes in gene expression [17]. Animal studies have shown that exposure to stress in pregnancy may alter the hypothalamic-pituitary-adrenal (HPA) axis, leading to higher levels of HPA hormones including corticotrophin-releasing hormone (CRH) [18]. CRH acts as a "placental clock" causing the restriction of uteroplacental perfusion together with the induction of labor, resulting in LBW and PTB [19].

Moreover, in utero exposure to maternal stress may have negative neonatal consequences even in the absence of adverse birth phenotypes such as LBW. According to this, a recent study demonstrated for the first time that prenatal IPV is independently related to infant cortisol reactivity and behavioral problems [20]. Future studies are needed to better clarify the impact of antenatal violence on epigenetic, infant adrenocortical reactivity and behavioral functioning.

Knowing the effects of IPV during pregnancy is important in order to prevent them and implement the required services for caring women experiencing violence and their children. Pediatricians should be informed and aware of the possibility of IPV as an underlying factor in newborn's ill health.

32.2 Children Exposure to Intimate Partner Violence

According to a recent report by the World Health Organization, the prevalence of IPV among women is about 30% [1]. United States (US) population-based estimates indicate that between four and six million women are physically or sexually assaulted annually by either a current or former intimate partner [21]. The extreme consequence of IPV is the homicide of woman: up to 39% of female homicides worldwide are perpetrated by an intimate partner, while only 6% of murdered males are killed by a partner [22]. The National Survey of Children's Health conducted in 2012 by the National Center for Health Statistics estimated that 7% of US children witness domestic violence in the home each year [23]. An adult retrospective self-report found that 10–20% of children are at risk for exposure to domestic violence [24]. Witnessed violence is still an underestimated type of child abuse. It depends on the close relationship between the abuser and the victim, the difficulty of the woman to denounce the partner, and the unawareness of the impact of IPV on children who could not be present at the moment of violence. However, it is well documented that exposure to domestic violence can have adverse effects on the mental health of children and adolescents [25] and increase the risk of developing psychopathology [26, 27].

Several studies have found a significant association between post-traumatic stress disorder (PTSD) diagnosis in children and exposure to domestic violence [28–31]. The prevalence rates of PTSD in children exposed to IPV vary widely in the different studies, ranging from 13% to 60% [32–35]. Furthermore the risk of suffering other type of additional maltreatment increases in children exposed to IPV, suggesting that many children who witness domestic violence have also directly experienced child abuse; the most strongly linked has been with physical neglect and psychological maltreatment [36]. When there is a coincidence of different types of abuse, a cumulative effect almost doubles the risk of PTSD diagnosis [37].

Children's perception of IPV varies with age, and the effect of exposure could manifest in a different way according to the developmental stage of the child [26]. Some children adopt unconsciously the characteristics of the abusive parent becoming disrespectful, aggressive, and sometimes threatening and violent toward the victim parent. Others line up with the last one because they know only two possible models to identify themselves: perpetrators or victims. It has been reported that the association between exposure to IPV and externalizing symptoms is stronger for boys than for girls. This can contribute to intergenerational cycle of violence, a phenomenon whereby victimization and offending are strictly linked to one another [38].

There are a wide range of serious consequences of children's exposure to IPV including emotional, behavioral, physical, social, and academic problems [39, 40] (Table 32.2). In extreme cases children are involved in physical violence between caregivers till their own death, or they experience the multiple losses when a parent kills the other one [41, 42].

A child exposed to IPV may develop problematic attachment behaviors as role inversion, when he tries to console and protect the mother to ensure continuity of the family not revealing the abuse, or hyper-adaptation, when he renounces to his self-affirmation. Moreover the child can deny violence to preserve his security sense, and this may lead to future evaluation mistakes in relationships being enable to recognize reliable people [43]. Finally, IPV also affects maternal mental health and maternal parenting quality negatively, which have been associated with behavior problems in children exposed to the violence [44].

Table 32.2 Consequences of children exposure to IPV

Image of self	*Regulations of emotions*
Disorders of the body image Low self-esteem Experiences of shame and guilt	Difficulty in describing internal experiences Understand and describe internal moods Communicate needs and desires
Attachment	*Cognitive function*
Problems with personal boundaries Distrust and suspicion Interpersonal difficulties Difficulty in tuning into the emotional states of others Difficulty in assuming a point of view Difficulty in recognizing others as allies	Altered design and forecasting capacity Learning difficulties Anxiety Difficulty of attention Lack of curiosity Difficulty in concentrating and solving tasks Language development difficulties
Behavior	*Physical health*
Poor ability to modulate the impulses Self-destructiveness/aggressiveness Sleep disorders Eating disorders Use of substances Excessive complacency/opposition Animal cruelty Difficulties in understanding and respecting rules and regulations	Somatization Wide-ranging health problems (pelvic pain, dermatitis, bronchial asthma, immunological problems, etc.)

Screening adult women for IPV in healthcare setting is mandatory to identify children exposed to domestic violence; signs and symptoms of children's exposure have to be assessed by clinicians, teachers, and other professionals working with youth. Primary prevention generally refers to educational programs for teens or media campaign that attempts to increase awareness or change attitude about IPV [25].

Children exposure to IPV is a well-established form of maltreatment with harmful and long-term consequences for both health and well-being. Nevertheless, some children develop resilience, the ability to overcome serious hardship, while others do not [45]. Thus, it is essential that all children exposed to IPV undergo through a diagnostic assessment to determine if any intervention is needed. It is also important to assess whether exposure to IPV is still ongoing.

Interventions that have shown benefits include psychotherapeutic interventions such as child-parent psychotherapy, trauma-focused cognitive behavioral therapy or community-based group therapies, parenting skills and training, and advocacy plus psychoeducation [25]. Recently anti-violence centers for abusers who want to stop their violent or abusive behavior toward their family members had been organized with promising results [46].

Another important form of witnessed violence is the children's exposure to violence within a community (i.e., being present when a person initiate a fight or robs someone), a common problem in urban communities with low socioeconomic backgrounds, ethnic minorities, and high crime rates [47]. Community violence exposure can negatively impact multiple domains of functioning, including academic outcomes, and lead to conduct disorder.

Finally, a widespread form of violence is the screen entertainment media violence (i.e., television, video games, and the Internet), which increases the likelihood of aggressive and violent behavior and leads to desensitization to violence, making children less sensitive to the suffering of others [48].

Exposure to domestic, community, and media violence can have harmful effects on children. Different forms of violence often co-occur; thus it is important to understand that is the accumulation of negative experiences and the relative lack of protective factors that lead to develop emotional, behavioral, or social problems in children exposed to the violence. Pediatricians, educators, and other professionals who work with children should be aware of this in order to prevent witnessed violence and promote the necessary interventions and services for caring mothers and their children.

References

1. World Health Organization. Global and regional estimates of violence against women: prevalence and health effects of intimate partner violence and non-partner sexual violence. Geneva: WHO; 2013. p. 52.
2. World Health Organization. Global plan of action to strengthen the role of the health system within a national multisectoral response to address interpersonal violence, in particular against women and girls, and against children. Geneva: WHO; 2016. p. 60.
3. Goodwin MM, Gazmararian JA, Johnson CH, Gilbert BC, Saltzman LE. Pregnancy intendedness and physical abuse around the time of pregnancy: findings from the pregnancy risk assessment monitoring system, 1996–1997. PRAMS Working Group. Pregnancy Risk Assessment Monitoring System. Matern Child Health J. 2000;4(2):85–92.
4. Bacchus L, Mezey G, Bewley S. Domestic violence: prevalence in pregnant women and associations with physical and psychological health. Eur J Obstet Gynecol Reprod Biol. 2004;113(1):6–11.
5. Campbell J, Garcia-Moreno C, Sharps P. Abuse during pregnancy in industrialized and developing countries. Violence Against Women. 2004;10(7):770–89.
6. Salari Z, Nakhaee N. Identifying types of domestic violence and its associated risk factors in a pregnant population in Kerman hospitals, Iran Republic. Asia Pac J Public Health. 2008;20(1):49–55.
7. García-Moreno C, Jansen HA, Ellsberg M, Heise L, Watts C. WHO multi-country study on women's health and domestic violence against women: initial results on prevalence, health outcomes and women's responses. Geneva: World Health Organization; 2005.
8. Devries KM, Kishor S, Johnson H, Stöckl H, Bacchus L, Garcia-Moreno C, et al. Intimate partner violence during pregnancy: prevalence data from 19 countries. Reprod Health Matters. 2010;18(36):1–13.
9. Shamu S, Abrahams N, Temmerman M, Musekiwa A, Zarowsky C. A systematic review of African studies on intimate partner violence against pregnant women: prevalence and risk factors. PLoS One. 2011;6(3):e17591.
10. World Health Organization. Intimate partner violence during pregnancy. Geneva: WHO; 2011.
11. Alhusen JL, Ray E, Sharps P, Bullock L. Intimate partner violence during pregnancy: maternal and neonatal outcomes. J Womens Health (Larchmt). 2015;24(1):100–6.
12. Bailey BA. Partner violence during pregnancy: prevalence, effects, screening, and management. Int J Womens Health. 2010;2:183–97.
13. Shah PS, Shah J. Knowledge synthesis group on determinants of preterm/LBW births. Maternal exposure to domestic violence and pregnancy and birth outcomes: a systematic review and meta-analyses. J Womens Health (Larchmt). 2010;19:2017–31.

14. Alhusen JL, Lucea MB, Bullock L, Sharps P. Intimate partner violence, substance use, and adverse neonatal outcomes among urban women. J Pediatr. 2013;163:471–6.
15. Coker AL, Sanderson M, Dong B. Partner violence during pregnancy and risk of adverse pregnancy outcomes. Paediatr Perinat Epidemiol. 2004;18:260–9.
16. Yost NP, Bloom SL, McIntire DD, Leveno KJ. A prospective observational study of domestic violence during pregnancy. Obstet Gynecol. 2005;106:61–5.
17. Wadhwa PD, Buss C, Entringer S, Swanson JM. Developmental origins of health and disease: brief history of the approach and current focus on epigenetic mechanisms. Semin Reprod Med. 2009;27(5):358–68.
18. Takahashi LK, Turner JG, Kalin NH. Prolonged stress-induced elevation in plasma corticosterone during pregnancy in the rat: implications for prenatal stress studies. Psychoneuroendocrinology. 1998;23:571–81.
19. Kalantaridou SN, Zoumakis E, Makrigiannakis A, Lavasidis LG, Vrekoussis T, Chrousos GP. Corticotropin-releasing hormone, stress and human reproduction: an update. J Reprod Immunol. 2010;85:33–9.
20. Levendosky AA, Bogat GA, Lonstein JS, Martinez-Torteya C, Muzik M, Granger DA, von Eye A. Infant adrenocortical reactivity and behavioral functioning: relation to early exposure to maternal intimate partner violence. Stress. 2016;19(1):37–44.
21. Heise L, Ellsberg M, Gottemoeller M. Ending violence against women, Population reports, Series L, No. 11. Baltimore, MD: Johns Hopkins University School of Public Health, Population Information Program; 2013.
22. Stöckl H, Devries K, Rotstein A, Abrahams N, Campbell J, Watts C, Moreno CG. The global prevalence of intimate partner homicide: a systematic review. Lancet. 2013;382(9895):859–65.
23. Sacks V, Murphey D, Moore K. Adverse childhood experiences: national and state-level prevalence. Child Trends: Research Brief. 2014. Publication 28.
24. Carlson BE. Children exposed to intimate partner violence: research findings and implications for intervention. Trauma Violence Abuse. 2000;1(4):321–40.
25. McTavish JR, MacGregor JC, Wathen CN, MacMillan HL. Children's exposure to intimate partner violence: an overview. Int Rev Psychiatry. 2016;28(5):504–18.
26. Evans SE, Davies C, DiLillo D. Exposure to domestic violence: a meta-analysis of child and adolescent outcomes. Aggress Violent Behav. 2008;13:131–40.
27. Wood SL, Sommers MS. Consequences of intimate partner violence on child witnesses: a systematic review of the literature. J Child Adolesc Psychiatr Nurs. 2011;24:223–36.
28. Carpenter GL, Stacks AM. Developmental effects of exposure to intimate partner violence in early childhood: a review of the literature. Child Youth Serv Rev. 2009;31:831–9.
29. Crusto CA, Whitson ML, Walling SM, Feinn R, Friedman SR, Reynolds J, Amer M, Kaufman JS. Posttraumatic stress among young urban children exposed to family violence and other potentially traumatic events. J Trauma Stress. 2010;23:716–24.
30. Graham-Bermann SA, De Voe ER, Mattis JS, Lynch S, Thomas SA. Ecological predictors of traumatic stress symptoms in Caucasian and ethnic minority children exposed to intimate partner violence. Violence Against Women. 2006;12:662–92.
31. Levendosky AA, Bogat GA, Martinez-Torteya C. PTSD symptoms in young children exposed to intimate partner violence. Violence Against Women. 2013;19:187–201.
32. Rossman BB, Hughes HM, Rosenberg MS. Children and interparental violence: the impact of exposure. Philadelphia, PA: Brunner/Mazel; 2000.
33. McCloskey LA, Walker M. Posttraumatic stress in children exposed to family violence and single-event trauma. J Am Acad Child Adolesc Psychiatry. 2000;39:108–15.
34. Mertin P, Mohr P. Incidence and correlates of posttrauma symptoms in children from backgrounds of domestic violence. Violence Vict. 2002;17:555–67.
35. Chemtob CM, Carlson JG. Psychological effects of domestic violence on children and mothers. Int J Stress Manag. 2004;11:209–26.
36. Hamby S, Finkelhor D, Turner H, Ormrod R. The overlap of witnessing partner violence with child maltreatment and other victimizations in a nationally representative survey of youth. Child Abuse Negl. 2010;34:734–41.

37. Castor LE. The impact of additional traumatic events on trauma symptoms and PTSD in preschool-aged children exposed to intimate partner violence (IPV). Ph.D. Thesis, University of Michigan, Ann Arbor, MI; 2010.
38. Reckdenwald A, Mancini C, Beauregard E. The cycle of violence: examining the impact of maltreatment early in life on adult offending. Violence Vict. 2013;28(3):466–82.
39. Bair-Merritt MH, Blackstone M, Feudtner C. Physical health outcomes of childhood exposure to intimate partner violence: a systematic review. Pediatrics. 2006;117:e278–90.
40. Lourenço LM, Baptista MN, Senra LX, Adriana AA, Basılio C, Bhona FMDC. Consequences of exposure to domestic violence for children: a systematic review of the literature. Paideia. 2013;23:263–71.
41. Jaffe PG, Campbell M, Hamilton LH, Juodis M. Children in danger of domestic homicide. Child Abuse Negl. 2012;36(1):71–4.
42. Alisic E, Groot A, Snetselaar H, Stroeken T, van de Putte E. Children bereaved by fatal intimate partner violence: a population-based study into demographics, family characteristics and homicide exposure. PLoS One. 2017;12(10):e0183466.
43. MacMillan HL, Wathen CN. Children's exposure to intimate partner violence. Child Adolesc Psychiatr Clin N Am. 2014;23(2):295–308.
44. Levendosky AA, Leahy KL, Bogat GA, Davidson WS, von Eye A. Domestic violence, maternal parenting, maternal mental health, and infant externalizing behavior. J Fam Psychol. 2006;20(4):544–52.
45. Kitzmann KM, Gaylord NK, Holt AR, Kenny ED. Child witnesses to domestic violence: a meta-analytic review. J Consult Clin Psychol. 2003;71:339–52.
46. Stover CS. Fathers for change for substance use and intimate partner violence: initial community pilot. Fam Process. 2015;54(4):600–9.
47. Kersten L, Vriends N, Steppan M, Raschle NM, Praetzlich M, et al. Community violence exposure and conduct problems in children and adolescents with conduct disorder and healthy controls. Front Behav Neurosci. 2017;11:219.
48. Anderson CA, Bushman BJ, Bartholow BD, Cantor J, Christakis D, Coyne SM, Donnerstein E, Brockmyer JF, Gentile DA, Green CS, Huesmann R, Hummer T, Krahé B, Strasburger VC, Warburton W, Wilson BJ, Ybarra M. Screen violence and youth behavior. Pediatrics. 2017;140(Suppl 2):S142–7.

Suggested Reading

Callaghan JEM, Fellin LC, Mavrou S, Alexander J, Sixsmith J. The management of disclosure in children's accounts of domestic violence: practices of telling and not telling. J Child Fam Stud. 2017;26(12):3370–87.

Drury SS, Mabile E, Brett ZH, et al. The association of telomere length with family violence and disruption. Pediatrics. 2014;134(1):e128.

Nowakowski-Sims E, Rowe A. The relationship between childhood adversity, attachment, and internalizing behaviors in a diversion program for child-to-mother violence. Child Abuse Negl. 2017;72:266–75.

Pantell RH, Committee on Psychosocial Aspects of Child and Family Health. The child witness in the courtroom. Pediatrics. 2017;139(3):e20164008.

Peek-Asa C, Saftlas AF, Wallis AB, Harland K, Dickey P. Presence of children in the home and intimate partner violence among women seeking elective pregnancy termination. PLoS One. 2017;12(10):e0186389.

Pérez-González A, Guilera G, Pereda N, Jarne A. Protective factors promoting resilience in the relation between child sexual victimization and internalizing and externalizing symptoms. Child Abuse Negl. 2017;72:393–403.

Part VI

Histories and Epilogues

The Association of the Teachers of the Bologna University (AdDU): A Story of Increasing Consciousness

33

Paola Monari

Key Points
- Academic positions: Professor Emeritus
- Gender studies
- University of Bologna
- Women teachers
- Women association: AdDU University of Bologna Women Teachers Association

1. The paper tells the adventure of a group of women professors of the University of Bologna who in 1991 decided to join in order to change the still very sexist culture within the University. They have imposed their presence in academic roles and their scientific expertise in research. Since then, the change has been fast. Today there are many women teachers who are part of the academic bodies and who run departments or schools in a climate of consolidated collaboration. This experience, started by a group of women of good will, has become the daily experience [1–4].

   The history of the university teachers' association (Associazione delle Docenti Universitarie, AdDU) of the University of Bologna is still a short story, but it deserves to be remembered in its most significant stages, above all to give value to those academic women who are committed to achieving a true equality of opportunities in the world of scientific research [5, 6].
2. In the first months of 1991, a small group of women university professors, solicited by Maria Luisa Altieri Biagi and by Paola Monari, met to discuss the opportunity to create, within the University of Bologna, an association of women teachers and researchers. A previous experience of aggregation among women

P. Monari (✉)
University of Bologna, Bologna, Italy
e-mail: paola.monari@unibo.it

I. Tarricone, A. Riecher-Rössler (eds.), *Health and Gender*,
https://doi.org/10.1007/978-3-030-15038-9_33

professors belonging to different disciplinary sectors contributed to this project. This experience was created during the celebrations for the IX Centenary of the University of Bologna, during the writing of the book *Alma Mater Studiorum: The Presence of Women from the 18th to the 20th Century* (Clueb, Bologna, 1988) [7, 8].

In June 1991, this letter was sent to all the women professors of the University of Bologna:

Dear Colleague

we are thinking about the possibility of creating an Association of the Teachers of the University of Bologna. The association, unrelated to any political and trade union perspective, should have three main purposes:

(a) *To promote the circulation of ideas and the exchange of information on research and teaching activities, in an attempt to modify the current situation of separation between the Departments and Faculties;*
(b) *To promote the activity of anyone within the University, who has given and demonstrates scientific seriousness and didactic commitment, favoring the achievement of the right goals by those who deserve it; in particular, to reflect on the historical reasons for phenomena that still affect the activity of women in the academic world, and on the ways to overcome this conditioning;*
(c) *To discuss university problems as they arise, in order to be better informed about them, more attentive to their development, and more proactive in relation to their solution.*
(d) *If you are interested in it, we ask you to attend a first meeting, to which all the women teachers and researchers of the University are invited, and which will be held on 14 June, at 5 pm in the hall of the VIII Centenary kindly granted by the Rector.*
The promoter group
Maria Luisa Altieri Biagi, Rosanna Benassi, Paola Rossi Giovanardi, Laura Guidotti Lenzi, Paola Monari, Gabriella Poma, Fosca Veronesi Martuzzi.

3. The first meeting of the new Association was held in the VIII Centenary Hall of the University and saw a notable attendance of women professors from all the Departments. These women teachers are considered the promoter members of the Association of Women University Professors whose Italian acronym is AdDU.

The establishment of a club of women teachers, first in Italy, arouses interest not only in the University. A local newspaper *Bologna. Yesterday, today, tomorrow* published an article signed by Gianni Renoldi, with the picturesque title "Beware, beware of the witches are back!" subtitle "Career women also in the chair: an idea, born almost by chance, can dye the University of Bologna in pink (taken as a model, as usual)."

In reality, the article contained an interview with Paola Monari, in which the issues of the University were exposed on which the teachers of the AdDU proposed to reflect, giving positive contributions.

In March 1993, at the opening ceremony of the academic year, for the first time in the history of the nine centuries of the University, the masterly lecture was given by a woman, Maria Luisa Altieri Biagi, who was also the President of AdDU.

On 25 January 1995, the AdDU organized a meeting on the theme "Designing the University of 2000." In that context, the final report of the survey on the opinions of members of the AdDU on essential aspects of university life was presented and illustrated by Paola Monari. The event, in the presence of the Rector Fabio Roversi Monaco, receives considerable interest not only among academics but also in the local community; witness the articles on the meeting, which appear on the pages of major newspapers.

The report, with the title "Reflections of the Bolognese teachers on their University" is published in the Bulletin of the University of Bologna.

4. On 11 May 1995, in view of the election to the Office of Rector, the AdDU inaugurated a tradition that has been consolidated over time to date, and organized a meeting with the candidates for the office of Rector. Paola Monari will moderate the meeting.

In January 1996, the AdDU, in collaboration with the Club FIDAPA (Italian Federation of Professional Women) of Bologna, gives two study awards to two young Senegalese scholars for remembering the colleague Franca Marcato Falzoni, owner of the first chair in Italy of Literature Francophone, who prematurely disappeared.

It is also the year in which the AdDU proposes to the academic management the institution of a kindergarten for the children of university employees. This proposal was welcomed with skepticism and disbelief and then met with increasing approval.

In October 1996 elections were held for the renewal of the teachers' representatives in the Academic Senate and in the University Board of Administration: the AdDU supports the candidacies of three women professors, all of whom were elected.

After those first years of consolidation, the Association has continued. Many Presidents have succeeded. And in all the most important moments of academic life, AdDU has always been present and has strongly contributed to change a still very sexist culture. This has created a strong solidarity between women and, it seems a paradox, even with male colleagues [8, 9].

Today there are many women teachers who are part of the academic bodies and who run departments or schools in a climate of consolidated collaboration.

This experience, started by a group of women of good will—some now gone—today is no longer news. It has become the daily experience [10].

References

1. Alma Mater Studiorum. La presenza femminile dal XVIII al XX secolo. Bologna: CLUEB; 1988.
2. Deem R. Gender, organizational cultures and the practices of manager-academics in UK universities. Gender Works Organ. 2003;10(2):239–59.
3. Luppi E. Representations of leadership within a gender perspective among secondary school students. Formazione Insegnamento. 2013;2:109–28.
4. Rettaroli R. Ricercatrici e docenti nell'Alma Mater Studiorum, Università di Bologna: situazione e prospettive. In: Eredi di Laura Bass. Milano: Franco Angeli; 2014.

5. Fortunati V, Morisco G, editors. The representation of the self in women's autobiography. Bologna: Erasmus Publications; 1993.
6. Fortunati V, Lamarra AM, Federici E, editors. The controversial women's body: images and representations in literature and art. Bologna: Bononia University Press; 1993.
7. Monari P. Le donne nell'Università di massa. In: Alma Mater Studiorum, editor. La presenza femminile dal XVIII al XX secolo. Bologna: CLUEB; 1988.
8. Monticelli R. Theories and gender studies in a transnational perspective. In: Fortunati V, Catani F, editors. Questioning the European Identity/ies. Deconstructing old stereotypes and envisioning new models of representation. Bologna: Il Mulino; 2012.
9. Showalter E. Introduction: the rise of gender. In: Speaking of gender. New York: Routledge; 1989.
10. Sartori F. Differenze e disuguaglianze di genere. Bologna: Il Mulino; 2019.

The Vase of Flowers: A Tale for Preschool Children on Mothers' Chemotherapy Side Effects

34

Michela Rimondini

Key Points

- Parents' cancer is a highly stressful life event for both parents and their children. An open and honest dialogue helps the expression and elaboration of emotions and concerns.
- Storytelling and the use of narratives is an effective way to promote healing and to integrate the relational and psychological dimensions associated with illness.
- The *Vase of Flowers* tells a story in which the most frequent chemotherapy side effects are described in 15 watercolor painting boards. The short verbal elements accompanying the images allow to tailor the amount of information to the needs expressed by the child during the reading process.
- By describing a story of external transformation, this picture book conveys also a symbolic message of internal transformation: the underlying therapeutic goal is to enhance readers' ability to accept change and to recognize its potential positive value.
- Public and private clinical centers which decide to offer their patients this instrument represent concrete examples of commitment in promoting humanization of care and patient-centered medicine.

A report of the National Cancer Institute indicates that about 5% of all cancer diagnoses in the United States is delivered to young people, aged between 15 and 39 years [1]. According to these data, cancer in young women can be considered infrequent, and, consequently, the presence of this health condition/disease in women during the years following their pregnancy is even rarer.

M. Rimondini (✉)
Section of Clinical Psychology, Department of Neuroscience, Biomedicine and Movement, University of Verona, Verona, Italy
e-mail: michela.rimondini@univr.it

I. Tarricone, A. Riecher-Rössler (eds.), *Health and Gender*,
https://doi.org/10.1007/978-3-030-15038-9_34

Nevertheless, when this condition occurs, it has a strong impact on the psychological well-being of both mothers and children. Experiencing such an illness at a stage of life that is dedicated to maternity and to nurturing young children confronts women with specific challenges [2]. Most of the patients face difficult questions such as the following: what is going to happen in the next future? Will I have enough energy for taking care of my children's needs? When should I tell my children what is happening? Which words can be used to guide and support them in an experience that will change the dynamics of the whole family?

Emotional distress and supportive care needs of mothers facing cancer have been investigated in the last decades, showing high rates of anxiety, depression, and stress-response symptoms [3].

Parents' illness is an issue affecting also children's psychological functioning [4]. Studies examining emotional distress among cancer patients' children and adolescents suggest that their negative feelings tend to be underestimated and that an open and honest dialogue between parents and children is effective in reducing these reactions and favoring adaptations to parents' health conditions [5, 6].

However, dealing with preschoolers' emotions might require a diverse approach, considering that they are at a different step of their emotional and cognitive development and have therefore specific explanatory and emotional needs.

The literature offers good evidence of the efficacy of interventions aiming to manage psychological reactions of cancer patients and their families [7]. In particular, the use of narratives in clinical practice and education is described (also known as *Narrative Medicine*) as an effective way to promote healing and to integrate the relational and psychological dimensions that accompany illness [8]. Storytelling in childhood is considered by pedagogues and psychologists one of the most powerful communication tools. Picture books, in which colored images are accompanied by short, simple phrases, stimulate the visual-verbal channel, encourage creativity, and enable the development of an affective relationship between the parent and the child starting from a very early age [9].

Moving from these premises, a team composed of a psychotherapist (involved in research and clinical practice in a public university hospital), a painter, an illustrator, and a graphic designer created *The Vase of Flowers* in 2016 (Picture 34.1) [10]. This picture book is for preschool children and their mothers who are undergoing chemotherapy treatment, and it is principally aimed to promote their resilient attitude by fostering and facilitating their emotional communication. Its pages tell a story in which the most frequent chemotherapy side effects (e.g., hair changes, fatigue, vomiting) are described in 15 watercolor painting boards. Painting techniques, the range of colors and nuances, the symbolic value of the images as well as the content of the commenting text were attentively discussed by the team. The short verbal elements accompanying the images are not mainly aiming to deliver information but are rather meant to be stimuli for further discussion between the adult and the child who are reading the book together. For this reason, the picture book allows to tailor the amount of provided information to the needs expressed by the child during the reading process, reaching in this way different levels of informativeness and explicitness.

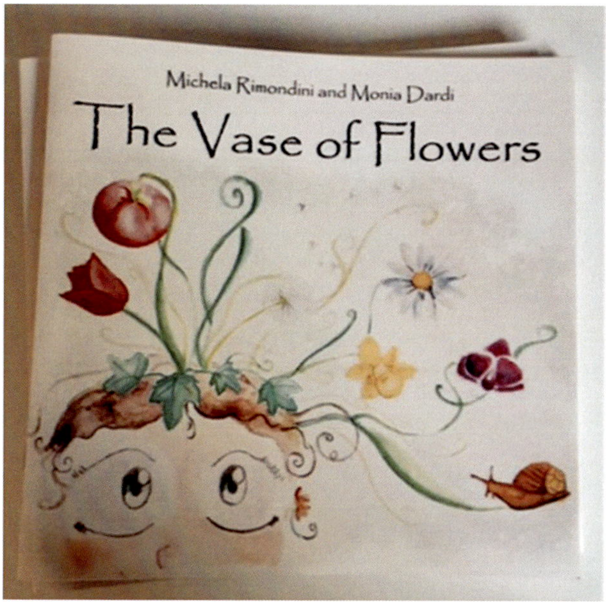

Picture 34.1 *The Vase of Flowers*. Picture book for preschool children whose mothers are undergoing a chemotherapy treatment

By describing the external transformation occurring when the mother is losing her hair, the book conveys a symbolic message of internal transformation. The underlying therapeutic goal is to enhance the readers' ability to accept change and to recognize its potential positive value. Many patients define their resilient attitudes as the product of a process of transformation: initially, they accept to change parts of their psychological functioning in order to better cope with the new challenges imposed by the illness (e.g., personal beliefs about health), and, successively, they accomplish a more structural change that involves elements of their personality and interpersonal style (e.g., life core values).

Through a dialogue between a mother and her son, in which the child has to imagine how the mum may look like after the loss of her hair, three messages are conveyed to the readers:

1. At first glance, change might seem a daunting task, but it can be tackled.
2. Mothers and children are not alone in this process, since there are a lot of people willing to support them (e.g., fathers, family, teachers, healthcare providers).
3. The relationship between mothers and their children is infinite and cannot be threatened by the challenges that will have to be faced in the process of care.

Several patients' associations offered support for this project, financing the distribution of the picture book to all Italian oncological units that wished to receive copies for their patients. The picture book, originally written in Italian, has been translated into English and can also be translated into other languages upon request, such as German, French, or Spanish. Public and private clinical centers, which decide to offer their patients this instrument, represent concrete examples of commitment to promoting humanization of care and person-centered medicine.

References

1. Adolescents and young adults with cancer. Report of National Cancer Institute. https://www.cancer.gov/types/aya.
2. Semple CJ, McCance T. Parents' experience of cancer who have young children: a literature review. Cancer Nurs. 2010;33(2):110–8.
3. Compas BE, Worsham NL, Epping-Jordan JE, Grant KE, Mireault G, Howell DC, Malcarne VL. When mom or dad has cancer: markers of psychological distress in cancer patients, spouses, and children. Health Psychol. 1994;13(6):507–15.
4. Moore CW, Rauch PK. Addressing the needs of children when a parent has cancer. In: Holland JC, editor. Psycho-oncology. 2nd ed. Oxford: Oxford University Press; 2010. p. 527–31.
5. Morris J, Martini A, Preen D. The well-being of children impacted by a parent with cancer: an integrative review. Support Care Cancer. 2016;24(7):3235–51.
6. Kroll L, et al. Cancer in parents: telling children. Br Med J. 1998;316:880. Academic OneFile.
7. Chong Guan N, Mohamed S, Kian Tiah L, Kar Mun T, Sulaiman AH, Zainal NZ. Psychotherapy for cancer patients. Int J Psychiatry Med. 2016 Jul;51(5):414–30.
8. Charon R. Narrative medicine. A model for empathy, reflection, profession, and trust. JAMA. 2001;286(15):1897–902.
9. Whitehurst GJ, Falco FL, Lonigan CJ, Fischel JE, DeBaryshe BD, Valdez-Menchaca MC, Caulfield M. Accelerating language development through picture book reading. Dev Psychol. 1988;24(4):552–9.
10. "Il Vaso di Fiori" web site. https://sites.google.com/site/ilvasodifiori/home/english-version.

Suggested Reading

Bleyer A, Barr R, Ries L, Whelan J, Ferrari A. Cancer in adolescents and young adults. 2nd ed. New York: Springer; 2017.

Charon R. Narrative medicine: honouring the stories of illness. New York: Oxford University Press; 2006.

Charon R, Montello M. Stories matter: the role of narrative in medical ethics. New York: Routledge; 2002.

Evans J. Talking beyond the page: reading and responding to picture books. London: Routledge; 2009.

Nikolajeva M. Picture books and emotional literacy. Read Teach. 2014;67(4):249–54.

Taylor D. Tell me a story: the life-shaping power of our stories. Berlin: Bog Walk Press; 2001.

Welch A, Wadsworth M, Compas B. Adjustment of children and adolescents to parental cancer. Parents' and children's perspectives. Cancer. 1996;77(7):1409–18.

Women at School

35

Francesca Frascaroli

Key Points

- A gender gap in teaching has led women to become key figures in education and at the same time face growing workloads.
- Women increasingly been applying for tenured teaching positions, but there has not been a corresponding flow of men into education.
- Girls are better students than boys.
- Female teachers should be mentored to be more selective in their service-related choices.

When I was asked to take part in this project and to consider my life and work experiences from the point of view of women's health, I realised that teaching has always been at their heart. I could read at 5, so I started my career unknowingly, by telling my friends stories they loved to hear or babysitting for younger children. Later on, I tutored my classmates and younger students at high school, Liceo Classico Statale "Marco Minghetti" in Bologna. Liceo Classico is a 5-year secondary school type, one of the few European schools where ancient languages (Latin and Ancient Greek) are taught together with current ones (mostly English). Among the other subject matters are Mathematics and Physics, History and Philosophy, Chemistry, Biology, Natural Science, and Art History. Classes are generally formed by 20–25 students, most of whom typically progress to HE (higher education).

And that is what I did: I chose to study Modern Languages and Literatures, then spent some years working at the Comparative Literature Department of the University of Madison, Wisconsin. I was sometimes homesick and felt vulnerable, since I was the only non-native speaker student attending PhD courses, but I was lucky enough to meet a competent advisor and a wonderful teacher, Mary Layoun, whose enthusiasm and dedication helped me through those years.

F. Frascaroli (✉)
Liceo Classico Marco Minghetti, Bologna, Italy

I. Tarricone, A. Riecher-Rössler (eds.), *Health and Gender*,
https://doi.org/10.1007/978-3-030-15038-9_35

While studying Comparative Literature, I was also teaching French and Italian and often found encouragement and support from my students—they eased even my most tiring or challenging classes. I can still remember their faces, and, thanks to social media, I keep in touch with some of them, as well as with my American colleagues. The approval and support of my students have always been the main reason why I consider my profession as a true gift.

However, teachers often face fatigue, disillusionment and boredom. They have to cope with their own and their students' successes and failures. Sometimes they are tolerated and in other cases rejected or even despised and feared. Sylvia Plath's well-known poem, "Daddy", deals with the legacy of the poetess's father and frames the image of a strict parent and severe teacher.

The first time I read it I was attending classes at the English Department, together with other female students, and we were all deeply struck by the feelings of painful rage and hopeless despair Plath conveys—together with a vain wish for love and tenderness, for a welcoming and not rejecting father and, possibly, teacher. Both as a daughter and a teacher, I deemed the lines quoted below peculiarly meaningful:

> I have always been scared of you,
> With your Luftwaffe, your gobbledygoo.
> And your neat mustache
> And your Aryan eye, bright blue.
> Panzer-man, panzer-man, O You—
> Not God but a swastika
> So black no sky could squeak through.
> Every woman adores a Fascist,
> The boot in the face, the brute
> Brute heart of a brute like you.
> You stand at the blackboard, daddy,
> In the picture I have of you,
> A cleft in your chin instead of your foot
> But no less a devil for that, no not
> Any less the black man who
> Bit my pretty red heart in two.
> I was ten when they buried you.
> At twenty I tried to die
> And get back, back, back to you.
> I thought even the bones would do.

Plath underlines how scared she was of her father Otto, a German professor of Biology at Boston University, pro-Nazi and "brutal".

The feelings shown in the above lines are exactly the opposite of mine: trust, protection and safety are the keywords to describe my feelings towards my father, my first guide in life, a safe presence, constantly reliable but never judgmental. In my adult and professional life, as a mother and a teacher, I have struggled to be that kind of presence, aware that parents, such as professors, can easily become critical, intrusive and overbearing.

My field of activity in Italy is guaranteed by an institutional framework for gender equality. Nevertheless, over the last few decades, a gender gap in teaching has led women to become key figures in education and at the same time face growing workloads. Not only have women increasingly been applying for tenured teaching positions, but there has not been a corresponding flow of men into education. Particularly, men have been put off applying for jobs in nursery schools and primary schools, as working with young children is considered a woman's profession. Therefore education, given women's role of caregivers and educators, is still one of the few "safe" careers for them. Not always safe in terms of service loads, though.

According to the data provided by ISTAT (*Istituto Nazionale di Statistica*, National Statistical Institute) and MIUR (*Ministero dell'Istruzione, Università e Ricerca*, Ministry of Education), women represent 79% of teachers—rising to almost 100% in nursery schools, 95% in primary schools and 85% in middle schools. In other words, women largely accept responsibility for and relatedness to their pupils. Their workload tends to become limitless and unmanageable. In terms of gender equality, secondary school education is more balanced. Female educators are 59% of the total, but these percentages depend on the types of secondary schools (teacher training schools or technical colleges, for instance, see a different balance of female and male teachers).

On the other hand, ISTAT's data state that girls are better students than boys. The latter are not always seriously involved in the learning process and often merely reach passing grades (21%), while the former are better students (86% girls score higher than passing grades). Thirty-three percent of boys attend remedial courses, while only 26% of girls need these. At university level, 24% of women graduate against 15% men, between 30 and 34 years of age.

The gender gap in teaching further decreases at university, where female and male research assistants show an even split. Women in academic careers, however, are less likely to hold tenured—or full—professor positions, and, according to Miur's recent survey, only 5 out of 78 faculty deans are women.

After almost 20 years of teaching English language and literature at secondary school in Italy and years of teaching abroad, I have witnessed some of the underlying problems the above data hint at. Although they outperform their male colleagues in terms of service, female teachers still have to face disproportional service loads. When I came back to Italy, after studying and working as a teaching assistant at the University of Madison, I found strong evidence that—even at university level—women faculty perform more service than male, participating in internal rather than external service. This imbalance leads to a disproportionate workload, which affects teachers' lives both professionally and privately.

The same pattern can be found in secondary schools, where female teachers should be mentored to be more selective in their service-related choices and improve their ability to say no to requests. To fix service imbalances, institutions should emphasise gender monitoring and promote gender education policies.

All through these years I have been listening to my colleagues' complaints about workloads that are getting harder and harder to handle. At the same time, I have been trying to become an unintrusive guide for students who face the demanding phases of growth. I have been trying to avoid spending too much time "at the blackboard" and being the kind of stern and controlling educator Sylvia Plath's father must have proved. I have been reading with my students, listening to them, finding answers with them.

My hopes for the improvement of women's health lie in the educational chances female teachers can be offered to contribute to a culture of kindness, generosity and support towards women. This culture should have gender equality as its aim.

I experience the strength and support of the girls I work with at school and wish that equal opportunities will soon be offered to women from all over the world. The answer to some of the weak points in education can be found in the way women are trained (even to say no, sometimes), in the way they can help their students to access culture without compromise, in the way they can promote access to good-quality education regardless of gender bias.

Suggested Reading

http://www.istat.it/en/.
http://www.miur.gov.it.
http://www.miur.it/guida/guide.htm.
http://www.tandfonline.com/doi/abs/10.1080/13608740408539574?journalCode=fses20.
http://www.tandfonline.com/doi/abs/10.1080/00223980.1993.9914889.

When the Daughter is a Doctor

36

Ilaria Tarricone

It is a pleasure and an honour to conclude this intense work, which I began some years ago, with a special memory dedicated to my father. My father was the person along with my mother who most encouraged my love for study and research. I remember when I was a child sitting on the sofa at home with my sister and my brother, and my father would read a favourite school book which he felt strongly about, one on human anatomy. He showed us the bones of the skeleton and, as an excellent chemist, aroused our curiosity for what we cannot see but sustains our lives.

My father unfortunately left us shortly after I started writing this book, struck down by a dramatic and quick-moving cancer in only 3 months, it being diagnosed when it was already far advanced. And so, while 3 months before he was still the head of his company, driving me and my mother and sister to my second PhD ceremony at King's College London, 3 months after diagnosis, he was gone and, apart from anything else, failed to see this work finished. What comforts me is that he would have liked it anyway, being able to choose, if he had been confronted with the dramatic choice of how to end his intense existence: a little time to organize greetings, fight and believe until the end and then, when the doctors decreed it was time to go, leave, surrounded by his loving family. And it happened just that way. Let me tell you about it.

The departure of my father, has painfully allowed me to mature some reflections on the end of life, in particular on how important it is to maintain a sensitive alertness to the patient's medical relationship and his unique cultural and gender identity, especially when, in circumstances such as this, the main focus of all our skills becomes precisely the doctor-patient, physician-family relationship. The condition of being close relatives of a person nearing death and at the same time doctors

I. Tarricone (✉)
Bologna Transcultural Psychosomatic Team (BoTPT), Department of Medical and Surgical Sciences, Alma Mater Studiorum, University of Bologna, Bologna, Italy
e-mail: ilaria.tarricone@unibo.it

I. Tarricone, A. Riecher-Rössler (eds.), *Health and Gender*,
https://doi.org/10.1007/978-3-030-15038-9_36

forces us into a dramatic exercise of reconciling the two sides of medicine, scientific technique and human understanding of suffering, when the doctor, as Jaspers said, "must dispose of knowledge not as a landowner in relation to his territory, but as a traveller to his way" [1].

I will try to summarize here some comments that arose in accompanying my father to his departure, hoping as I now do that the remarks expressed in this text by so many scholars and colleagues on gender differences in the medical field may strengthen the growing sensitivity and cultural awareness in the doctor-patient relationship.

Given the diagnosis, and in keeping with my father's character, we tried in every way to get the best treatment and whatever offered some hope of improvement. Shortly before starting chemotherapy, my father's blood tests showed severe thrombocytopenia. I will never forget how one of the day-hospital oncologists attending my father scientifically examined all the possible causes of that thrombocytopenia. Thus, it was possible to prove that the cause was a severe and rare paraneoplastic complication.

The serious complications mentioned above slowed the beginning of "chemotherapy" and made us lose sight of the fact that in a situation of such severity as we were living through with my father, the treatment was not, or only part partly, chemotherapy but rather palliative care to support the person's quality of life. We awaited "the treatment" in clinics full of patients, all waiting together for the verdict of the blood tests, in appointments always delayed by the complexity of a reality that, as in the case of my father, lengthened the duration of consultations in an exasperating way. Our expressed emotions went sky high, unfortunately. My father was then finally subjected to some cycles of chemotherapy. However, the presence of intestinal diverticulosis and inflammation due to constipation led unfortunately to perforation of the diverticula and, in spite of emergency surgery, to death.

In those few very painful weeks, I received from my father, my colleagues and my life four precious teachings that I would like to summarize here.

I will never forget how comforting it was in the event, and given the dramatic turn of events, that one day the head of the oncology department realized how important it was to speak to me frankly. "We may not have said anything yet clearly," he told me, "but I should tell you that your father's life expectancy is about three months". No words were more wisely spent, given the dramatic evolution of the clinical picture: my father died about 3 months later due to perforation of the intestinal diverticula. Knowing that, maybe not because of that dramatic complication, my father's illness would presumably lead to him dying around that time point was the only consolation for us at such a distressing moment.

The second most important lesson came directly from my father. On the days before his death, he was extremely debilitated but lucid; he insisted to me that if evacuation were resumed normally, the situation would be solved. His attention to this bodily function seemed rather bizarre yet he was absolutely right. Despite help with evacuation, he did not recover enough to avoid perforation of the diverticula, which proved the fatal complication.

The third lesson came from contact with colleagues at the hospital when intestinal perforation was diagnosed. My father was lucid and focused, although prostrated by pain and fatigue. The doctors decided, given the gravity of the situation, to ask us immediately to consent to an operation. We were facing one of the most painful decisions of our lives. Nothing would have changed in the evolution of the clinical picture if, instead of giving us that point-blank communication, we had been given a different setting in which to reflect and "waste" a few more minutes. Once again, I painfully learned how important it is to respect the timing of the relationship even in an emergency situation. We chose to proceed with surgery because none of us, including my father, could have borne the thought of not having done everything possible to save his life, as he would have done with us. And for our having accepted that choice and therefore intervened—no obvious event, given my dad's "terminally ill" condition—we are grateful to the medical-surgical team of the hospital.

The last lesson came from the last scenario of departure, that of resuscitation, the department where my father was hospitalized for three days, after undergoing intestinal resection. These last hours of my father's life taught us how fundamental pain therapy is in these situations, meaning both the physical pain of the patient and the moral pain of the family. We must never forget that, despite the sedation and obnubilation, the person at the end of life feels and understands everything. On awakening from surgery, which went well, my father could not speak because he was intubated, but he was lucid and smiled his congratulations when I gave him my good professional news. Unfortunately, the third night was complicated by myocardial infarction. That night an anaesthetist colleague invited me to go home to rest. I went away reluctantly, so as not to annoy the colleague who appealed to me to "trust" him. After a few hours' sleep, I arrived in time to be with him at the last. And my mother, my brother, my sister, my son, my nephew and sister-in-law also made it. My father was happy to see his loved ones around him before leaving, his family gathered around him, as used to occur every Sunday evening. My father died shortly after the doctor on duty, at the bedside, had confessed there was nothing more to be done. We learned that a loved one can leave, holding hands, in a wonderful Pietà setting, thanks to the generous support and discretion of nurses in the intensive care unit.

It is not easy to generalize from my experience, nor do I wish to make this epilogue a treatise on end-of-life medicine. But, in a nutshell, I believe that there are four aspects of care to be borne in mind in every treatment, even in the most serious conditions: (1) clearly communicating a diagnosis and prognosis with a view to clarifying that diagnosis and prognosis are two perspectives linked to best medical practice but not infallible; (2) listening to the person suffering and placing his or her illness at the centre, as something that can be treated even when the disease is "terminal"; (3) respecting the doctor-patient relationship and patient-family relationship at every juncture, even and especially in emergencies; and (4) finding room for psychological support of the patient, his family and the caring team.

Finally, it is certainly thanks to the love and trust of my family, my friends and my colleagues that I managed to remember to be first and foremost a daughter, sister, mother and friend who happens to be a doctor and researcher. And together with all of them including my father Antonio, it is my heartfelt wish that the coming generations will be brought up in a humanitarian vocation, respectful of gender and culture differences in the healing professions.

Reference

1. Jaspers K. Der Arzt im technischen Zeitalter. Monaco: R. Piper; 1986.